MARKETING
AND NURSING

A CONTEMPORARY VIEW

Marketing and Nursing

A CONTEMPORARY VIEW

MARY SAYRE TILBURY, RN, EdD
Vice President of Administration
Director of Nursing Practice
Rochester General Hospital
Rochester, New York

TREVOR A. FISK, MSc
Associate Executive Director
   for Marketing and Planning
Thomas Jefferson University Hospital
Philadelphia, Pennsylvania

National Health Publishing
A Division of Williams & Wilkins

Published by
National Health Publishing
99 Painters Mill Road
Owings Mills, Maryland 21117
(301) 363–6400

A division of Williams & Wilkins

Printed in the United States of America
First Printing

Acquisitions Editor: Elizabeth Jane Kramer
Copyeditor: Michael Treadway
Production Coordinator: Karen Babcock
Designer: Sandy Renovetz
Compositor: Absolutely Your Type
Printer: Edwards Brothers

ISBN: 1–55857–005–5
LC: 88–063449

Contents

List of Figures

Preface

This book was written in response to suggestions by a variety of nursing leaders. They pointed out the need for an introduction to marketing that was relevant to nurses.

The nursing profession faces a number of complex challenges. Each depends for its solution, in part, upon using marketing concepts, strategies, and skills. Among those challenges are:

1. How can we continue to recruit enough able young men and women into the profession in the face of expanding alternative career opportunities?

2. How can we retain existing personnel in the profession, instead of training them and giving them their early practical experience, only to see them hired away for their most productive years into other fields?

3. How can we best train nurses to combine their clinical responsibilities with the skills needed to respond to the growing "consumerism" of patients?

4. How can nurses self-promote their clinical skills and aspirations to their colleagues in other health professions?

5. How can the nursing profession secure better public and payer recognition of their contemporary roles as health care providers?

6. As nurses increasingly find themselves part of a team responsible for the planning and profitability of health services, how can they best apply marketing to those tasks?

7. As nursing administrators increasingly find themselves involved in debate with hospital executives conversant in principles, how can they make their contribution effective?

8. As nurses find themselves increasingly engaged in health education and community outreach efforts, how can they apply marketing skills to those duties?

9. As more nurses go into health-related businesses as entrepreneurs, what do they need to know about marketing?

10. As nurses find their professional knowledge sought out by enterprises as varied as insurance companies, drug companies, medical equipment manufacturers, and new types of health providers, how can they relate effectively to the market-driven culture of those organizations?

One way to learn how marketing can help with specific nursing issues is to attend specific skills seminars (e.g., "How to Recruit Nurses" or "Marketing Home Care"). Such seminars play a useful role, but they also have two significant deficiencies. A little learning can be a dangerous thing. Marketing, like nursing, is a science in its own right, with its own analytical concepts, its own developed techniques, its own ways of looking at problems and trying to produce solutions to them. A superficial knowledge of it can be misleading. Further, such brief learning experiences often leave participants uncertain as to how knowledge is transferred to other issues they face.

This book offers an alternative approach to helping clinicians, educators, and administrators acquire marketing expertise. It introduces the reader to the most important concepts and skills of marketing, with continual reference to the familiar environment of nursing. It can be used as an ad hoc reference, as a self-administered study course, or as a textbook.

As described in this book, marketing requires a three-step process. Skipping any one step is dangerous, and each step is difficult to do well. Chapters 1 and 2 set the stage by describing the new need for marketing skills in nursing and introducing the general philosophy of marketing. Chapters 3 through 6 prepare the reader for the first essential step in marketing: understanding how consumers view health services and approach their use. Their goal is to enhance the reader's ability to take any idea and analyze it from the consumer's viewpoint, since rarely, if ever, does the consumer see a service as its provider sees it. Chapters 7 through 9 prepare the reader for the second step of marketing: evaluating an idea in light of possible consumer reactions, modifying it to maximize its chances of success, and getting it into final shape for its market launch. Chapters 10 through 12 are intended to refine the reader's skills in the third step of marketing: communicating the availability of a service to its intended market and handling consumer response. Finally, Chapters 13 through 16 illustrate the application of these concepts in a variety of nursing environments through actual case studies and the use of these concepts by nurses in a wide variety of positions and settings.

The test of any marketing effort, like any nursing activity, is a simple one. Does it work? The same test should apply to this book. Can it give its reader a reasonable proficiency in the complexities of marketing? To test this proposition, much of its material was used by one of the authors as the basis of a course offered in the spring of 1988 at the College of Allied Health Sciences of Thomas Jefferson University.

At the outset, the students showed minimal proficiency both in routine marketing skills and in more complex analytical tasks. By the end of the course, each participant exhibited increased knowledge and enhanced skills. The projects they produced reflect in many respects the creativity and innovation demonstrated by the contributors featured in Chapters 13 through 16.

This book is not "Marketing Made Easy for Nurses." An oversimplified introduction to marketing would be unwise. The book requires effort and commitment on the reader's part. The authors believe that by the end of the book the effort and energies invested will have paid off.

Acknowledgements

The completion of this manuscript involved a number of individuals who deserve recognition for their skill, creativity, support and loyalty. Carmheil Brown, Janet Brunham, Mary Ann McGinley, R.N., M.S.N., Elizabeth Kramer and Bob Krapfel contributed invaluable ideas which we incorporated. Deirdre Crandall, Barbara Naftal, Tricia Riebel, Trish Stahl and Donna Turner checked our math, spent hours in the library with literature searches and research, and coordinated production from concept to completion. Finally, to our families — who did all those things that help when you would like to be with them and can't.

Part I

An Introduction to Marketing

Chapter 1

Why Marketing?

The Marketplace

Marketing as a concept or as a topic of regular discussion is unfamiliar to most practicing nurses. Indeed, only recently has marketing become a major focus in health care. One could appropriately ask: Why should nurses involved in clinical practice, administration, education, and research be concerned with an array of activities more commonly associated with sales charts, coupons, commercials, and advertisements?

Yet, current health care literature is dominated by an often unfamiliar marketing jargon that speaks of joint ventures, efficiency, productivity, corporate restructuring, and customer relations. Operational performance is increasingly linked to profit motives and economic indicators such as payback periods, return on investment, cost-benefit analysis, and contribution margins. Case-mix management, strategic planning, and market research now dominate feasibility studies and justification proposals.

These signs point to the fact that fundamental, uncompromising change is the order of the day in health care. Other signs and symptoms of the transformation include decreasing inpatient admissions, major reductions in length of stay, prospective rather than cost-based payment methods, and the growth of alternative delivery systems such as health maintenance organizations (HMOs) and preferred provider organizations (PPOs).

Nursing, in terms of sheer numbers, represents the largest component of the health care team. It can ignore the current environment and hold to traditional knowledge and skills, or it can respond and retool to proactively and successfully participate in the developing health care system. Change creates opportunity. Individuals and groups that respond effectively advance; those who resist action

3

decline. The future of nursing as a profession depends, at least in part, on its response to change.

This introductory chapter seeks to provide a brief overview of the current health care environment, identify and describe major forces shaping the change process, specify how and why marketing fits in, and identify how marketing applies to professional nursing roles. The factors at work are complex. It is appropriate to begin with a general discussion of where the system has been, its current state and where it is likely to go.

Economic Environment

Health care is the second largest employer and third largest area of consumer spending in the United States. In 1950, health industry expenditures comprised 5% of the gross national product. In 1984, they approached 11% ($387 billion), or more than $1 billion a day. If this trend continues, each man, woman, and child in the United States will spend approximately $2,600 annually on health care needs alone by 1990 (Califano 1986).

Although we think of patients as the system's focal point, their role in health care purchase decisions is vastly different from that played in the usual exchange between buyer and seller. In the past, health care consumers have not been directly influenced by cost in acquisition decisions. The two major purchasers of health care are the corporations and governments that provide for the reimbursement of goods and services, through employee benefits and social programs such as Medicare and Medicaid. In the corporate sector alone, health care costs and insurance premiums paid by employers increased from $4 billion in 1960 to $110 billion in 1984, a 2,600% increase in 24 years. General Motors for example, pays more for employee health care than for the steel used in manufacturing its primary product (Califano 1986).

The number-one consumer of health care services, however, is the federal government. Federal budget deficit problems and legislation designed to strictly control federal spending have focused the attention of budget analysts on Medicare spending rates. In 1984, the federal government paid $112 billion to cover the costs of its primary programs and employee obligations — including Medicare and Medicaid; benefits for active military personnel, their dependents, and veterans; and research activities at the National Institutes of Health. These figures do not include contributions made by local and state governments, which add another $50 billion to the expense side of the balance sheet.

Corporations and governments act as purchasing agents for their subscribers and employees. They are strategically positioned in the health care marketplace to drive down health care costs. Corporations large and small are increasingly turning the mechanisms such as utilization review, second and third opinions, and employee-based financial incentives as means of control. In 1986, for example, General Motors reported a 9% decrease in health care costs, which the company attributed to the introduction of better health care management techniques for employees and their families (Califano 1986).

The federal government also has the ability to profoundly influence health care economics. In 1983, it took a major step in that direction. Historically, Medicare inpatient services have been reimbursed on the basis of reasonable cost. In order to curb future expenditures, the government introduced a prospective payment system for Medicare recipients. Commonly referred to as DRGs (diagnosis-related groups), this payment mechanism created a system whereby hospitals would receive predetermined amounts for specific illness episodes or DRGs, rather than according to the traditional cost-based method. In other words, the newly developed system determined, on the basis of several indicators, what the government would pay for a specific illness. If the hospital provided the service for less than the predetermined amount, the difference was theirs to keep; if not, the loss would, it was hoped, be recovered from a more profitable patient service or product. In the future, the government plans to include capital equipment reimbursement in the predetermined DRG payment, and major alterations in the Medicare physician payment model are under consideration.

The effect of these initiatives has been profound. In 1984, the national average daily hospital census was 970,000; in 1986, it was 883,000. A study by the Department of Health and Human Services revealed that average length of stay at hospitals dropped 22% from 1980 to 1985. In 1980, patients stayed an average of 7.35 days, but this number dropped to 5.71 days in 1985. However, the trend seemed to be ending in 1986 (Staff 1988). In 1985, the average facility occupancy rate was 64.8%, a 10.5% decline from a 72.5% industry low in 1984 (American Hospital Association 1987). These figures would have been more dramatic if the hospitals had not taken 18,000 beds out of service in 1985. Some of the bed reduction resulted from the closure of 61 hospitals during 1985—49 community and 12 specialty facilities—while other hospitals closed patient care units. A Touche-Ross survey reported that an additional 83 hospitals closed during 1986, and 43% of the respondents reported that they were at risk for closure (in Porter-O'Grady 1987).

Predictions regarding reductions in occupancy rates are even more dramatic. For example, the Rand Corporation studied 1,132 medical records of adults hospitalized between 1974 and 1982, and found that 23% of the admissions were unnecessary and could have been provided on an outpatient basis. An additional 7% had surgery that could have been done on an outpatient basis. When these figures were applied to the overall inpatient business, it was revealed that as many as 40% of current hospital stays may be unnecessary (in American Hospital Association 1986).

Hospital admissions, rather than length of stay and percentage of occupancy, are now the critical indicator of performance. What has been lost as a result of shorter stays can be recovered by increasing the number of admissions. Hospitals are now concentrating on how they can keep their empty beds filled, by attracting larger numbers of patients who need health care services.

Economic factors alone, however, are not responsible for the restructuring of the health care system. Social, technological, and political forces also play major roles, an understanding of which will help to answer the question: Why marketing?

Social Environment

Three major social changes have combined to shape health care marketplace dynamics. First, the supply of physicians has dramatically increased; second, consumers are playing a major role in purchase decisions; and third, individuals are assuming increased responsibility for their health status.

Physicians, once a scarce commodity, have markedly increased in numbers. In 1963, there were 143 practicing doctors for every 100,000 U.S. citizens; in 1985, there were 227. The U.S. Department of Health and Human Services projects that this ratio will increase to 235 in 1990 and to 260 by 2000 (Califano 1986). One third of the physicians now practicing medicine graduated during the 1980s and current medical school enrollment is not significantly down. Physician services should be readily available in the foreseeable future (Califano 1986); (Coddington and Moore 1987).

The half-million physicians practicing medicine today are key players in the provider network and strategically important elements in the hospital marketplace. On the other hand, they must also struggle with the changes in their own marketplace. The economic laws of supply and demand indicate that a buyer's market for physician services will dominate. More intense competition among physicians for patients in urban areas and lower fees are natural market responses. These changes are already evident, according to Coddington and Moore (1987). They report higher concentrations of specialized physicians — such as anesthesiologists, diagnostic radiologists, and child psychiatrists — in rural settings, as doctors attempt to effectively distribute themselves to lessen competition for service fees. In the future, physicians will alter their customer/patient service patterns, become more cost conscious, and establish joint ventures and alternative financial arrangements, such as fee reductions, in order to gain access, for example, to HMO-based patients. Regarding the latter, although the HMO concept is almost 40 years old, it would seem that its time has come, along with other alternative delivery systems, such as PPOs. Consumers now have a number of service options available, and they are actively participating in the selection process.

Corporations and the federal government foster the development of HMOs because these organizations place greater emphasis on keeping members out of the hospital and controlling length of stay for those admitted. These practices effectively reduce costs associated with employee and subscriber health care. Consumers, however, may choose not to belong to an HMO because they lose the individual doctor-patient relationship. In response, another alternative delivery system, the PPO, overcomes this perceived deficit by allowing members to select their physician from a list of approved health care providers. In order for a doctor to appear on the list, the doctor must pay a provider fee.

Employers, who offer the options, and employees, who elect membership in PPO and HMO arrangements, pay a periodic fee, similar to insurance plan premiums. The fee covers necessary services such as office visits and hospitalization, and may cover items such as prescriptions and eyeglasses. HMO and PPO care goals emphasize consumer education and wellness, rather than the traditional illness-oriented, inpatient perspective. Smoking cessation, weight control, nutritional consciousness, and physical fitness dominate today's health care scene. These movements reflect the wellness orientation of society and complement the goals of developing alternative delivery systems.

In 1970, alternative delivery systems such as HMOs had only 3 million members and were available in fewer than 15 states. By 1984, 41 states and the District of Columbia offered these options to consumers, and enrollments had increased by 22%. Predictions call for 30 million members by 1990 (Califano 1986). As these organizations become more consumer oriented, their market share should increase. In addition, government and corporate buyers are developing attractive incentives designed to persuade more consumers to select these less expensive options.

The net effect of these delivery systems is decreased inpatient utilization and increased ambulatory care services. Hospitals and physicians are forced to vie for patients. Consumers' and employers' willingness to "shop" presents major marketing opportunities for health plan brokers and insurance companies. Competition is the order of the day.

Technological Environment

At the beginning of this century, physicians carried medical technology in a small black bag. Today, the black bag has all but disappeared. The production and general distribution of highly sophisticated technological advances has dramatically affected the health care system. Technology will continue to play a key role in shaping the marketplace.

Over the years, the acquisition and use of sophisticated techniques moved from the physician's office and research lab into the hospital. Although technology has led to increased costs, it has attracted new patients and has satisfied perceived physician needs. In many respects, benefit has exceeded cost. For instance, the role of the computed tomography (CT) scanner in making exploratory brain surgery unnecessary or that of chymopapain in treating ruptured disks.

New medical technologies are usually adopted when two conditions are met: first, product safety and appropriateness in treatment are validated; and, second, third-party payers accept the technology, allowing financial reimbursement. In the future, technological development and acquisition by hospitals will be influenced by three factors: specialization and regionalization of highly expensive technologies, such as positron emission tomography (PET) scanners; incentives to develop outpatient and home care services, such as total parenteral nutrition; and service growth opportunities, such as organ transplantation.

Technology often increases cost while it enhances health care services, but it can also save valuable dollars. Until very recently, for example, tubal ligation required a 2- to 3-day inpatient stay. This service is now provided safely and effectively on an outpatient basis. Almost overnight the development, acquisition, and use of laparoscopes changed gynecological health care. As another example, the lithotripter, which uses sound waves to pulverize kidney stones, has reduced the need for painful surgery and lengthy periods of hospitalization. A similar approach is being tested to treat gallstones. CT scanners, magnetic resonance imaging (MRI), ultrasonic devices, and fiberoptics all facilitate early diagnosis, intervention, and treatment.

The health care industry has yet to see the full impact of drugs designed to prevent atherosclerosis or to treat myocardial infarction; or the effect of genetic splicing in the treatment of sickle cell anemia; or the full-scale preservation and implantation of human organs. Some of these developments will increase the movement of inpatients to outpatient markets, while other developments, such as organ transplantation, will enhance the creation of new and larger inpatient markets. The demand for inpatient services will also be affected by how extensive the AIDS problem becomes.

Political and Legal Environment

The formulation of government policy and legal activities will also continue to play a major role in shaping the marketplace. As previously noted, Medicare reimbursement will be tightly controlled, as the federal deficit problem is addressed. Reimbursement, on the other hand, is likely to allow altered payments based on some method of measuring severity of illness and quality of care such as the experiment currently under way in Rochester, New York (Fortney 1988). This development would improve reimbursement for tertiary providers and reduce payments in less complex settings.

Legislation and regulations will include stringent peer-review requirements as a means of identifying low-cost, high-quality providers at the service level. Requirements for certificate-of-need applications and reviews will decrease, in order to conform to the accepted characteristics of a free market. Finally, malpractice insurance premiums will influence relationships among physicians, hospitals, and the marketplace. Hospitals, for example, may elect to underwrite malpractice insurance premiums for obstetricians and anesthesiologists as a means of maintaining market share and providing essential community services. Legislation to place limits on malpractice awards can also be anticipated. Market responses, however, will continue to be influenced by actual and potential legal actions and threats.

Implications for Nursing

Rising costs, disgruntled government and corporate buyers, technologies of the brave new world, changing social attitudes, DRGs, alternative delivery systems, and an oversupply of physicians have all combined to spawn revolutionary reform. Health care, once a social service, is now big business. Community hospitals, traditionally a sort of cottage industry and the backbone of the delivery system, are threatened with negative balance sheets and acquisition and competition from large hospital systems.

From a social service to a business, from a cottage industry to multimember hospital systems, from being provider driven to being economically driven, from a system based on cooperation to one based on competition — all of these factors indicate that health care services are increasingly managed as economic products, like airline travel or kitchen appliances, which are most appropriately and efficiently distributed in competitive markets.

To return to this chapter's main question: What has all this fundamental change got to do with nursing? After all, nurses are concerned with providing highly skilled services in a number of different settings, not with competition, conflict, and market share, right? Wrong. Health care system restructuring has brought hospitals, physicians, and nurses face to face with competition. Traditional relationships among patients, providers, and insurers are breaking down, and hospitals, the major consumers of nursing services, face an uncertain future.

The nursing community will experience this revolution with the same immediacy and impact as hospitals and doctors. Just as the patient's and society's view of the physician's role has changed markedly, so, too, nurses are being called upon to think and act in ways that seem foreign. The act of nursing means many things to nurses, patients, and physicians alike. Nurses have been and will continue to be, first and foremost, principal caregivers. Patients have more contact with nurses than with any other provider type. The quality of care provided by the professional nurse will continue to be measured in both medical and human terms. But new dimensions are being added. Increasingly, nurses are expected to view their efforts as a product — a product that is part of a larger array of services.

The implications of this new way of thinking are profoundly unsettling. Nurses are not educated to focus their concern on anything other than patient welfare. Now, nurses, especially nursing leaders, are being asked to consider whether particular DRGs or clinical specialties are "growth areas" in patient and revenue terms. Some types of patients are seen as more desirable than others, not because of their need for service or likelihood of recovery but because of the costs expended to provide the service to them.

While the merits of these changes are debatable, the probability of their occurrence is not. For nurses and nursing, the issue is not whether costs, profits, and market dynamics will dominate the agenda, but how nursing will respond and react. The number and type of positions in nursing will inevitably undergo significant restructuring, as nursing deals with external marketplace factors and its own internal market dynamics.

For one thing, the availability of clinical services will be shaped by demographics and consumer demand, as well as by technological development. Access to more desirable types of employment will be limited not only by technical competence and proficiency but by the individual's ability to be part of a team that is market driven. Administrators and clinical leaders will be selected and evaluated on the basis of their business savvy as much as by their supervisory and clinical skills. The forces producing these changes are well under way, and their momentum is great.

Marketing concepts, principles, and skills are vital in the environment just described. What precisely is marketing? Some will say advertising, others product line management. Both are partially right. Marketing can be described as a process by which an organization or individual determines a consumer need and develops a product or service to meet that need.

That health care is embracing marketing is readily apparent. In 1985, the industry spent $125.6 million on television advertising, representing a 40% increase over 1984 totals and an amount five times that spent in 1980. In 1987, the average hospital marketing budget exceeded $236,000; nationwide, the hospital industry spent $1.38 billion on marketing activities, including staff salaries (Droste 1987; Powills 1986).

Marketing departments have been created in hospitals and frequently include a sales force; communications personnel, such as physician referral services and "Ask A Nurse" programs; as well as separate groups who manage various hospital products. Specific market segments, such as obstetrics, women's services, emergency services, outpatient surgery, and geriatric programs are receiving special attention by marketing personnel, owing to their size and the choices consumers can make in these areas. Response to these markets can be seen in the spending patterns of marketing departments. Commercial advertising expenditures per hospital jumped 43% between 1986 and 1987, to an all-time high of $146,000. Predictions called for hospitals to spend $726 million on advertising in 1987, with no indication that the rate would level off or decline in the foreseeable future.

In California, package pricing for obstetrical services has been introduced. Some consumers select the short-stay programs costing $600, while others choose a $3,500 package featuring a 4-day hospital stay, supplemented by a home visit from a registered nurse specializing in obstetrical care. The ultimate in marketing know-how is the 14-bed unit that recently opened in Bethesda, Maryland, offering first-class surgical service. Patients are picked up by limousine at their home on the day of admission, meals are catered by a gourmet French restaurant, and the staffing complement is 100% registered nurses. The hospital's physical environment looks more like a classy hotel than a hospital. Indeed, there is a waiting list to get in!

While hospitals are the major players utilizing marketing techniques, they are certainly not the sole focus of application. Free-standing emergency centers, birthing centers, midwifery services, home health care agencies, HMOs, PPOs, and individual physician and nursing practices are services that can utilize the marketing process.

So why should nurses be interested in marketing? They should be interested because those adept at marketing themselves and/or their agencies will fare relatively better in an increasingly competitive world. Similarly, nursing administrators and managers in various settings should be adept at marketing concepts and applications because they must lead the engineering of patient and employee satisfaction at every distribution point. Nursing educators, too, should be informed about the importance of marketing because they transmit the professional culture, its knowledge and skills, via the curriculum, and because marketing concepts and principles are vital in student recruitment.

In addition, clinicians in all walks of professional life — nurse practitioners, nurse midwives, clinical specialists, staff nurses, community health nurses, and physician office nurses — should be aware of marketing theory and practice because they play a vital role in shaping programs to attract patients. Finally, nursing researchers should be interested in marketing because the assessment of need and the evaluation of effect are vital to the marketing plan and to the development of the service offered to the customer.

In conclusion, as this book will demonstrate, nurses should embrace marketing because they are in a strategic position to assess, plan, implement, and evaluate marketing proposals designed to influence customer behavior and shape public perception. The outcomes of the health care revolution are by no means clear. Nurses, individually and collectively, have an opportunity to respond and participate, not only on behalf of their own interests but on behalf of those of the patient as well. Marketing is a nursing imperative.

References

American Hospital Association. 1986. Rand study claims up to 40 percent of hospital stays are unnecessary. *Hospital Week* 22: 46.

Califano, J.A. 1986. *America's health care revolution.* New York: Random House.

Coddington, D.C., and K. Moore. 1987. *Market driven strategies in health care.* San Francisco: Jossey-Bass Publications.

Droste, T., ed. 1987. Marketing budgets increase a modest 4%. *Hospitals* 61: 22.

Fortney, D.L. 1988. Hospitals exploring linkage of payments to patient outcomes. *Healthcare Financial News* 2: 3.

Porter-O'Grady, T., ed. 1987. Take note. *Aspen's Advisor for Nurse Executives.* 3: 1.

Powills, S., ed. 1986. Marketing budgets on the rise. *Hospitals* 60: 5.

Staff. 1988. Hospital briefs. *Healthcare Financial News*, (July): 2

Review Questions

1. The development and implementation of the Medicare prospective reimbursement system was a primary factor in the generation of a competitive marketplace. How is non-Medicare reimbursement for acute care services

being handled in your state? How has it affected marketplace dynamics? How will services be reimbursed 5 years from now? How will the future payment system affect the marketplace?

2. Alternative delivery systems such as HMOs and PPOs develop contracts with facilities to provide acute care services for their members. What role should nurse clinicians and administrators play in the acquisition and retention of these agreements?

3. The current nursing shortage has been called the most severe health care personnel crisis in this century? If you agree, how has the impact affected the marketplace and how have individual facilities utilized this environmental factor in a marketing strategy?

4. What impact has the competitive marketplace had on other distribution points for nursing services, such as nursing homes, occupational health, and community health? Identify the marketing implications for nursing?

5. Identify future trends in reimbursement, identify marketplace implications, and the implications for nursing.

Chapter 2

The Philosophy and Science of Marketing

Marketing as a Philosophy

Marketing, as discussed later in this chapter, is an organizational science. Marketing manages the relationship between providers of products and services and their existing and potential customers. It does so by applying basic scientific concepts — diagnosing problems, deciding how to "treat" them, implementing that treatment, and monitoring its effect. In addition to being an organizational science, marketing is also a philosophy. How can anything be both a science and philosophy? Consider medicine itself. What doctors and nurses do is mostly a science — they diagnose a problem, plan treatment or therapy, implement the treatment, and monitor its outcome.

Those actions are guided, however, by a philosophy — that pain and suffering should not be accepted as the "will of God" or "the luck of the draw" and that a deliberate effort should be made to arrest or reverse the consequences of illness. This philosophy also holds that it is the duty of health professionals to respond to emergencies rather than to "look the other way"; that health professionals should, while taking sensible precautions, place themselves among the infectious rather than distance themselves from them; that a patient once accepted should not be abandoned; that health professionals should "first do no harm," and so on.

This philosophy of medicine is so ingrained in the medical professions that it is often taken for granted. Yet, one can easily cite examples in recent history demonstrating that adherence to this philosophy is not guaranteed — for example, the medical "experiments" conducted by doctors in the Nazi concentration camps, or the psychiatric treatment of political nonconformists in the Soviet Union. Therefore, without a guiding philosophy, the science of medicine loses its sense of direction.

Marketing, also, requires a guiding philosophy. What is the marketing philosophy? One noted marketing authority (Kotler 1972) defines it as "a customer orientation aimed at generating customer satisfaction as the key to satisfying organizational goals." This simple definition sounds like a universal truism, not unlike the components of the philosophy of medicine until one asks two crucial questions: Is this marketing philosophy really followed universally? and, Even where it seems to be followed, is it just being given lip service, or does the person or organization involved really mean it? The answer to these two questions is, "No, the marketing philosophy is not universally followed or always followed thoroughly." There are three common situations where it is ignored. These occur in connection with a production orientation, a sales orientation, and an "I'm the expert" orientation. Each situation is discussed next.

The Production Orientation

In the production orientation, a person or organization pursues an idea simply on the basis of personal preference. The crucial question of whether enough people will want or have a need for the product to make it viable is not addressed.

Take the ill-fated videodisk, for example, RCA's potential rival to videotapes. RCA's research and development staff pursued the idea as an exciting challenge to their electrical engineering and production skills. The videotape market was booming and was expected to continue to do so. RCA did at least address whether a market existed. They did not, however, ruthlessly pursue the question, "Is this what enough people want?" The product fared poorly, lacking the flexibility and reusability of videotape. Eventually, RCA withdrew the product, incurring a multimillion dollar loss.

RCA was a major corporation, but small enterprises are just as likely, perhaps more likely, to be driven by the production orientation. In the health care field, where personnel often do not have formal business education, potential for failure is greater. According to the traditions of medicine, physicians and nurses focus on mastering their professional knowledge and skills. In the process, many of them identify a field of strong personal interest in which they become personally engrossed. They identify an idea that they want to pursue, and do not pause to ask whether enough patients can be attracted to it to render it viable.

To cite an actual example, several years ago, a young neurologist joined the faculty of one of the smaller medical schools. His personal field of interest was seizure disorders. The medical school hospital agreed to investigate with him the creation of a regional epilepsy center. The initial analysis was promising—the program could cover its costs if it attracted 500 patients. Since epilepsy is a chronic condition with most patients requiring periodic lifetime care, the program would need only to attract a few new patients in each subsequent year to make up for those who moved away or died.

The medical school started developing a marketing strategy to attract these 500 patients. The first disconcerting discovery was that the incidence of epilepsy in the population is low. In fact, the neurologist was unable to quote it—his whole concentration had been on understanding the etiology of the disease and available treatment regimens. It emerged that there were only 5,000 probable cases within a 50-mile radius of the center. Thus, the new program would need a 10% market share to break even. Next it was realized that, because epilepsy is a chronic condition, most patients were already in some pattern of care in their communities. The number of new cases diagnosed annually within a 50-mile radius was probably less than 100. The new center would therefore need to attract many established patients away from their existing care providers, a challenge made greater by the fact that, for many of them, the center was considerably farther from their homes.

The neurologist was then asked to define two or three reasons that might convince a potential patient or referring physician to switch from existing care resources to this center. The neurologist explained that he was researching improved treatment protocols, but as yet had no proven methods to offer that were not likely to be available through more local resources. Although some community physicians have traditionally been willing to refer some patients to physicians for research programs, this appeal was unlikely to draw more than a small portion of the needed 500 patients.

The next issue reviewed was how to directly reach families with epileptic members, since possibly some of them might self-refer just because the center was new and, through time, might offer hope of a better treatment. The neurologist suggested that the local chapter of the Epilepsy Foundation might agree to give the center use of its mailing list to reach such families. A call to the foundation revealed, however, that it only had 200 people on its mailing list and was uncertain whether it would share it with the center for this purpose. It appeared that the only viable way to attempt to reach these 5,000 families with a message strong enough to attract 10% of them would be by a major media advertising campaign. Such a campaign could cost in excess of $80,000 and would be a risky venture, given first, that most patients already had other, closer resources available; second, the center could not really claim that it had a "better" product; and, third, a 10% response would be ambitious for any advertising campaign.

In light of all these barriers to success, the decision was made not to launch the center. The neurologist eventually developed a more general neurology practice along more conventional lines.

There is, of course, an element of tragedy here. A new and more effective treatment for epilepsy might possibly have been acquired if this young neurologist had been able to pursue his idea. It was, however, the right idea in the wrong circumstances. At another medical school, with more senior colleagues sharing his interest and more capability to attract research funding, the neurologist might have been able to pursue his goals without having to attract an unattainable volume of patients. This case does, however, demonstrate the production orientation—pursuing an idea without regard to whether enough people will use it.

> *The marketing philosophy recognizes that circumstances do not necessarily support every idea and venture. To satisfy your own or your organization's goals, you must also be able to satisfy the goals of enough customers. Whereas production orientation focuses upon the delivery of a product or service, the marketing philosophy focuses on creating a mutual exchange of goals and the means to satisfy them.*

The Sales Orientation

> *The sales orientation recognizes that products and services have to be sold. In this respect, it complements more the philosophy of marketing than the production orientation. It still fails, however, to ask the critical question: "Will we have to modify*

*our product or service, or the way we present it, to maximize its
appeal?"*

To take again an example from industry, when Du Pont
launched the Teflon pan, it followed the sales orientation, attempting to capitalize on the low amount of fat required to cook with
Teflon. However, sales were so poor in the first 6 months that Du
Pont seriously considered withdrawing the product. First, however,
it decided to ask some of the people who had bought Teflon pans
why they had done so, and discovered that the main benefit was easy
cleaning—"the nonstick pan." Had Du Pont made a greater initial
effort to find out what really mattered to homemakers, they might
well have avoided this costly initial mistake. As it happened, they
did not have to modify the product to maximize its appeal, but only
change their sales message.

Frequently, the modifications needed to create a matching of
goals between a supplier and the potential customer are drastic, en-
tailing modifying the product or service itself, or the way it is
delivered. Consider now an actual example from within health care.
Several years ago a hospital recruited to its staff an andrologist
(specialist in male infertility). It already had on staff a reproductive
endocrinologist (specialist in female infertility). The andrologist
asked the hospital to help in promoting his program. Two other
local hospitals already had both andrologists and reproductive endocrinologists on staff and over the years had developed strong
reputations for infertility management. The hospital marketing staff
asked how this new program could be given a clear and distinctive
appeal. How could "new" also be promoted as "better"? The
reproductive endocrinologist reported that he had received calls in
the past from patients dissatisfied with the existing centers. It appeared that the main source of grievance was that the andrologists
treating the man and the reproductive endocrinologists treating the
woman at these other centers saw patients in their own separate office suites and maintained separate files on each partner. There was
no coordination between the andrologist and endocrinologist in
each center, raising the suspicion in couples' minds that the separate
treatments might not be aligned to maximize the prospects of conception.

These reports led the physicians and the marketing staff of the
new program to develop a center focusing mainly on infertile
couples, with both physicians seeing these patients in one of their of-

fice suites, and with scheduling such that the couple could, if they wished, come in for appointments at the same time and have joint discussions with both doctors if needed. In addition, a combined medical record would be maintained so that each physician could easily see what the other was doing. Although none of those proposals was difficult to implement, each violated traditional methods of medical practice and involved major concessions from the physicians. The doctors did agree to all these steps, however, and the new center quickly gained patients despite the competition from two longer established and better-known alternatives.

This case illustrates that it may often be necessary to go beyond a sales orientation to achieve a real matching of goals between providers and customers. It is rare that a service, as conceived by its providers, exactly matches what a significant number of people want. Yet even if some customers will accept "second best," there is a hidden danger in letting them do so. Satisfaction results when service meets or exceeds expectations. If a service falls short of expectations, customers may spread negative reports of it to their friends and further handicap the program in achieving its sponsors' own goals. That is the greatest danger of the sales orientation. By promoting a product or service that is not close enough to what people want, a supplier may draw more first-time customers but also inflate the number of dissatisfied customers. It may almost be possible to sell anything once, but it is not possible to sustain the sales of a "second best" product or service. The sales orientation focuses on that selling task, whereas the marketing philosophy, defined earlier by Kotler, focuses on generating and sustaining "customer satisfaction."

Another example may help to illustrate this important distinction. A medical practice implemented an extensive marketing program to attract more patients with a variety of pain syndromes. Its volume rose, as a result, by some 20%. It was pleased with this growth until it conducted a satisfaction survey and discovered that 10% of all patients left with very negative feelings about their visit. Further study showed that the main reason for this dissatisfaction was that these patients had chronic, intractable problems that the practice could not treat or alleviate, making the patients feel that their visit had been a waste of time. The practice responded by screening patients more carefully when they called and by trying to identify alternative resources for those whom it was unlikely they could help. In so doing, it was consciously lowering both its patient volume and revenue in the short run in order to have a success rate closer to 100% and more positive word-of-mouth testimonials circulating in the community. The strategy succeeded; 6 years later, the practice is now four times as large as it was before the survey and is very well regarded in its service area.

The sales orientation would have resisted such a deliberate lowering of sales despite an increase in customer satisfaction. The marketing philosophy, on the other hand, would regard it as an unusual, but entirely logical step, because it recognizes high satisfaction among customers as essential to continuing to match its goals with theirs.

"I'm the Expert" Orientation

The "I'm the expert" orientation asserts that the supplier, whether an individual or an entire organization, knows what is best for customers and expects them to conform. It never asks the critical question: "To what degree can we give the customer choice?"

The best example of this orientation is illustrated by Henry Ford's ill-fated proclamation that the customer could have a Model T in "any color as long as it's black." Ford dominated the early mass market for automobiles by being the first to develop assembly line production and to offer an auto at a price affordable to the average family. However, as Alfred P. Sloan gradually organized and expanded General Motors, his company posed an increasing threat to Ford by offering more variety and choice. Henry Ford was reluctant to abandon the formula of low price but rigid standardization that had worked for him in the past. He thought he was "the expert" on mass marketing of automobiles, because he had invented it.

The "I'm the expert" phenomenon is illustrated in health care in the case of a hospital nursing department that had made a major commitment to both the primary nursing approach and holistic care. It was proud of its accomplishments, and this pride was highest on its obstetrics units. Then a detailed study of patient satisfaction throughout the hospital produced the disconcerting finding that the obstetrics floor had the lowest level of patient satisfaction in the hospital. What had gone wrong?

The nurses had genuinely developed sensible protocols for the holistic care of the patient and newborn, covering issues such as use of birthing rooms, "rooming in," visiting hours for family and relatives, sibling presence at delivery, child birth education, and so forth. The shortcoming of this approach, however, was that it did not accommodate potential differences in patients' desires or involve the patients in any significant decision making regarding their care. A matching of goals was not taking place in the minds of at least some patients, who did not want "what was best for them" to be determined unilaterally.

How, then, can one reconcile the marketing philosophy of responding to what the customer wants with the profession's inherent responsibility to do no harm or even to waste time on nonefficacious placebos? The answer to this apparent dilemma is that the customer is not always right.

> *The marketing philosophy asserts that a matching of goals should form the basis of any enterprise, not that a provider should subordinate his or her goals totally to those of the customer. That is not a matching but a surrender. The marketing philosophy does entail offering the customer reasonable choice where it does not eradicate the value of the service.*

The obstetrical nurses just discussed responded professionally to the new input about patient satisfaction. They identified which elements in their protocols were essential to good care and which were discretionary. They then introduced a nursing assessment process that included actively presenting choices to patients on discretionary issues and soliciting their preferences. In other words, they embraced the marketing philosophy.

Recent literature on the marketing philosophy has underscored that successful marketing requires individuals who can exercise on-the-spot judgment regarding how to balance customer satisfaction with organizational or professional policies, who know how to bend the rules without breaking them to improve customer satisfaction. For instance, in *In Search of Excellence*, Peters and Waterman (1983) concluded that the most important element in excellent companies was the presence of lots of people who believe in flying in the same direction, but not necessarily in formation.

It has been pointed out, however, that nurturing such a marketing orientation also calls for a special organizational culture — one that demands quality and professionalism but puts the customer first from the top down and does not punish people for poor judgment so long as they were endeavoring to promote customer satisfaction. Buck Rodgers, in *The IBM Way* (1986), one of the most revealing insider accounts of life in a successful enterprise, recounts how, as a new IBM executive, he arrived late for a meeting with the company chairman and several vice-presidents. As he walked into the room, the chairman proclaimed that he demanded punctuality at meetings. Rodgers spoke up and explained that he had been detained talking to a customer. The chairman told him that he had "the right priorities" and never again raised the punctuality issue.

The marketing philosophy, therefore, requires both individuals who will reach beyond the "I'm the expert" orientation when customer satisfaction is at stake and senior managers who will allow them to honor that priority.

The differences between the marketing philosophy and the other three orientations analyzed here do not usually relate to goals. People and organizations, regardless of which orientation they possess, are likely to want to:

1. Realize their own potential — to be all that they can be

2. Strive for and take pride in the quality of what they do

3. Provide a service — to do good for those who buy their products or use professional services

What distinguishes a marketing orientation from the other orientations relates to the *means* of achieving those objectives. According to the earlier-cited definition by Kotler (1972), marketing is founded on the philosophy that the only way to satisfy your own or your organization's goals is through finding, attracting, serving, and satisfying customers. To do so, you must be prepared to:

1. Invest time and effort to understand as much as possible about what people want, how they prefer to get it, and what makes them satisfied or dissatisfied with a product or service experience

2. Modify the details of what you do and how you do it to fit in best with customer needs and desires

3. Invest time and effort to publicize what you offer, because people have multiple alternatives available to

them to satisfy most of their needs, and you must compete for their attention

These characteristics sound simple enough, but they have enormous implications for satisfying individual needs.

All occupations, including professional jobs, entail developing standard ways to approach situations. The marketing philosophy expects such standard approaches to clash at times with the unique needs and opinions of specific customers. It asserts that suppliers of services should be willing, wherever possible, to change the way they do things in order to maximize customer satisfaction, so long as the quality and efficacy of the service are not compromised.

Marketing as a Science

As noted at the beginning of this chapter, marketing is a scientific process guided by a philosophy. It is a science in that it examines and seeks to address issues by following a scientific process — attempting to diagnose an issue, identifying an appropriate line of action, implementing it using specialized skills, and monitoring its impact.

For example, a hospital launched an internal guest relations program emphasizing the need for courtesy, friendliness, and a quick response to patient requests. It did so following a patient survey that suggested a need for improvement in these areas. The program appeared well designed and well executed, but a follow-up survey showed that it had achieved little impact. A resulting investigation revealed that many of the hospital's nurses had grievances concerning the condescending attitude displayed toward them by many senior physicians at the hospital. They had responded by trying to emphasize the technical and clinical aspects of their work — to demonstrate to the physicians that the modern role of nursing extended well beyond attending to routine patient needs. The "guest relations" priorities struck them as focusing on the least professional aspects of nursing, and they had, therefore, largely ignored the new program.

The hospital thus discovered that before it could expect its nurses to match goals more fully with patients, it must first more adequately match goals with them. The hospital's original market research was flawed in that it took for granted that the nurses would support the program. Faulty diagnosis had led to a flawed prescription for the program, ineffective implementation, and a lack of positive results. As a science, marketing follows a scientific process to address issues, including, as this example illustrated, measuring outcomes and rediagnosing if results are less than desired.

Also, in common with other sciences, marketing seeks to establish laws and models of how things work. These laws and models have been developed through past observation or through prior formal experimentation. Their role is to allow practitioners to predict what will happen in given circumstances.

Medical and nursing practice are among the fields of knowledge in which such laws and models are most abundant. That is what makes medicine such an advanced science — it now has a high rate of success in accurate differential diagnosis and in predicting the impact of different therapies on differing disease states.

Marketing is a less exact science than medicine, principally because it deals with a form of human behavior — relations between suppliers and customers or products and services. The laws and models of an organic science such as medicine tend to be more reliable than those of a behavioral and organizational science like marketing. This is so because in medicine it is usually possible to isolate the limited phenomena being considered more completely from other variables that might affect the validity of the law or model. A simple example is a patient's drug regimen. When necessary to maximize the therapeutic value of a medication, it is possible to control the intake of other drugs, the intake of chemicals in food or the purity of the air the patient breathes.

It is rarely, if ever, possible to completely isolate the effect of a behavioral or organizational action, since its precise consequences are conditioned by many factors that are uncontrollable. Consider an action so simple as writing a letter to someone asking them to do something. How it will be received depends upon many variables, including the recipient's mood when he or she receives it, how much other mail he or she receives that day, and whether other letters command his or her attention to the exclusion of yours.

Despite these limitations, however, marketers through the years have developed a set of laws and models to help them understand

and predict how people behave as customers. As an example, there are well-established rules dealing with even so limited an aspect of marketing as how to maximize the probability of direct mail responses. Marketers have developed these rules by trial and error as well as by conscious experimentation. Research into marketing has, for several decades, consumed close to $1 in every $150 spent in the United States. It has grown into such a major field of spending because the success of so many enterprises depends upon it (Twedt 1968).

Do the laws and models of marketing apply to health care? After all, the practical experience from which marketing laws were developed has largely occurred outside of health care. It is reasonable, therefore, to question whether these laws apply to consumer decisions about health care. In fact, the science of marketing has been developing now for approximately 100 years, and while the many laws and models of marketing may have first been observed in relation to one type of supplier-customer relationship, when tested in other fields, they have been found to have similar applicability. One of these laws, the unique selling proposition was developed decades ago by Dik Twedt, a then leading theorist of advertising techniques. The unique selling proposition holds that, to succeed, an advertising slogan must focus on something of real benefit to the purchaser, it must be believable, and it must be something that competitive products cannot claim or are not choosing to claim. Two of the early applications of this law led to the two slogans "Get a Piece of the Rock" (for Prudential Life Insurance, a mutual insurance firm that has no stockholders and that is thus "owned" by those who buy policies from it) and "Peanut M & M's Melt in Your Mouth, Not in Your Hand." Before those campaigns, the conventional wisdom was that life insurance sold by virtue of the cost-per-thousand-dollars of coverage obtained and candy sold by price and taste. Note that neither of these slogans mentions these benefits at all. Yet these two campaigns were among the most successful in the history of advertising, and the phrase *unique selling proposition* is now part of the working vocabulary of every advertising executive.

One reason, therefore, to believe that marketing laws and models also apply to health care is that they were developed from experience in a wide variety of settings, from candy to steel, from life insurance to vacations, from electronics to home repairs. If health care is just one type of situation in which suppliers and customers interact to achieve an exchange of goals, it is probable that at least some of the laws and models found to apply across these other markets also have applicability in health care decisions.

It is, nevertheless, still possible to argue that health care is different because it is a highly complex field in which the customer lacks sufficient knowledge to make as informed a decision as he or she can in selecting soup or toothpaste, for example. However, health care is by no means the only field in which the customer is confronted by a knowledge barrier. As is pointed out in subsequent chapters in this book, most customers for automobiles, stereo equipment, home repairs, services of a travel agent, or even soup or toothpaste, to name but a few examples, are not equipped to make a comprehensive technical assessment of the product or service. This does not mean that they refrain from making choices. Each of us, as customers for complex products and services, has developed methods of managing a relationship with suppliers, of making choices, of evaluating this experience, and of making future judgments based upon it.

The fact that health care is complex does not put it in a category of marketing all by itself. Countless other marketing situations raise equivalent complexities for customers. Yet customers tend to handle them in broadly similar ways.

Again, one might claim that the role of doctors as intermediaries in health care decisions make the field different from other markets. In actuality, however, many marketing situations involve intermediaries who have more expert knowledge than the customer — travel agents, architects, lawyers, car salespersons, insurance brokers, realtors, investment advisers, electricians, plumbers, and so on.

The typical customer is used to situations in which an expert intermediary, such as a doctor, health professional, other professional, counselor, salesperson, or adviser helps to shape his or her precise service utilization patterns. This is a common marketing situation, not one unique to health care.

Finally, one might contend that any laws and models that apply to "typical" supplier-customer relations are set aside by patients, because they are dealing with matters of life and death. In fact, more than 90% of all patients visiting doctors' offices and more than 80% of all patients admitted to hospitals do not have life-threatening conditions that would lead them to set aside their normal customer behaviors. Those behaviors apply to most health care encounters.

The precise manner in which the laws or models of marketing as a science apply to different types of patients in differing circumstances will vary, but they still are applicable as a scientific basis for understanding and managing the marketing relationships that arise in health care.

References

Kotler, P. 1972. *Marketing management.* 2nd ed. Englewood Cliffs, NJ: Prentice Hall.

Peters, T., and R. Waterman. 1983. *In search of excellence.* New York: Warner Books.

Rodgers, B. 1986. *The IBM way.* New York: Harper and Row.

Twedt, D. 1968. *Survey of Marketing Research.* Chicago: American Marketing Association.

Review Questions

1. What are the main differences among the production orientation, the sales orientation, the "I'm-the-expert" orientation, and the marketing orientation?

2. "Medicine is both a science and a philosophy, and so is marketing." Comment.

3. What are the essential elements of any scientific process, and how do they apply to marketing?

4. "The things that marketers have found to be true about other products and services just don't apply in health care." Comment.

Part II

Understanding Health Care's Customers

Chapter 3

Recognizing the Need for Health Care

The previous chapter repeatedly referred to the "customers" of health care. Marketing scientists use that term much more precisely.

Customers

The customer of a product or service is the person who initiates the purchase, decides which supplier to use, makes the purchase, and pays for it. In many marketing situations, the customer is thus just one person. For instance, a homemaker shopping in a supermarket may play each of the four customer roles just described. In numerous other marketing situations, however, these roles are divided among different people. A nurse, for instance, who requests a new supply of record forms for a nursing unit initiates the process. However, the nursing administration may well decide which forms and therefore which supplier to use, a purchasing department may order new stock from that supplier, and a finance officer may arrange for payment.

As another example, a patient referred to a specialist's office by a primary care doctor has initiated the process by taking the problem to the first doctor. The primary care physician was the decision maker in the referral. If the referral was discretionary and the primary care doctor presented it as an option to the patient, both were decision makers. The primary care doctor's office staff, or the patient personally, may have made the purchase by actually contacting the specialist.

Readers may be wondering about what happened to the "consumer" aspect of this definition of *customer*.

Marketing draws a distinction between a "customer" and a "consumer"; they are not always the same person.

Consumer

The consumer of a product or service is the person who uses and derives benefit from the product or service. Often the customer is also the consumer, but frequently they are different people, as when a homemaker does the weekly food shopping knowing that he or she personally will consume only part of the purchases. A parent bringing a child to an emergency room plays most of the roles of the customer—initiating, deciding on the supplier, making the purchase, and possibly paying at least part of the bill. The child is the "consumer." However, just as more than one person can share the role of customer, more than one person can also share the role of consumer, if each derives a meaningful *benefit* from the experience. In the emergency room example, the child is the primary consumer of the service rendered, but the parent also may derive a less tangible benefit of reassurance, relief from anxiety, and help with parenting in a medical emergency.

Three other types of people may be parties to a purchase decision without being either a customer or a consumer (Reibstein 1985):

Influencer

As the word implies, an influencer helps to shape the views of a customer or consumer, but plays the role of neither in the purchase or encounter.

Now that health care consumes about $1 in every $9 spent in the United States, it also employs a significant percentage of the work force. As a result, most people know, or are related to at least one person who works directly in health care and they therefore turn to them as influencers of their own health care decisions. Even more frequently, people also seek advice from relatives or friends who may themselves have had similar health care needs and who influence the health customer's decisions.

Surrogate

A surrogate makes a decision to purchase a product or to use a service on behalf of someone else who will be the actual consumer. Parents often thus act as surrogates for their children. Some adult customers, when faced with technically complex decisions, also pass the task of decision making to someone whom they regard as more qualified.

Note the distinction between an influencer and a surrogate. An influencer does not make the decision on behalf of the customer, but only shapes his or her decision. A surrogate actually chooses the supplier on behalf of the customer.

There has been much debate in recent years about the relative roles of the primary physician and the patient in health care decisions—such as which hospital to go to, which specialist to see, or which other type of health service or agency to consult. Numerous surveys of patients have been published suggesting that a growing minority of patients see themselves as having chosen a hospital, agency, or specialist independently of any primary physician's influence. These patients therefore see themselves as the customer and consumer of these health services. Many of them admit that friends or relatives have been influencers in those decisions. Another minority of patients—and a group that appears to be diminishing in size—report that they leave all such decisions to their primary care physicians, who thus act as their surrogates.

The majority of patients fall between these two extremes—they see hospital or specialist selection as a joint decision reached with their primary care physician. These patients treat their primary doctors, therefore, as neither influencers nor surrogates but as cocustomers for the hospitals' or specialists' services.

Gatekeeper

A gatekeeper limits the choices available to a customer. Gatekeepers thus have more power in the transaction than influencers but less than surrogates. The gatekeeper concept has become familiar to health care in recent years through the spread of health maintenance organizations (HMOs) which only allow enrollees to access a specialist via referral from a primary care physician. The term has long been used in marketing, however, to describe the role of intermediaries who control the flow of information to customers about products and services, or who limit the options among which customers can choose. Many hospitals, for instance, require vendors to first contact a purchasing office or materials management department rather than letting them "run loose" around the facility. Even if such gatekeepers do not have the final power of decision on which precise supplies the hospital will buy, they do have considerable control over which vendors get access to the decision makers. Investment brokers, librarians selecting books, and hospital medical staffs who add or delete drugs from formulary are all examples of this gatekeeper role.

Agent, Representative, Salesperson

An agent, representative, or salesperson works on behalf of a producer or supplier. His or her role is to identify, advise, persuade, and ultimately introduce customers to the producer or supplier.

The influencers, surrogates, and gatekeepers just discussed do not work for the producer or supplier whose products or services they recommend, select for a consumer, or offer as one option to a consumer. By contrast, agents, representatives, or salespersons are employees of a producer or supplier. Customers do not expect them to be impartial. Their job is to provide information about their organization, persuade customers to select it, and help them to access it.

A common example outside of health care is that of life insurance. A life insurance agent represents his or her company's "products" only, not those of other companies. By contrast, an insurance broker acts as a gatekeeper, limiting the options offered to someone wanting a policy and advising on the merits of the different policies and insurance companies with which the broker deals.

In health care, a physician's office staff, a hospital information service, or the health agency staff who respond to inquiries about services act as agents, representatives, or salespersons.

The following real-life case example illustrates the lengths to which some patients now go in hospital selection. As you read the case, make a list of the different people involved and try to define which of the roles described (customer, consumer, influencer, surrogate, gatekeeper, agent) each played. Remember that, as with the parent bringing a child to an emergency room, any person can play more than one of these roles.

The patient learned that she was pregnant. Her sister, a nurse, advised her that the quality of obstetric services varied widely among hospitals, even for an apparently routine delivery. The patient had a regular gynecologist who also practiced obstetrics. Her first thought was, therefore, to go to one of his hospitals. He advised her that he delivered at three different hospitals in the town. The patient, stimulated by her sister's advice, called each of those hospitals and asked to speak with the nurse who supervised the labor and delivery suite, the postpartum unit, and the normal newborn nursery. One of the three hospitals refused to connect her but tried to divert her call to the patient representative. Another of the hospitals explained that three different senior nurses were responsible for these areas and connected her with each. She like the manner and specific answers given to her questions by two of these nurses but found the nurse in charge of the normal newborn nursery rather aloof. The third hospital connected her with the director of nursing, who did not seem able to answer her more detailed questions about sibling visiting, rooming-in, and so on.

Unhappy with any of these hospitals, the patient decided to extend her search beyond the town to other hospitals within an hour's drive. After asking for advice from several friends with small children, she identified four further possibilities. She repeated the process of telephoning the supervisory nurses, and based on these calls, she now selected a hospital. She telephoned the hospital again and requested a list of its most active obstetricians. When this list arrived, she reconsulted the friend who had first suggested that hospital; her friend reported positively on her obstetrician. The patient then called that practice and arranged to visit it. Impressed by her visit, the patient called her gynecologist, informed him of her search, and told him that she was going elsewhere for her obstetrical care.

Who played which role or roles in this case? The patient herself acted as the *customer*, initiating the decision-making process, deciding among the hospitals, making the purchase by going to that hospital when in labor, and paying for the service. Although she carried medical insurance, her policy only provided for minor coverage for routine obstetrical care. Her insurance company could thus be regarded as a copayer and therefore as also sharing in one aspect of the customer role.

The patient was also the *consumer*. She personally used the obstetrical services involved, but she was not the only consumer.

Her unborn child benefited from the prenatal care provided by the obstetrician and from the care during and after birth at the hospital. Her child was thus also a *consumer*. The patient herself acted as a *surrogate* for her child.

The patient's gynecologist attempted, unsuccessfully in this case, to act as a *gatekeeper* by trying to guide the patient into choosing among the hospitals where he practiced.

The patient's sister acted as an *influencer*. Even though, in this case, she did not recommend a specific hospital, she influenced the path that the patient followed to that choice. The friends whom the patient consulted also acted as *influencers*.

All the nurses with whom the patient spoke at the various hospitals were acting, during those telephone conversations, as *salespersons*, *representatives*, or *agents* of a supplier. Each of them acted on behalf of her hospital to attempt to answer questions and to offer reasons why the patient should prefer her organization over its competitors. The hospital that the patient finally selected acted as a *gatekeeper* when it supplied the list of its affiliated obstetricians. It presented a limited choice to the patient from which to choose.

When the patient was eventually admitted, her obstetrician also became a *consumer* of the hospital's resources and services. The hospital enabled him to realize certain "benefits" — to discharge his professional responsibilities to his patient, to earn his fee, to receive the support of its nursing staff, and so on. In this particular case, this obstetrician was not a *customer* of the hospital. He neither initiated the process, selected the hospital for the patient, took the action that brought the patient to the hospital, or paid for her stay.

> *Decisions to buy products or use services are often complex and involve more than one person in the role of customer, consumer, influencer, surrogate, gatekeeper, or agent (or representative or salesperson).*

The Service Selection Process

How do customers approach making such decisions? Again, marketing science has developed a general model of the purchasing or service selection process.

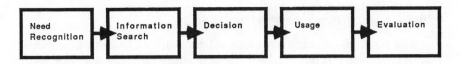

Figure 3-1 The service selection process.

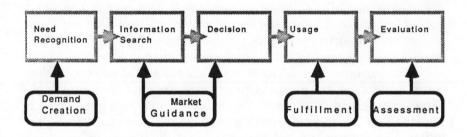

Figure 3-2 Marketing roles in the service selection process.

The customer for a product or service follows a five-step process of decision making (see Figure 3-1):

1. Recognition of need

2. Search for information on options

3. Purchase or usage decision

4. Experience or use

5. Postpurchase or postusage evaluation

Active marketing efforts by service providers can influence customer behavior at each step of this service selection process, as Figure 3-2 illustrates.

The remainder of this chapter is devoted primarily to a discussion of needs recognition. The other steps in the service selection process are discussed in subsequent chapters.

How Customers Recognize Needs

The process of using a service starts with recognition of a need. In the case just discussed, the patient learned that she was pregnant and realized that she would need a hospital for the delivery. The idea that service selection starts with needs recognition sounds obvious. In practice, however, many enterprises and programs fail to attract sufficient customers precisely because they do not analyze this step in the process. Often they are confused about the meaning of the word *need*. To a marketing scientist, a customer or consumer *need* is expressed in *obtaining a desired benefit*. Too often suppliers of products or services think of products or services as though they were ends in themselves, and not means to satisfy a need.

Does anyone "need" an automobile? An automobile maker would answer yes, but a marketing scientist would answer no. People perceive a benefit from being able to get quickly to a place that is too far to walk without depending on some other mode of transportation. The automobile just happens to be the means of satisfying that need that currently commands most customer support.

Does anyone "need" a hospital bed? Again, health planners would say yes, but a marketing scientist would say no. Some people perceive a need to help alleviate pain, to overcome a life-threatening condition, to improve the shape of their nose and thereby their self-esteem, to have a healthy baby, and so forth. Currently, the most expeditious and efficient way to meet those needs may be to put patients in hospitals beds. If better alternatives were available, no one would "need" a hospital bed. The bed is a means of obtaining a benefit, not a need in itself.

> *Defining precisely the benefits that the customer seeks in any service, and not confusing them with the means to achieve those benefits, is essential to arriving at the matching of goals basic to successful marketing.*

Often, a customer may seek more than one benefit from a particular product or service. Marketing science refers to such combinations of benefits as *benefit bundles*. A simple example is a diet — the user is seeking both to satisfy his or her need for food and to improve appearance and self-image by losing weight. Meals are often also family and social occasions, so the dieter may be looking for a diet plan that does not unduly disrupt these social needs.

How does a customer recognize the need to obtain a benefit? What triggers the service selection process? Marketing scientists draw heavily upon the study of psychology to answer those questions.

The benefits that any individual customer or consumer seeks to obtain are a product of:

1. Basic human needs

2. Values, attitudes, and perceptions

3. Knowledge

4. Experience

5. Social influences

6. Age factors

7. Gender factors

8. Life-style

The best-known model of basic human needs is Abraham Maslow's hierarchy of needs (Maslow 1954). Maslow argued that each person has five levels of need:

1. Physiological needs—for life, absence of hunger, thirst, pain, freedom from disability

2. Safety needs—for a sense of security and an absence of fear

3. Social needs— for affection and belonging

4. Esteem needs—for status and recognition by others

5. Self-actualization needs—for fulfillment of personal goals

Basic Physiological Needs

The principal purpose of most health services is to address the basic physiological needs in the Maslow hierarchy. The customer typically, however, also has other needs in the benefit bundle that he or she seeks to satisfy. In the obstetrical case discussed in Chapter 2, the nurses attempted to define the "ideal" approach to each aspect of the childbirth experience as an expression of their own needs for professional esteem and self-actualization. Unfortunately, their patients wished for greater scope for personal choice as part of their personal self-actualization — or fulfillment of their personal goals for childbirth.

Values, Attitudes, Perceptions

Different customers bring different values, attitudes, and perceptions to the service selection process. These may be general cultural values, attitudes, and perceptions, which influence customers' behavior in many aspects of life, or they may be specific values, attitudes, and perceptions about what matters to them in service settings.

Variations in *general* cultural values, attitudes, and perceptions may, for instance, help to explain preferences for natural versus anesthesia-assisted childbirth; or the use of secular versus church-related hospitals or a hospital that a patient's family has always used; or ideas about health fitness, and the value of medical intervention. One study (Ziff 1971) found that people fall into one of four groups in regard to their ideas about health and health care:

1. Fatalists, who see health and longevity as largely matters of luck, have little faith in doctors, and tend to underuse medical care

2. Realists, who value health care, but also accept its limitations and tend to heavily use over-the-counter drugs

3. Authority seekers, who value medical care and also want the assurance that comes with consulting health professionals

4. Hypochondriacs, who abuse medical care by taking even minor ailments to a physician

Recent research (Gonnella, Holbrook, and Louis 1984) has also shown that people's willingness to seek medical care may partially explain whether they are admitted to a hospital early in the course of their disease, when inpatient care may not yet be warranted; at a timely stage of the disease; or at a late stage, when they require major medical or surgical intervention.

A commonly observed variation in *specific* service-related values is the extent to which patients demand placement in a hospital "close to home" versus one that may be farther away but superior in its clinical care or personal service. (Of course, this preference could be considered a reflection of a general cultural value if the person constantly chose to stay in his or her own community for all activities rather than venturing farther afield.)

Knowledge

Consumer needs are also shaped by their knowledge. The patient with a history of a chronic disease, for example, is usually more alert to further benefits that medical care might confer, because often he or she has deliberately tried to become informed about the condition.

Among well people, their level of interest in health matters and the degree to which they educate themselves about health and fitness vary widely. Providing appropriate patient education is becoming an increasingly complex area of nursing responsibility. Yet information is an essential element of the benefit bundle that most patients seek. The patient's prior knowledge about medical matters thus shapes the level of information and degree of explanation that providers offer, in addition to influencing their expectations about the clinical content of their care.

Experience

Experience also shapes customer needs. Customers will seek to repeat a favorable experience and improve upon an unfavorable one. They may also be strongly influenced by reports of others or experiences acquired with them. If, for instance, a pregnant woman has had a positive experience with midwife delivery for a previous childbirth, or has personally witnessed a sister or friend undergoing such a positive experience, her personal benefit bundle for her own labor and delivery may well include elements retained from that experience.

Social Influences

Social influences also have an impact on customer needs. These influences may be "lessons" learned from parents, opinions of friends and acquaintances, peer pressure to conform to group norms, or notions spread via the mass media that something is in vogue. For example, a July 1984 press release by the American Academy of Facial, Plastic and Reconstructive Surgeons was widely reported in the media. It stated that more than 2 million Americans annually now undergo plastic surgical procedures. The news undoubtedly influenced at least some patients to proceed with plastic surgery, by demonstrating that it was a "normal" event. (At the same time, it may have influenced others, who prefer not to be trend followers against plastic surgery.)

Age and Gender

Age and gender have a self-evident impact on need recognition. Health care is not alone in having customer needs that are age- and sex-related. However, most marketing experts have learned to be very cautious about potentially exaggerating their impact or stereotyping people by age and sex.

For instance, is the statement that "older people are less likely to switch physicians than younger people" true or false? Studies conducted at Thomas Jefferson University (Fisk 1987) suggest that this statement is true as a generalization but is misleading. These studies showed that older people tend, as might be expected, to visit physicians more frequently. However, a significant minority of the older people interviewed had not visited a physician for several years, and they had no strong loyalty to those physicians. Conversely, those younger people who had visited particular physicians frequently were generally loyal to them. Thus, loyalty to a physician may well be less related to a patient's age than to frequency of visit. Incidentally, market research in relation to other products and services has shown the same pattern. Customers switch brands least for products that they use frequently (Engel, Blackwell, and Kollat, 1978).

For a gender-related example, consider the statement, again on the basis of surveys by this author and others, "Men acknowledge that their wives decide which hospital emergency room to take a child to." This statement, again on the basis of surveys by this author and others, seems to be false. Men do seem to acknowledge that their spouses make more health decisions for their children. In emergencies, however, men claim that they often call the shots. Whether they actually do or not is unclear, but they certainly claim to do so. These examples should serve as a caution against overplaying the role of age or gender in how customers recognize needs.

Life-style

Life-style can also have a major impact on how customers recognize need. What are the components of life-style? One marketing expert defines it as "the choices that reflect self-concept . . . within the constraints of everyday living" (Reibstein 1985). Each person is "constrained" by income and by the daily demands of work, family, or social contacts. Yet most people can exercise a wide range of choice, within those constraints, regarding the products or services that they will buy or how they will spend their leisure time. For example, a different perspective on life-style is what leads one family to build a pool in their backyard, while another family would regard a pool as a limitation on their freedom to use their spare time. Similarly, what leads one obstetrical patient to ask if her other children can attend the birth, while another patient does not even want her spouse there? The answer again may well be different life-styles — the one with a strong sense of family sharing of experiences, the other with a sense of childbirth as a very personal and private occasion.

Because so many Americans are sufficiently affluent to have a wide range of life-style choices available to them within their personal, financial, and daily constraints, some marketing scientists argue that life-style is the single most important determinant of how each individual recognizes his or her needs as a customer. A method for identifying which type of person is most likely to be interested in what type of benefit bundle, and, consequently, in any given service or product, has been developed using the life-style concept. It is known as VALS (for "values and life-styles"). Several types of VALS analyses are now available. One, for instance, holds that each person fits into 1 of some 15 major life-style categories. (The home-entertaining, child-centered, pool owner fits into one such category.) For any given service or product, the inventors of the VALS model will advise on the type of person most likely to be interested.

Consider *the pulse meter* for instance. An electronics company introduced several years ago a wristwatch-style pulse meter. The company directed its advertising to people over 45 year of age, who they assumed would be most worried about their heart rate. However, sales were very disappointing. A VALS analyst then advised that defining the audience by age was much less helpful for such a product than defining it by VALS. The analyst concluded that the people most likely to buy this product were "strivers" — younger people who were still trying to "make it," and worried about their jobs, money, personal security, and health. A new advertising campaign featuring such people using the pulse meter produced much higher sales.

There are even now some standardized VALS profiles designed to categorize patients of health services (Endresen 1987). One recent VALS study (Elkis 1987) of pregnant women found that they tended to fit into one of five broad categories (the risk-conscious, the carefree, the naturalists, the assurance seekers, and the escapists). These life-styles extended beyond their preferences for childbirth settings. They also explained many of their other attitudes toward health and the health professions.

The fact that VALS analysis can produce important insights into how customers recognize needs is not to say that this method should be relied on exclusively. In addition to life-style, the other sources of influence already described — basic human needs; values, attitudes, and perceptions; knowledge; experience; social pressures; age and gender — also can play an important role in shaping a customer's initial identification of an "unfulfilled need" or an "unrealized benefit."

Note how closely Reibstein's definition of life-style — "the choices that reflect self-concept within the constraints of everyday living" — relates to Maslow's idea of "self-actualization needs" for fulfillment and self-realization. Maslow arranged human needs in a hierarchy because, he argued, they must be satisfied in sequence. Only when a person has fulfilled basic physiological needs for food and health does the person focus on safety needs, then social needs, then esteem needs, and finally, self-actualization needs or selection of a preferred life-style.

Implications for Health Care Providers

These ideas have several major implications for providers of health services and for how those services are marketed:

1. People differ in their perceived needs. These differences are shaped not only by variations in knowledge, experience, social influences, age, gender, and income, but by variations in chosen lifestyle — in how people pursue personal fulfillment and self-actualization and in the relative values that they attach to different benefits.

2. In a relatively affluent society where most people have some discretionary income after satisfying basic needs, the pursuit of lifestyle, or Maslow's self-actualization needs, assumes a higher priority. These latter needs tend to shape the approaches that people take to satisfying more basic needs, including their physiological needs for health. When someone is sick and needs health care, he or she expects the same range of choice and level of personal attention and service as are provided in all of his or her activities as a modern customer and consumer. Even in satisfying a need as basic as that for food, which Maslow ranks with health as among the most basic of all types of human need, consumers are accustomed to heavy advertising, to wide choice, and high standards of service while shopping. They do not, therefore, surrender their normal expectations as customers when they become patients.

3. Within our modern, affluent society, there is still, of course, a significant minority of disadvantaged and poor people, who are also customers for health services. A simple interpretation of the ideas discussed here could lead to the assumption that these individuals are "less demanding" in their approach to health care. With less discretionary income, it may be argued, they have a narrower life-style and lower expectations of choice and of service. It must be remembered, however, that disadvantaged peoples' attitudes have been shaped by many of the same social influences that affect the affluent. They see the same choices presented in advertising; they often shop for food in the same stores as the more affluent, and although they may shop more prudently, they are used to the same service standards (the store is clean, food they want is in fact available, and clearly priced, employees answer any questions in a helpful and friendly manner, and so on.) They have also matured in an era when politicians have articulated the idea of "entitlement" for the less affluent to the satisfaction of their more basic needs. It is there-

fore, imprudent to assume that such individuals approach services with lower expectations or radically different benefit bundles.

4. Nurses, physicians, and other health professionals have the same hierarchy of needs as do patients. They work not just to earn the income necessary to pursue their "chosen" life-styles after work. The average person, with an average life span, spends the equivalent of 17 years of his or her life at work or school. Sleep is the only activity that consumes more time — the equivalent of 24 years. As a result, most people hope to realize at least some of their safety needs, social needs, esteem needs, and self-actualization needs within their time at work. Indeed, it can be argued that professional careers tend to attract those people with the greatest personal need for fulfillment and self-realization. A major challenge to medical leaders, and to hospital and nursing administrators lies in trying to satisfy the personal needs of health professionals in ways that also promote the greatest possible fulfillment of customer needs. The potential for conflict between employee and customer needs is always present. The marketing philosophy discussed earlier seeks to reconcile this conflict by seeing "customer satisfaction" as the means through which individual suppliers and enterprises fulfill their own goals.

5. Contemporary health care is concerned with satisfying more than the lowest level of need in Maslow's hierarchy — the physiological need for health, life, absence of pain, and an ability to function. As society has grown more affluent, customers for health services have increasingly turned to doctors, nurses, and hospitals to help them achieve more advanced needs in Maslow's hierarchy. At the same time, expanding medical knowledge has made it possible to respond more to those demands. Consequently, in today's health care system, services that principally address physiological needs for life, fitness, and functionality — such as cardiac care, trauma medicine, stroke treatment, cancer therapy, high-risk obstetrical care, and rehabilitation medicine — still represent the most *intensive* application of medical resources, but many patients now turn to health care for help with *safety, social, esteem,* and even *self-actualization needs.*

Two case histories may help to further explain these last two points, for nurses and other health professionals.

Owing to an increasing nursing shortage, a hospital's nursing administrator sought the advice of marketing professionals for help in recruitment. They began by discussing why people choose nursing as a career and, following Maslow's hierarchy of needs concept, agreed that the primary motive was "self-actualization." For many people, nursing allows them to realize personal goals—for responsibility, continued learning, challenge, and helping others. The nursing administrators and marketing experts jointly developed a new style of recruitment advertising, focused on how the hospital helped nurses to achieve their personal goals. The result was an influx of applicants, many with high qualifications (the ads had helped to screen out people who did not have high needs for self-actualization). Several months later, a large number of newly graduated nurses joined the staff. The nursing director noticed on her rounds the great variety of uniforms, hairstyles, and makeup of the reporting nurses. This lack of conformity in dress code had probably existed in previous years but was now more noticeable because of the large intake of graduate nurses. The nursing director faced a dilemma. On the one hand, she knew that nonconformity in dress, hairstyle, and makeup, has always been a major means of self-expression and with society's acceptance of a multiplicity of individual life-styles, the choices for personal dress and appearance are growing even more diverse. On the other hand, the nursing director knew that one of the two or three main attributes that patients seek in nurses is that they "seem experienced." The variety of dress and appearance, including some punk hairstyles, might convey an impression to patients that some of these young nurses were less highly trained, less experienced, and less motivated than they really were.

The nursing director's decision was a wise one that reflected an appreciation of the concept of a hierarchy of needs. She invited representatives of the nursing force to help define appropriate dress codes and to participate in selecting a range of approved designs allowing for individual choice and self-expression within mutually agreed upon standards. She thus gave the nurses the opportunity to participate in a higher form of "self-actualization" than exercising variations in appearance—the right to share in defining the rules under which they lived. The process largely removed the more extreme dress variations and also increased the nurses' sense of professional involvement and pride. If the director had unilaterally outlawed some of these forms of self-expression, she would have lowered the nurses' convictions that their safety needs, social needs, esteem needs, and self-actualization needs were being met through nursing at that hospital. Such an action might also have led some of the nurses to feel threatened, disliked, disrespected, and regimented.

The following case example illustrates the diversity of patient needs that contemporary medicine seeks to fulfill. A nursing school lecturer began every new class by asking the students to introduce themselves and to say something about their reasons for selecting nursing as a field of study. Invariably, a high percentage of the students would state that they felt a vocation to help people who were sick, in pain, or disabled. This answer both encouraged and troubled the lecturer. It showed that nursing still, as always, attracted young people with a strong sense of service to those in adversity. The lecturer also knew, however, that modern health care addresses many patient needs that are more esoteric. The lecturer wanted neither to discourage the students' sense of altruism, nor to risk their later disillusionment if they found themselves caring for patients whose life and health were not on the line. The lecturer decided to talk them through Maslow's hierarchy of needs. He went to the blackboard and asked the class to help him identify at least one health service that principally addressed each of the types of need that Maslow identified. He also asked the class to define the major benefit that each service delivered, to show that it clearly related to that type of need. Here is the list that they developed.

Physiological Needs Radiation therapy for cancer — "keeping the patient alive, or at least reducing pain in a terminal patient"

Safety Needs Well-baby care — "protecting the infant against possible health risks and reassuring the parent"

Social Needs Fertility management — "assisting couples, where one or both partners have an organic barrier to conception, to achieve their shared goal of having a child as fulfillment of their love for one another"

Esteem Needs Speech therapy — "helping someone to overcome or reduce a speech impediment that he or she perceives as a barrier to status and recognition by others"

Self-Actualization Needs Counseling of chronic diabetics — "helping someone whose diabetes is under medical control to master methods of coping with the disease so that it interferes as little as possible with his or her desired life-style"

The lecturer then pointed out to the class that each of these examples involved assisting people to satisfy important needs, of which the basic physiological needs for life and health were only a part; and that, therefore, to define the reasons for pursuing a nursing career wholly in terms of meeting such physiological needs was to take too narrow a view of human beings and their needs. Therefore, the health professional who wants to help others should seek to help them in whatever way his or her knowledge and skills permit, to meet this complete range of needs. The nurse who provides patient education to a diabetic trying to pursue his or her own life and career goals is as altruistic as the nurse assisting in open heart surgery.

Patients, thus, often recognize complex needs at the outset of their search for health care. Those needs are shaped by many influences, ranging from basic physiological needs to intangible, but very important, needs for self-fulfillment.

Role of Marketing in Needs Recognition

Marketing scientists argue that these personal needs already exist in individual customers or consumers before something triggers people to do something active to meet these needs. These needs are part of each person's human nature and personality. In that sense, marketing cannot "create" preexisting needs. Marketing efforts can, however, help to nudge people into taking action to satisfy these needs in several ways:

1. *Publicizing solutions. Marketing can inform people that there is a solution available to a need when they may not have realized it.* For example, media publicity given to Alzheimer's disease has created an impression in many older people and their adult children that all memory loss is attributable to Alzheimer's and that nothing can be done to help Alzheimer's victims. The facts are that 60% of memory loss cases are related not to Alzheimer's but often to treatable conditions, and that patients with Alzheimer's itself, although not yet curable, can still be assisted to lead fuller lives.

2. *Publicizing alternatives. Marketing can inform people that alternative solutions to needs are available.* For example, in recent years,

several alternative therapies to radical mastectomy for breast cancer have been developed, but public knowledge has often lagged behind these medical advances. The American Cancer Society currently holds that these alternatives often compare with radical mastectomy in effectiveness, making choice of procedure a matter of informed patient decision. Marketing has helped to promote awareness of this choice.

3. *Motivating prompt action. Marketing can influence people to take action now to realize a particular need, rather than postpone it, by reminding them of it and publicizing a means of addressing it.* For instance, there is increasing public awareness of the value of baseline mammography before age 40, but many women do not follow that recommendation. Marketing can remind them of the need and of how to fulfill it.

Demand Generation

Marketing

These three activities — publicizing solutions, publicizing alternatives, and motivating prompt action — are at the heart of "demand generation," marketing's main contribution to the need recognition phase of the service selection process. The concept of generating demand is the source of one of the most frequent criticisms of marketing: "Marketing persuades people to buy products or use services that they otherwise would not have wanted." This criticism is perhaps voiced more often in relation to health services than to other types of purchase. "Patients as laypersons," it is argued, "are misled into seeking health services that they do not actually need. This problem is exacerbated because most people have health insurance and are not, therefore, wasting their own money if they pursue unnecessary health services. Health providers overdiagnose or overtreat such cases, either out of greed or because of fear of malpractice suits."

Marketing experts defend themselves against this criticism in several ways. First, they argue, marketing activities do not create needs, they only help generate demand for specific solutions to those needs. The needs themselves must preexist and remain unfulfilled, in order for people to respond to the marketing efforts.

Second, they argue that customers frequently have to make judgments about products and services about which they lack complete technical knowledge. To claim that people are led astray in such situations is to insult the average customer. Because they are used to assessing complex products and services (from insurance to banking services, from foods with additives to automobiles with differing engineering efficiencies and safety features), they have developed certain approaches to doing so. They are no more likely to seek an unneeded health service out of limited knowledge than they are to buy a faulty life insurance policy. Most people do not consciously try to waste their time and money.

Third, marketing experts claim that there are many checks and balances against "unnecessary" health services, including those of medical ethics and the elaborate utilization review, precertification, and second opinion procedures required by health insurance carriers. Indeed, many health care providers would contend that patients are now better informed of their health care choices and of their right to ask questions before agreeing to treatment than they are about the scope of their health insurance coverage.

The authors of this book do not seek to take sides on this issue. Because it is a matter of controversy, the best advice that a health care provider can heed is to be aware of the issues and to carefully analyze the ethical basis for any marketing effort that seeks to generate demand. Will it tend to motivate customers to seek unnecessary medical attention, or is it clearly designed to explain how important customer needs can be effectively met?

In any event, marketing plays a much less active role in generating demand in the needs recognition phase of the service selection process than do three other sources of influence — media reports, family or friends, and health professionals.

Mass Media

As the mass media have paid more attention to health matters in recent decades, they have become the major means by which many people become aware of possible health needs that may have otherwise remained obscure to them (General Mills 1979). Earlier comments in this chapter, however, have warned against reading too much into such general statements about health consumers. They have noted that people vary widely in their values, attitudes, and life-styles, as well as in the attention they pay to reports about health matters in the mass media.

About 60% of adults in the United States have a high latent interest in health matters; while another 20% have only moderate interest; and a final 20% have only a low interest (Roper Organization 1985). These statistics demonstrate that health is a popular topic for media coverage. That is why the mass media have become such a force in creating public awareness of health needs and in triggering some individuals to advance to the next step in the service selection process.

Family, Friends, and Acquaintances

After the mass media, the next most frequent sources for health care referrals are family, friends, and acquaintances. Partly because of the relatively high level of latent interest in health matters, health is recognized as a widely acceptable topic of conversation among friends and acquaintances, and displaying concern about each other's health has always been a commonly accepted role of family members. People do, therefore, pass on health information to each other and even provide health advice more easily than they will converse about many other topics of mutual interest.

Health Professionals

Doctors and other health professionals rank as only the third most common "triggering mechanism" for seeking health care. That health professionals hold third place is partly a function of the comparatively lower accessibility of doctors and other health professionals for routine advice. These individuals are less easy to consult than the media or friends. There has also been a decline in the number of people who have a primary care physician whom they visit for periodic checkups even if they are feeling well, which may partly be a function of how lax some employers are in insisting that employees undergo regular physicals. Studies quoted earlier in this chapter indicated that many people are fatalistic about their health and that significant numbers may be seeking medical intervention at an unnecessarily late stage in the development of disease. Noncompliance with recommendations for regular checkups probably contributes to this situation.

Thus, patients start the service selection process by recognizing an unmet need. That recognition must be translated into actual generation of demand for a solution. That demand is most frequently triggered by mass media; by family, friends, or acquaintances; by a physician discovering a problem during a checkup, or lastly by an active marketing initiative by a health care provider. It is, of course, possible for more than one of these triggering mechanisms to influence a particular customer into action.

As an aid to remembering these different triggers to generating demand for health services, consider the reasons given by people for enrolling in a smoke cessation program:

The Mass Media as Demand Generators "I finally saw on TV a picture of the inside of a smoker's lung. That did it for me. Of course, I already knew it was risky, but somehow I couldn't imagine what it was actually doing to me."

Family as Demand Generators "My spouse had always nagged me about it, but when the kids started lecturing me too, that did it."

Friends and Acquaintances as Demand Generators "I noticed that fewer and fewer people who I work with were smoking. Often I was the only person lighting up at a meeting. Then some of them banned smoking in their own offices and pointedly told me not to light up there. Finally, the company took part in the Great American Smoke Out day, and two of my own staff gigged me into participating. I was the boss; I couldn't look weak-willed."

Doctors as Demand Generators "I had a checkup that included a lung function test and I scored below par. I work out a lot and thought I had strong lungs, but this thing said that I was below average, and my doctor told me why."

Marketing as a Demand Generator "I'd seen a lot of ads about ending smoking. They all claimed it was easy. If it was easy, I'd have done it long ago. I knew it would be tough, so all those ads seemed baloney to me. Then a nurse gave a talk at my workplace and started by saying that quitting was tough. At last someone was talking my language, so I enrolled to give it a try."

The preceding quotations illustrate some of the ways in which nurses and other health professionals can influence potential patients in their needs recognition. Try making your own more comprehensive list and then compare it with the one that follows:

1. Contact with patients during nursing assessment, patient education, and explanation of discharge instructions and ideas for follow-up care can directly influence patients' perceptions of their needs.

2. Patients are likely to talk about their care to family and friends, based upon their interactions with nurses, doctors, and others, thus influencing their perceptions of needs.

3. Contact with family and visitors may well broaden patients' abilities to communicate their knowledge to other friends and acquaintances with similar needs.

4. In hospitals with semiprivate rooms, one patient may indirectly learn about a roommate's disease and treatment and discuss it with others after discharge.

5. Patient education materials developed by nurses may be taken home and shared with others.

6. Public health education sessions, screening programs, participation in health fairs, and formal wellness programs can influence needs recognition.

7. Communication by nurses with doctors about services and nursing procedures can influence the information that they share with patients.

8. Nurses as private citizens have their own family and social contacts whom they can influence regarding health needs recognition.

9. In their private contacts with friends, nurses may often be more influential than non-health professionals in stimulating needs recognition, because they are regarded as more informed sources of opinion.

10. Nurses can have input into marketing materials (brochures, mailings, advertisements) and thereby influence customer needs recognition.

11. Nurses share information informally with nursing colleagues, which in turn may influence what they tell others.

12. Nurses share information formally with nursing colleagues which influences what they impart to patients, personal friends, and others.

References

Elkis, J. 1987. Nursing care and consumer selection of health care services. Paper presented at Annual Nursing Research Conference, Nov. 5-6, Nashville, TN.

Endresen, K. 1987. *HealthStyles*. Seattle: Endresen Research.

Engel, J., R. Blackwell, and D. Kollat. 1978. Consumer behavior. Hinsdale, IL.: Dryden Press.

Fisk, T. 1978. Communicating effectively to older adults. Paper presented at the Ireland Corporation Seminar on Marketing to Older Adults, May 28-29, Denver, CO.

General Mills. 1979. *Family health in an era of stress*. Minneapolis: General Mills Corporation.

Gonnella, J., M. Holbrook, and D. Louis. 1984. Staging of disease: As case mix management. *JAMA* 251: 637-644.

Maslow, A. 1954. Motivation and personality. New York: Harper and Brothers.

Reibstein, D.J. 1985. *Marketing: Concepts, strategies and decisions*. pp. 143, 144, 169. Englewood Cliffs, NJ: Prentice Hall.

Roper Organization, 1985.

Ziff, R. 1971. Psychographics for market segmentation. *Journal of Advertising Research* (April):

Review Questions

1. What are the differences among customers, consumers, influencers, surrogates, gatekeepers, and agents (representatives or salespersons)?

2. What is the first step in the service selection process? How can nurses influence patients during this step?

3. What is the difference between "needs" as health care providers think of them and "needs or benefits" as patients think of them?

4. "Each patient, as a consumer, is a unique person, yet we deliver them a standardized health care service." Discuss.

Chapter 4

Finding Out About Health Services

Information Search

Once a customer has recognized a need and generated demand for a solution to that need, he or she embarks on the second step in the service selection process, that of searching for information about alternative ways to meet that need. The search may range from being cursory and limited to considering alternative suppliers of one given answer to the need to being extensive and searching for different ways to satisfy the need (or "substitute services").

This definition of an information search appears to rule out "impulse" buying, by asserting that at least some level of investigation occurs. Based on extensive research into consumer behavior, marketing scientists believe that a customer only rarely learns about a product or service for the first time and concludes "I must have it." Even if the customer appears to do so, often he or she means, "I have always wanted one of those," or "That's just what I've been looking for." They recognized the need previously but have not been able to find an attractive way to meet it.

What determines how extensive the information search will be? One obvious theory is that more important decisions generate more extensive search processes. Current evidence does not, however, support that theory. Studies outside of health care indicate that the intensity of the information search does not increase for high-ticket purchases such as automobiles or major appliances (Newman and Staelin 1972). As a health-care-related example, in some focus groups of recent mothers organized by one of the authors of this book, there was evidence that friends and relatives are very influential in the information search preceding selection of a setting for

57

childbirth, but, on average, the women interviewed reported only seeking such information from one or two other women.

The major determinants of the extent of the information search seem to be:

1. *How risky the customer perceives the decision to be*

2. *How much the customer perceives quality to vary*

3. *How accessible credible advice seems to be*

4. *The customer's age and education (Hugstad, Taylor, and Bruce 1987)*

Thus, the customer who normally extends the information search farthest is one who sees the product or service as risky (does it really work?), who senses that there are wide variations in quality between the best and the worst suppliers, who does not have ready access to a source of advice that he or she trusts and who, by virtue of educational background and experience, is accustomed to making choices thoughtfully and analytically rather than trusting to his or her intuition (Hugstad, Taylor, and Bruce 1987).

In recent interviews with mothers of young children, for instance, the least extensive searches were made by those who perceived themselves at low risk, had a high faith in the medical profession as a whole, had easy access to a friend or relative (most favored was an older sister) who had recently undergone an identical experience and was therefore seen as an "authority," and who were younger and had the fewest years of formal education.

Sources of Information

How do patients, as customers, typically conduct an information search? The most frequently consulted sources of advice are family, friends, and acquaintances with similar families (e.g., with or without children, of a similar age). Such sources are consulted in about 70% of cases. A significant minority of patients do not consult acquaintances in selecting doctors or hospitals. Even in selecting a nursing home, only about half of the patients involve a family member or friend (Dove 1986).

If the patient is searching for a primary physician, or for an alternative to a current primary doctor, physicians themselves play a minimal role as an information source. People pay more attention to friends or, indeed, to advertising.

Coverage in the media, which played a major role in needs recognition, plays but a minor role in service selection. As might be expected, people who read or hear of a specific physician in the media do not store that information until they might need it. If they do recognize a need via the media and decide to act immediately *and* if the report happens to mention a particular nearby physician, they may contact him or her. It is unusual, however, that these three different events coincide.

> *By contrast with a random and unrepeated media report, well-run advertising campaigns are continuous and repetitive. They seek to keep the name of a particular provider in front of the public. As a result, advertising can play a role in many customers' search processes. For instance, approximately 1 in 10 reports consulting the Yellow Pages during his or her information search.*

If, instead, a patient does have a regular primary care physician and is seeking a further service — a specialist or a hospital — about 80% of patients report that they consult the primary care physician as an information source. This statistic may, however, overstate the influence that doctors have on many patients, since only about 20% of patients report that they follow their physician's recommendations without question. Forty percent of patients see themselves as sharing in the decision with their physician. They ask him or her for more than one recommendation to consider, or the physician automatically offers them more than one choice, or they balance the physician's recommendations against those of friends. Asked what they would do if they received contradictory advice from their doctor and from a close friend, about 20% of patients state that they would go with the friend's advice.

In summary, patients seeking health services beyond those of a primary care physician appear to take one of four courses:

> Twenty percent of patients accept their primary physician's recommendations of further sources of health care without challenge.

Twenty percent of patients will accept their primary physicians' recommendations of further sources of health care unless a close friend makes a contradictory recommendation.

Forty percent of patients see themselves as sharing in the choice of further sources of health care with their physician. They expect the physician to offer them a choice. Some of these patients are also influenced by friends, but will normally lean toward a doctor's recommendations in preference to those of friends. Others of this group do not consult friends at all.

Twenty percent of patients do not consult their primary physician at all in their information search about further sources of health care.

Even these comments tend to imply possibly a greater level of loyalty to primary care physicians than is the case. For instance, some 60% of patients claim to have switched primary care physicians within the last 3 years or so (*Medical Economics* 1985). Approximately 30% of patients report having consulted a chiropractor, faith healer, or other "alternative" type of primary care provider (Halpern, Fisk, and Sobel 1984; *Medical Economics* 1985). These patterns are not those of patients who have a blind and unswerving allegiance to established sources of primary care. Those patients who do exhibit long-term and unswerving trust in one primary doctor now seem to comprise only a minority of the population.

Thus, a significant number of patients do rely on physician input in their information search, but significant numbers do not, and many weigh physician input as one of several factors. Some of those who do rely heavily on primary care physician input have loyal relationships with them, while others only have a temporary relationship with them.

Determinants of Patient Loyalty

What determines how "brand loyal" a patient will remain to a physician or other source of health care? Four factors seem to play the largest roles:

Frequency. As already noted, consumers in all fields tend to remain most loyal to products or services that they use most often. The smaller the time intervals between visits to a doctor, the less likely is the patient to switch.

Venturesomeness. Some people are just more venturesome than others, that is, more likely to try alternatives. Interviews with recent mothers conducted by one of the authors revealed that many could recount at least one very upsetting experience with their obstetrician. Some intended to switch if they became pregnant again, but others, equally critical of their doctors, intended to remain in his or her care, the most common justification being that the patient had "invested a lot of time in developing a rapport and comfort level with that doctor and did not want to go through that again." A survey commissioned years ago by the *New York Times* found that about 50% of people were "very likely" to try an alternative primary care practice "staffed entirely by experienced nurses, as long as its fees were substantially lower than in a doctor's office." The other 50% were highly unlikely to try such an alternative. The two groups thus had very different levels of venturesomeness in their response to this new option for their primary care.

Satisfaction with Service. As customers, patients evaluate their experiences with doctors and may switch if dissatisfied. As the previous two paragraphs have shown, they will not always switch if dissatisfied, but some will. The *Medical Economics* reports (1985) quoted earlier found that most of the 60% of adults who had switched primary doctors in the 3 years prior had done so because of dissatisfaction, not because of their moving or because their doctor retired, or because they joined a health maintenance organization (HMO) in which their doctor did not participate.

Satisfaction with Referrals. Patients evaluate their experiences with doctors and hospitals to which their primary physicians or other primary care providers refer them and, if unhappy with those experiences, often blame the referrer. If this dissatisfaction is intense, they will switch primary providers.

Regarding the role of HMOs, it bears repeating that there do not appear to be sizable numbers of patients who switch their primary physician because they join an HMO in which he or she does not participate. The available evidence shows that the influence of HMOs on primary care selection is more complex. Some of those who join HMOs do so because they are dissatisfied with their current physician and the HMO offers an excuse to drop him. Others, having grown dissatisfied with their physician, lose confidence in their ability to make a wiser choice unaided and are attracted by the HMO's assurance that it has selected good doctors.

What matters most to customers of health services in their information search? What attributes do they most seek? The answers to these questions vary, depending upon the precise stage that the customer has reached in the health care services chain. The customer may:

1. Be contemplating membership in an HMO that restricts customers as to the primary physicians, specialists, and hospitals that they can use.

2. Be seeking a primary care provider

3. Be seeking a specialist

4. Be selecting a hospital, either for self-referral or to check a physician's recommendation

In each of these situations, customers of health services tend to perceive slightly different needs. They seek slightly different benefit bundles.

Benefits Sought from Health Insurance

The most frequently quoted reason why people join HMOs or PPOs is to save money. In recent years many employers have amended the coverage afforded employees by traditional health insurance options (e.g., Blue Cross and Blue Shield or a commercial indemnity plan like Travelers or Prudential). They have increased the deductibles or copayments that the employee must pay out-of-pocket before the coverage starts. They have taken these actions for two reasons: to keep the scope of coverage intact, while controlling costs to the employer, at a time when health costs have risen steeply, and in the belief that employees who must pay a larger share of any medical bill will be more thoughtful before seeing a doctor. HMOs or PPOs, it is argued, are an attractive option for employees who do not want to make this personal contribution and, in return, are willing to accept more restrictions on their freedom of choice. An HMO or PPO can offer such relief from deductibles and copayments because it has persuaded some doctors and hospitals to accept lower payments from them than they would get from more traditional health insurers. Since health care costs the HMO or PPO less, it shares some of these savings with its enrollees by not charging such high deductibles or copayments.

It would seem then, that customers seeking information about HMOs and PPOs would be principally concerned with how much membership will save them financially, taking into account their family size, age, and health care needs. However, only a minority of potential HMO or PPO members base their search wholly on price issues (Berki and Ashcroft 1984; Scotti, Bonner, and Wiman 1986). Another segment is concerned with both price and the perceived quality of the doctors and hospitals with which the plan works. The remaining segment, perhaps surprisingly, pays little attention to price in selecting an HMO. Their major concern is quality. Many of them, as already noted, are dissatisfied with their past experiences with doctors or hospitals and do not feel confident enough to make a sound choice unaided, a freedom afforded by more traditional forms of health insurance. They are attracted by the structured approach to health care that an HMO or PPO seems to offer. The most influential source of information in their search is the HMO salesperson, whom they meet at their workplace and who must appear authoritative and able to offer a credible plan.

It is this variation in customers' information search priorities that explains why different HMOs in major metropolitan areas (10 to 15 HMOs may be competing with each other in any one urban area, as well as with more traditional insurers) follow different marketing strategies. Some strive totally to "maximize coverage while minimizing cost" and are not particularly selective about which hospitals or doctors they will use. Such plans are pursuing the "price-driven" customers. Other HMOs follow a different strategy by being very selective about the hospitals and doctors they try to recruit (Fisk and Somers 1987), conducting extensive research to find out which hospitals are best regarded by corporate leaders and by the wider local public. Their goal is "the best hospitals and doctors at a price slightly lower than traditional insurers." Such plans aim for the "quality-driven" customers. Still other plans seek a middle ground—"moderate prices for medium quality"—to appeal to the segment of customers concerned with both. One common form of this middle strategy is to try to recruit the single most prestigious hospital in the area as the "flagship," along with the lowest-priced hospitals for most routine needs. These plans then market themselves as offering customers low-cost but convenient community hospitals for most needs, but "the best in town" for major diseases.

In their information search for health insurance options, customers do not share a standard set of goals or require the same benefit bundle. They tend to fall into one of six segments, as follows:

1. *Those with an almost exclusive goal of minimizing their likely out-of-pocket expenses for health care.*

2. *Those who are primarily concerned with freedom of access to the highest quality providers of health care and who will pay for that freedom.*

3. *Those who welcome the guided and structured approach to health care decisions that HMOs and PPOs offer and do not want the freedom of choice offered by more traditional types of insurance.*

4. *Those who are concerned with price, quality, and freedom of choice and try to strike a balance among these benefits. They look for an insurance option that best fits their defined personal benefit bundle.*

5. *Those who find the health insurance options available to them so confusing that they follow the lead of friends who seem better informed, or listen to agents of the various plans who make presentations at their workplace during the enrollment period and choose which seems most credible and convincing.*

6. *Those who are concerned with finding a health insurance option that has a simple and dependable claims process. They want minimal paperwork and maximum certainty as to which services will be covered.*

Because of the variation in the market for health insurance, competitive insurance plans do not try to look alike. Instead, each endeavors to make a strong appeal to one or more of these segments.

Benefits Sought in Primary Care

Numerous studies have been published on the attributes that patients seek in primary care providers (e.g., American Board of Family Practice 1987; Anderson, Fleming, and Aday 1981; Gochman, Stukenborg, and Feler 1986; Hall, Roter, and Rand 1981; Halpern, Fisk, and Sobel 1984). Together they show that four factors dominate the information that patients seek in the search process for primary care providers: Ability, availability, articulateness, and accessibility. These attributes are discussed in the subsections following.

Assessing Primary Care Providers' Abilities

Nearly all patients seek a primary care provider with ability. The only exceptions are a small minority who do not believe that quality in fact varies much from one provider to another. How do the majority of patients assess a doctor's or other primary provider's ability, when they know their own technical knowledge or medicine is limited?

First, it is important to remember that customers are used to making choices about products and services where their technical knowledge is restricted. This is a common, not a rare challenge to a customer.

Consider your own experience. Here are 10 types of purchases that many people make: buying auto insurance, buying a suit that you plan to wear quite often in situations where you should look well-dressed, buying a stereo system, buying a dishwasher, buying an automobile, selecting a type of savings account, getting someone in to service your heating system, buying a toothpaste, buying an over-the-counter analgesic for multipurpose use, buying shoes for a child. In which of these situations do you really have advanced technical knowledge? The typical person could not truthfully answer that they do in more than two or three of these situations at most.

Lack of detailed technical knowledge does not stop customers from making choices; it simply alters the way they go about the information search. The less technical knowledge they possess, the more likely they are to consult friends who have more knowledge of who have recently made a similar purchase; they may expand their search by reading up on the product or paying more attention to advertising; they will probably ask questions of salespersons; and they will likely use *proxies* or *labels* to help them judge technical quality indirectly. A proxy or label is something that a customer uses to assess the quality of a product. In selecting life insurance, for example, proxies may include whether the company's name is familiar and reputable and whether the agent seems honest and helpful. For durable business clothing, it may be the label or, indeed, the price.

When selecting a physician, a customer may consult a few friends; or an intermediary source such as a nurse whom he or she knows; or a hospital that offers a doctor referral service. The most commonly used proxies or labels seem to be the hospital(s) with which a doctor is associated, on the basis that "the better hospitals attract the better doctors," and evidence of special experience in the relevant field (e.g., board certification and reported areas of special interest). One label that seems to be considered by only a small minority of patients is where the doctor trained. Physicians themselves sometimes find this surprising, since place of training is a common attribute that doctors use in evaluating one another. For most patients, however, place of training seems less important than the doctor's experience and track record since graduation, a not illogical viewpoint.

Consider yourself faced with choosing between two lawyers, the first of whom went to Harvard Law School, has practiced alone for 5 years, appears to have no field of concentration, and has not represented anyone whom you know; the second of whom went to a law school you have never heard of but has practiced for 20 years with a large well-known local law firm, specializing in the field of law in which you now need help, and who has successfully represented a close friend with a similar problem who tells you that this lawyer has a reputation for winning tough cases. Which lawyer seems more qualified to assist you? Many patients would assess a doctor's quality the same way.

In summary, most patients do attempt to obtain information about a primary care provider's quality, even though they may not be able to judge it correctly. They listen to testimonials from friends, and they assess proxies or labels that may give some insight into a provider's attributes.

Assessing Primary Care Providers' Availability

Recent data (American Medical Association 1987) show that the average delay nationally in getting an appointment with a physician ranges from about 2 days in family medicine to some 12 days in certain specialties. Because these numbers are averages, they imply that some doctors can schedule patients more rapidly, while others are booked up even farther ahead. Indeed, a delay of over 4 weeks is not uncommon for some well-established and highly regarded doctors or groups. Many of these doctors will try to see real emergencies more rapidly. And family physicians will not necessarily make an established patient wait who feels in need of immediate attention.

Many specialists try to screen patients in order to see those in pressing need more quickly than others. Those with the least pressing problems must wait even longer than average, however. Thus, if it takes 12 days on average to see a specialist, but real emergencies are seen more rapidly, those without an immediate need must be waiting much longer than 12 days.

Will the patient wait that long? Some will, because they are familiar with a particular practice or have heard favorably about that doctor's ability and they put more weight upon ability than availability in their personal benefit bundle. Many others, however, will not regard seeing that particular doctor as worth a long wait. They will look elsewhere for a more available alternative even if ability is less well known.

Consider the hypothetical case of an island with only two doctors, one who has been there for many years and one who is a new arrival. It takes an average of 10 days to get an appointment with the older doctor, except in a real emergency, but only 2 days to see the younger doctor. What will happen in this situation? The answer depends on the relative importance that local patients attach to proven ability versus an early appointment.

If the entire local population values proven ability highly, but attaches no value to quick appointments, nothing will happen; they will remain patients of the older doctor. If, conversely, everyone on the island values an early appointment and is indifferent to proven ability, they will start switching to the younger doctor. This switching will stop when it takes as long to see the younger doctor as the older one.

Even if those patients attach equal importance to proven ability and early appointments, some will shift from the older to the younger doctor. They will accept less proven ability in their doctor in order to achieve more timely attention. However, the older doctor will still retain the majority of the population as his patients, and, in these circumstances where everyone on the island attaches equal weight to proven ability and early appointments, he will do so without cutting his scheduling delay to match that of the younger doctor. He only has to cut that delay to the point where his edge in proven ability compensates for the added delay in seeing him.

In the real world, patients do not all place the same weight on each benefit. Each looks, in his or her own information search, for a provider who best fits his or her own desired benefit bundle.

People thus differ in the importance that they attach to ability or availability. Each customer in his or her information search will look for a primary care provider who best fits his or her own benefit bundle.

How do patients find out about a doctor's availability? One obvious way is that they call the doctor's office and find out. Another is that they ask friends. Of course, the information they obtain may be erroneous, for a number of reasons. First, they or their friends may have called a doctor who tries to screen patients by level of urgency. A doctor may have been accessible for an apparent emergency but not for a less pressing case, or vice versa. Second, they may have called at an untypically easy or untypically difficult time of the year. Third, the doctor's "popularity" may have changed. Indeed, one risk for practices that reach a point where their scheduling delays are too long is that they become known as unavailable. People stop trying to reach them, the practice declines and they are left wondering what went wrong.

Marketing scientists see most markets as dynamic; they do not stand still. Consequently, the most difficult goal for any provider to achieve is that of a stable practice. Most suppliers are either growing or declining.

If delays in getting an appointment are a major factor in perceptions of availability of health providers, is the same true of waiting times once patients arrive for an appointment? National data (American Medical Association 1987) show national average waits in doctors' offices at around 20 minutes. Again, this is an average, so many people have shorter waits, while others have considerably longer waits.

Long waits appear to have a lesser impact upon patients' information search because it is harder to ascertain waiting time before actually seeing the doctor. One can find out about a delay in getting an appointment by calling the doctor's office, and at the same time asking the receptionist about typical waiting room times. Generally, however, the only prior information source about waits is from friends who have used that health service. But friends may have had an untypical experience, or they may be more tolerant of long waits, because of their loyalty to the physician.

Waiting times thus are of some importance in the way many customers react to health services, in their decision as to whether they will reuse a service, and in how strongly they recommend it to friends. They seem to be less important to the search process than either reports on a provider's ability or discovery of the likely delay before an appointment is available.

Is availability to talk to patients on the telephone an important aspect in the information search process? Some doctors will talk on the phone to established patients. Far fewer will talk to a customer during his or her information search. Several studies suggest that this service is much less important in the benefit bundle than such factors as ability, ease of getting an appointment, location, or communication skills. Telephone accessibility seems to play a much larger role in retaining established patients than in attracting new ones—because it increases the frequency of contact and affords some immediate response when an actual appointment may involve some delay.

Few doctors charge for a telephone "consultation." Those that do risk provoking patient resentment. Those who accept such calls but do not charge help to moderate any possible resentment caused by the fee for an actual visit, by showing that they do not demand payment for all their professional services.

Primary care providers who make house calls are assessed similarly by patients as those who are willing to talk on the phone. Only a small minority of patients seem to put any priority on whether the care provider makes house calls. For that minority, however, it is an important component. For the majority, this evidence of the doctor's availability may contribute to a positive image of the provider. However, for neither group is the availability of house calls important enough to compensate if the provider lacks an image of ability or if there are long delays in scheduling appointments.

While several aspects can thus contribute to a customer's over-all image of a medical service's availability, the most significant aspect seems to be how quickly the service is available when they need it. Nonetheless, individual customers differ in how much of a delay they will accept to see a reportedly able doctor or other health professional.

Assessing Primary Providers' Articulateness

The single most frequently mentioned attribute that customers seek in a physician is his or her ability to "explain things well" (Brown 1980). In one study, over 90% of patients named this characteristic among the top three attributes they desired in a doctor (Halpern, Fisk, and Brown 1983). There seem to be three reasons why health customers place such emphasis on articulateness.

1. Many patients today regard themselves well informed on health matters and expect both to ask questions and to get intelligible answers to help them participate in decisions about their care.

2. Seeking health care is a stressful activity and one that requires placing yourself "in someone's hands." Articulate explanation of what is being done and why reassures and helps to relieve anxiety.

3. An ability to articulate what you are doing is regarded by many customers as a proxy by which to judge ability. (For example, the auto repairman who can explain what is wrong with your transmission is seen as more likely to be able to fix it.)

Again, in the search process customers are primarily dependent upon secondhand evidence from friends to establish if any particular health provider has such skills. They cannot assess it directly until they meet with the doctor or other health professional. Nevertheless, it is in this aspect of the information search that a patient can be most influenced by advertising, direct mail, brochures, and other marketing communications. If those communications are clear and informative, it is a reasonable assumption that the provider is also. Even if the provider did not write them personally, he or she at least approved of them as conveying his message. The reverse, however, is also true. If a marketing publication is confusing, dull, full of jargon, or pompous, the customer is entitled to assume that it reflects the provider's style of professional communication.

This emphasis that health customers place upon articulateness makes the style of marketing communications that providers employ even more crucial than in other fields. It illustrates directly whether a health professional possesses one of the major attributes that the customer expects of him or her.

Patients searching for information about primary care providers place major emphasis upon evidence that the provider is articulate and "explains things well." They derive this evidence from the comments of friends. They also use a provider's marketing communications as evidence of whether he or she communicates well.

Assessing Primary Care Providers' Accessibility

Most patients will not undertake a long journey to reach an "ideal" primary care provider. They look for one close to home. There are practices with exceptional reputations that can draw primary care patients from slightly farther afield than their competitors. Even with such providers, however, it is easy to exaggerate their geographical pull. Most of their patients come from nearby. The hours that a practice operates also affects its perceived accessibility. That does not mean that extended hours are always attractive or important to patients. Many practices have experimented with variations in hours of operations, only to find that they have minimal impact on patient volumes. This decision is one that a practice must consider and, possibly, experiment with on an ad hoc basis. There is no general evidence that extended hours is a critical benefit sought by many patients. Conversely, however, there can be a danger in operating very restricted hours such as only half-days. Many patients who do not want or expect extended hours will, nevertheless, be put off by unduly restricted hours of accessibility.

In addition, many primary care providers strive to be in locations that afford easy parking for visiting patients. Other providers happen to be in locations, such as center city areas, where immediately adjacent parking is not feasible. How important is this factor? For most patients, it is far less important than the other attributes already discussed.

Most patients search for a primary provider who is able, can schedule appointments without a long delay, keeps waiting times within reason, has a reputation for being articulate, and is not too far from home.

Benefits Sought in Specialists

Do health customers seek different attributes in specialists than in primary care providers? With six exceptions, they appear to look for the same types of attributes in specialists as were just reviewed (Halpern, Fisk, and Brown 1983).

The first minor difference is that they seem to attach a little more weight, in assessing a specialist's ability, to certain labels such as board certification. Although health customers may have an imperfect knowledge of the types of additional training and certification that specialists receive, they are generally aware that these processes exist, and they look for evidence of them in a specialist's credentials.

The second minor difference in information searches about specialists is that some health customers seem to consult slightly more friends. Particularly if they require surgery, some patients try to speak with one or more people who have actually used a particular surgeon. Some surgeons who have observed this tendency now maintain lists of past patients who have consented to be available to answer questions from people inquiring about the practice.

The third difference concerns price. Because the cost of specialist consultation and treatment is high in comparison to primary providers' visit fees, some patients investigate costs more actively. This occurs most for procedures that may not be extensively covered by health insurance, such as cosmetic surgery or some types of psychiatric care.

The fourth difference is that many patients are strongly influenced in their choice of a specialist by a primary provider's recommendation. However, both the percentage of patients who refer themselves directly to specialists and the number who cross-check a primary provider's recommendation with friends seem to be on the rise.

The fifth difference concerns the importance attributed to a specialist's bedside manner. Patients seem just as concerned that specialists be articulate and explain things well, but they are slightly less concerned that the specialist be likable. There is still a prevalent realization that a surgeon's technical skills may not be reflected in his personality. Patients do, however, expect a surgeon to explain things and to answer their questions.

The sixth difference concerns accessibility. Many patients will travel farther to see a specialist, because they see the need as more critical and, also, as likely only to be temporary. Again, however, this willingness to travel should not be exaggerated. Each of the leading medical centers in the United States can quote examples of patients who journeyed long distances to consult one of their specialists. The number of patients involved, however, is quite small when viewed against the 30 million or so patients admitted to hospitals each year. Most people will not travel long distances for their care.

Health customers searching for specialists put even more emphasis on evidence of ability than they do in searching for primary providers. For some patients, costs are also of more interest in a specialist search. They still want providers who are articulate, but they are slightly less concerned, than in their search for primary providers, with personality, which many realize is not a valid proxy for measuring a specialist's technical skill.

Benefits Sought in Hospitals

It would appear that, in the majority of cases, the patient now plays at least some part in the selection of the hospital to which he or she will be admitted. Depending on the study consulted, the percentage of patients reporting that they left the selection completely to a physician ranges from a low of 20% to a high of 45%. The most important attributes that patients seek in a hospital are advanced technology, good doctors, good nursing, and closeness to home. The precise order of priority among these four attributes is difficult to ascertain, again varying slightly according to the surveys consulted.

Benefits Sought in a Hospital's Technology

In assessing a hospital's technology, health customers are most influenced by two sources: family or friends and the hospital's own marketing communications and media relations. In addition, health customers vary considerably in the status of their own knowledge about medical technology. Thus, the information that a hospital has a computed tomography (CT) scanner may impress the person who is unaware of how widespread CT scanning has become, but may fail to impress someone else with more up-to-date knowledge. As hospital marketing efforts increase, health customers may indeed become more confused, as each hospital will refer to its technology as being on the leading edge.

The health customer who makes but a cursory information search may not compare the technology claims of rival hospitals. He or she may study just one hospital and be sufficiently impressed by its claims to look no further. The hospital that really does have a technological lead in some field thus faces a special challenge in reaching the public with this message.

In the true sense of the word, *technology* is not simply advanced equipment. It consists, according to *Webster's Dictionary*, of "a technical method of achieving a practical purpose." Technology has become equated, through use of the term in the mass media, with up-to-date equipment. Hospitals have themselves fostered this notion by their own emphasis in media relations upon reporting major acquisitions of medical hardware. Many of today's most advanced medical "technologies," however, are not embodied in high-tech equipment. Some of them rely on advanced know-how but employ commonplace equipment. Trauma centers, for example, have dedicated operating rooms (ORs) but they do not look very different from other ORs. The technology of a trauma center lies in its organized systems of rapid and multidisciplinary medical and surgical care. Medical genetics is among the most advanced of health technologies but is largely conducted in laboratories that look only slightly different from those in a high school. The same applies to *in vitro* fertilization.

In their search for information about advanced hospital technology, health customers tend to be most influenced by reports about equipment, which they equate with "high technology." They may often be out of date in their knowledge of medical advances. Because they tend to equate technology with equipment, they may also overlook evidence of advanced clinical methods that employ standard equipment, but do so in new ways. Hospitals with such state-of-the-art programs thus face particular marketing challenges in communicating their benefits to potential patients.

Benefits Sought in a Hospital's Doctors

Most health customers prefer a hospital with a reputation for a high-quality medical staff. As mentioned earlier in this chapter, many health customers also regard the hospitals with which a doctor is associated as a useful proxy measure of the doctor's own ability. It would appear, therefore, that many health customers believe that "good hospitals have good doctors, and good doctors get admitted to the staff of good hospitals." There is an element of logic in the belief that the better doctors gravitate toward the better hospitals and, in so doing, maintain their high standards over time. By inference, many also believe that "The not-so-good hospitals attract the not-so-good doctors."

How are these beliefs formed? The answer lies in the elusive concept of "reputation." Certain organizations develop, over time, an aura of competence. This reputation has a halo effect on those who work for them, as well as on other products or services that the hospital introduces. Such reputations are not built overnight, but through decades of adherence to quality products or services. Take, for example, the images of major national corporations such as IBM or Campbell's Soup. There may be particular attributes of these organizations that individual customers dislike, but hardly anyone disputes that they stand for ability and quality in their fields. Many people also assume automatically that the people who work for them are exceptional. Through decades of achievement and of reasonably consistent high standards of service, these companies have acquired a positive image (Fisk 1987).

No hospital rivals these major corporations in having a positive image on a national scale. Hospitals work in local service areas or, at best, in regional markets. Within those regions, however, there are hospitals that rival national corporations as a household name for quality, that have a widespread and positive regional or local image. There are also at least two or three hospitals in many regions that have a questionable or negative image. Again, this image was not created overnight by a single, well-publicized and negative event, but more often was created through a long period of slightly questionable quality. In between these two extremes are many hospitals that lack either a strongly positive or a strongly negative image.

Hospitals develop such images — good, poor, or neutral — because they are highly visible organizations in their service areas. They are widely reported in the media and have large annual volumes of "visitors." Including inpatients, their visiting friends and family, outpatients, and patients visiting closely associated doctors' offices, a 500- or 600-bed hospital may well receive more than 400,000 visitors annually. A larger university medical center, with its additional flows of students and their friends and family, may well exceed 800,000 annual visitors. In addition to the publicity that they attract, hospitals are, therefore, experienced first-hand by large numbers of people in their service areas.

A strong image — positive or negative — is not easy to acquire. It takes time and reasonably consistent high or questionable quality to establish it. It is also not easy to lose, precisely because it is so embedded in the beliefs of the local population. A detailed study of the comparative images of some 80 hospitals in a major metropolitan area found very few significant changes in any of their public images over a 2-year period, despite major image campaigns by many of those hospitals (Robinson and Fisk 1988). The same study showed that none of those hospitals had either a universally positive or a universally negative image. Even those that were highly regarded by a large majority of the population were perceived negatively by at least some people, and those with a negative image among a significant percentage of local people were well thought of by some others.

When health customers assert that they look for good doctors as evidence of a good hospital, some may mean that literally. They have no strong preference for a particular hospital and are trying to make up their minds. They may, indeed, call for literature about the hospital and look for information about its doctors. Other hospital customers, however, are really looking for confirmation of a belief that they have already established, from the media, from friends, or from marketing communications, about the quality of the hospital.

Benefits Sought in a Hospital's Nursing

The principal measures by which health customers seem to assess a hospital's nursing staff during their information search are:

1. Whether the hospital is adequately staffed with nurses
2. Whether there is evidence that the nursing staff is experienced

After patients have experienced a hospital for themselves, other aspects of nursing care enter into their assessment. More will be said about these aspects later. In their information search, however, patients seem most concerned with staffing levels and with experience.

The concern with staffing levels is a product of the media attention paid to the "nursing shortage." Many people are now concerned about this national problem. Their concern is also, however, a product of reports heard from friends and family who have been hospitalized. For instance, a slow response to a call button may often be attributed to the nursing shortage by nurses on short-staffed units. While imparting this knowledge to a patient is both understandable and honest, it should also be recognized that it increases patients' anxieties and may well be recalled in their reports to friends. In short, it is not good public relations.

Incidents reflecting a lack of nursing care that occur through short staffing can be used as a proxy of staffing levels. The experience of a nursing staff is more elusive for a health consumer to assess. Only a minority of consumers are sufficiently informed to understand or ask about the distinctions between L.P.N.s, R.N.s, first-degree, and masters-level nurses. Again, they rely most on reports from friends who have recently been hospitalized, and they listen for cues that may indicate an experienced nursing force or the lack of it.

Both in assessing staffing levels and in looking for evidence of an experienced nursing force, health consumers also rely upon their own experiences in visiting friends in hospitals. National data show an annual admission rate to acute care hospitals in the United States of 150 per 1,000 population. In other words, slightly more than 1 person in 7, on average, is admitted to a hospital each year. If each has an average of only 3 adult visitors during his or her stay, therefore, more than half the population would see inpatient units personally each year. In fact, the percentage is not quite that high because of the heavy admission rate among the elderly, some of whom have multiple admissions during a year and do not have friends or family to visit them. Even so, a large percentage of the population sees the inside of at least one hospital each year, as either a patient or a visitor. During those visits, they form impressions about the nursing staff from a wide variety of incidents, including the apparent orderliness of the patient's bed and any medical equipment, the response if the patient needs assistance during a visit, the helpfulness of nurses to their own requests as visitors, and what they casually observe of nursing behaviors when on a unit.

Health customers during their information search, are often interested in evidence of nurse staffing levels and of nursing experience in the hospital(s) they are considering. They acquire these insights predominantly from friends, but often from their own observations during visits to a friend in the hospital.

They place most of their emphasis upon technology, upon evidence of a strong medical staff, and upon evidence of good nursing standards. Some hospitals, however, have acquired a broad image — good or bad. Hospitals with such well-developed reputations are often assessed by their overall reputation rather than by specific evidence of competence.

Benefits Sought in a Hospital's Location

Health consumers prefer a hospital close to home, other things being equal. What may persuade a health consumer to bypass the nearest hospitals? Two major factors: poor quality or a poorly perceived neighborhood.

Many health consumers are willing to travel a reasonable distance if they perceive a hospital to offer significantly superior quality. A large minority of patients, however, do not see major differences in the quality of hospitals or their associated physicians, and they tend to use the closest hospital regardless of quality issues. Patients' willingness to travel should not, however, be exaggerated. Rarely do patients travel very long distances, such as from Florida to a hospital in Philadelphia. Conversely, large numbers of people will travel 50 to 100 miles to a perceived "regional medical center" offering specialized and high-quality services. Nonetheless, such patients represent but a small percentage of these hospitals' total admissions. Most people go to a hospital quite close to home.

By the same token, hospitals in badly perceived neighborhoods have special problems attracting patients. They may be able to overcome this drawback if they have a very strong image. Some of the best reputed hospitals in the United States are in less than ideal locations — either an undesirable neighborhood or a hard-to-reach location. However, even these hospitals have had to accept the reality that there remains a significant segment of the population who will not come to them whatever their reputation.

Health customers thus differ in the distances that they are prepared to travel for perceived superior care. A few willingly travel long distances. A significant number will travel some distance, bypassing nearer hospitals seen as being of lesser quality. Many people, however, place a major emphasis on proximity and do not see major differences in hospital quality. A poorly perceived or inaccessible location definitely prevents even a hospital with a strong positive image from attracting certain segments of the population.

One other hospital attribute may also play an expanding role in the information search of significant numbers of patients: evidence of specialized competence. As hospitals increasingly market themselves, many tend to focus upon certain areas of clinical strength. Some of them do so in the belief that proof of a few strong programs may have a halo effect on the institution as a whole. Marketing efforts centered on such "centers of excellence" may indeed have that impact on some health customers. These efforts, however, may also encourage customers to differentiate among hospitals for specific services. It appears that most health customers today have a preference for one particular hospital. Although the evidence is inconclusive, increasing numbers of health customers may, however, divide their preferences among several hospitals for different types of need, if varying marketing efforts succeed in convincing customers that different hospitals have differing centers of excellence.

Health customers who have elected an HMO or PPO for their health insurance have a more restricted choice of hospitals among which to select. As previously discussed, HMOs and PPOs obtain lower prices from hospitals precisely because they restrict the number of institutions with whom they contract. Those hospitals, therefore, theoretically will each get more patients than under a more traditional insurance plan where patients have unlimited choice. To illustrate, if a city has 10 hospitals and 50,000 people convert from a more traditional plan to an HMO that deals with only 5 of these hospitals, each of the 5 should see twice as many admissions from this population as it did before. The other 5 hospitals are now inaccessible to these 50,000 people. In practice, the impact of growing HMO enrollment on any hospital is more difficult to assess, but this simple example has broad validity.

There is also, in concept, an important difference between an HMO and a PPO. In an HMO, enrollees are restricted completely to contracted hospitals. They cannot go elsewhere. Under a PPO, patients can select nonparticipating hospitals, and the plan will pay up to the level that it would have paid a participating hospital. The patient is liable for the difference in costs. Despite this difference in concept between HMOs and PPOs, there is little evidence as yet that PPO enrollees often exercise their greater freedom of choice. Most health customers do not see a significant difference between HMOs and PPOs.

It is also easy to overstate the restriction on hospital choice that HMO or PPO membership in fact imposes on health customers. As previously discussed, people who join these plans vary in the relative importance they attach to price and quality. Those who join primarily for reasons of price and who attach little importance to quality would probably not engage in a very extensive information search among hospitals, even if they had the greater freedom afforded by more traditional insurance.

Those HMO or PPO enrollees who are concerned with quality considerations may well have checked to be sure that their chosen plan listed hospitals that they rated highly as part of their earlier search for a health insurance option. Cases have been reported in the media of people who joined an HMO or PPO only to find themselves denied access to a specialized resource at a nonparticipating hospital, but these cases seem to be the exception rather than the rule.

Although HMO enrollment restricts hospital choice, many HMO members are either price-driven and not very concerned with a wide choice of hospitals or are concerned with quality but selected a plan that listed hospitals of which they thought highly. Although PPOs in concept allow people more freedom to use nonparticipating hospitals if they will pay the difference in cost, there is as yet little evidence that many exercise this choice. Like most HMO enrollees, most PPO members are either not interested in a totally open choice of hospitals or have predetermined that their preferred hospitals were participants in their selected plan.

Market Guidance

The principal function of active marketing efforts in the information search phase of the service selection process is market guidance. The objective of market guidance is to steer customers to one supplier in particular and away from competitors. The techniques for achieving that goal are discussed in later chapters. Perhaps the important decision for a supplier in this effort, however, is to decide which types of customer to try to attract.

Although the previous discussion of the attributes that health customers seek from health insurance, primary care providers, specialists, and hospitals seems complex, there was an underlying pattern. In each case, health customers regard a quite limited number of attributes as important parts of the benefit bundles they seek. In seeking primary care providers, ability, availability, articulateness, and accessibility were of principal importance. The same factors were sought in specialists, but with slight variations in emphasis. In seeking hospitals, technology, good doctors, good nursing, and proximity were important, although specialized areas of competence may also be of growing interest to customers.

In this chapter's discussion of each of those attributes, two main conclusions emerged:

1. Different groups of people (or *segments*) attach differing degrees of importance to these attributes. For example, in searching for information about health insurance, some people are almost exclusively motivated by cost concerns, while others attach high value to freedom of access to any preferred specialist or hospital (Smith and Rogers 1986).

2. The measures by which people assess the degree to which a supplier possesses those desired attributes vary.

(For example, among persons who value accessibility in a primary provider, some might be more impressed that a particular supplier is willing to talk on the telephone, others with the fact that a provider makes house calls, and others with a convenient office location and convenient hours.)

Because of this phenomenon of a segmented market for health services, many providers do not have to attempt to appeal to everyone. They can prosper by identifying segments to which they can make a stronger appeal than many of their competitors, and then market to that segment. This process of selecting target segments and focusing marketing efforts on them is called, in marketing science, "positioning." Here are some easily recognized examples of positioning at work:

IBM does not claim to sell inexpensive computers, it claims to seek high-quality and state-of-the-art computers compatible with the widest choice of software. (Radio Shack adopts the inexpensive computer "position.")

Sears, Roebuck & Company does not claim to sell upscale and chic clothing. It claims to sell middle-of-the-road clothing of reasonable quality at a low price. (Bloomingdale's adopts the upscale, chic "position.")

ClubMed does not claim to be the ideal vacation resort for senior citizens, (even though its facilities and its prices might appeal to them). It concentrates on the young market. Palm Springs prefers the older vacationer and lives in dread of the Spring Break invasion of younger customers.

To solidify their marketing positions, individual providers and organizations seek to emphasize different attributes about their products or services, so that target segments identify with them more easily. This process of translating a *positioning strategy* into distinctive marketing messages is known as a *differentiation strategy*. Combining these three ideas, a differentiation strategy communicates a provider's intended positioning strategy to its targeted segments.

Consider the case of the new HMO in town. When this particular plan started up, its service area already had one strong preexisting HMO. This rival had succeeded in attracting blue-collar families who were concerned about unforeseen out-of-pocket expenses under more traditional forms of health insurance, but who were also not very alert to variations in quality among hospitals. These families also often had young children who needed more routine office visits to primary care providers than would young adults without children. This rival HMO positioned itself to appeal to this segment by having first-dollar coverage for office visits and no deductibles for hospitalization. It had deliberately contracted with the lowest-cost hospitals in the area to keep its prices as low as possible.

The new plan also wanted to compete with more traditional types of health insurance. In addition, however, it had to compete with this established HMO. It therefore decided to pursue a different segment—young professional families with small children, with high joint incomes (over $40,000), where both spouses have at least one college degree, who are aware that the quality of medical care varies, but whose spending priorities in their early career years are such that they want to be protected against major out-of-pocket health costs.

To implement this positioning strategy, the new plan, unlike the existing one, deliberately sought contracts with the best-regarded local hospitals. In so doing, it faced higher costs than the existing plan. It still wanted to avoid any deductibles for hospital care, but concluded that it could maintain a small ($5) copayment for routine office visits to doctors, which the other plan did not have, because its target segment was moderately affluent. The new plan was launched with a differentiation strategy of emphasizing the high quality hospitals with which it had contracted. This strategy proved effective.

The process of market guidance that providers can undertake during customer's information searches can therefore include three types of information:

1. *Factual information ("We have a service for . . . .";*
"We have the following technology . . . ."; "We have a
nurse-patient ratio in our ICU of . . . .")

2. *Positioning information ("If you are the type of person*
who . . . ."; "This service is designed with . . . in
mind.")

*3. Differentiating information ("Unlike many other prac-
tices . . . ."; "The only hospital in the region that . . . .")*

Chapter 3's discussion of the "needs recognition" phase of the
service selection process identified 12 ways in which nurses can influence demand generation. Each of those methods is also available
for nurses to influence the market guidance task once a health customer has recognized a need and begins to seek ways to satisfy it.

Nurses have one further opportunity in this information search
phase. Often they may find themselves acting, formally or informally, as agents, representatives, or salespersons. They may do so,
for instance, in home care agencies, in physicians' offices, in health
agencies, in commercial health-related programs, in wellness services, and counseling services. As hospitals expand their marketing
efforts, nurses are also being called upon increasingly to support
face-to-face "sales" efforts either for traditional hospital services or
for new forms of service such as satellites, geriatric centers,
hospices, and day hospitals.

Such "sales" activities are an important component of marketing
in many organizations. As a result, the art and science of successful
selling has been well researched, documented, and developed. Many
textbooks are available on selling techniques, as are a wide range of
training courses.

Understandably, many people in health care resist learning formal sales methods. They have been repelled by past experiences
with high-pressure sales tactics and have an image of salespeople as
manipulative and "unprofessional." A good salesperson, however,
does not have to use high-pressure tactics. Nevertheless, he or she
does have to understand the psychology of selling and how to conduct a structured sales discussion that wastes the time of neither the
salesperson nor the customer. The philosophy of marketing discussed earlier in this book is founded on the concept of creating a
matching of goals between a supplier and a customer. The best techniques of salespersonship focus on three tasks.

1. Discovering rapidly whether the potential exists for an
   exchange of goals

2. Providing information to help the potential customer
   structure a decision

3. Concluding the matching of goals (or "closing the deal")

A good salesperson discovers rapidly whether the potential exists for matching of goals by asking well-framed questions and listening to the answers. The objective is to hear the potential customers articulate needs or goals (in other words to clarify benefits they are seeking). The best feedback from the potential customer states two or three benefits of interest that the product or service offered can address. An example would be, "I want someone nearby who really knows something about Alzheimer's disease to help my aging mother, whose memory seems to be going." Wrapped up in that sentence are three desired benefits — the chance to do something about the mother's problem, the realization that someone with expertise might do her the most good, and the desire to find help nearby.

Why is more than one benefit statement desirable? As this chapter has shown, most health consumers do not make decisions around one single need or desired benefit. They seek benefit bundles. A matching of goals may be difficult if pursued as if the customer only has one objective, when he or she really has several that should be addressed. If a good salesperson does not identify two or three statements of desired benefits from a reasonably brief dialogue, he or she may well terminate the discussion as quickly and politely as possible, to invest time more usefully in talking to someone with more relevant needs. The salesperson may, however, try the tactic of asking a leading question (e.g., "You have explained that your company does not have any present plans to invest in employee wellness programs, but isn't it a topic that deserves some careful consideration?"). If this tactic works, the process is worth pursuing. If it fails to solicit a useful response, the discussion should be terminated — perhaps with a "leave behind" (written material that may remind the person if he or she discovers the need at a later stage).

If the potential customer does not articulate two or three relevant benefits that he or she seeks rapidly, the customer is not yet at the information search stage of the buying process; he or she has yet to recognize the need for those benefits. Is it worthwhile, therefore, for the salesperson to switch to a demand generation role — to try to convert the person into recognizing those needs. It may be worth a brief effort, but only a brief one, since the odds are against its working, and time may be better invested elsewhere.

This concept — that time is best spent with potential customers who already recognize needs that the product or service can meet — may be a difficult one for some would-be salespersons to grasp. Selling, however, is not education. It is not a missionary process to convert people or organizations (as in a company that is not very interested in employee wellness as a corporate goal). It is a process to find people with whom the supplier can most easily effect a matching of goals.

If a good salesperson does hear a potential client articulate a desired benefit bundle that the service can address, he or she rapidly switches to the second phase in selling—providing information to help the customer structure a decision. The salesperson often starts by repeating to the customer the two or three benefits that the customer said he or she wanted, and then asking for confirmation that these have been summarized correctly. The goal is to focus the subsequent discussion on that agreed "needs agenda."

The good salesperson then gives a brief description of the service and how it meets that needs agenda. The emphasis is on brevity, not a long prepared description. Why? Because someone may prove to be an "easy sell." He or she may neither need nor appreciate too long an explanation; indeed, it may raise new concerns or doubts. After a brief explanation, the experienced salesperson asks for confirmation that the service seems to meet the customer's stated needs.

The salesperson listens for one of four types of response to that question. If the customer seems *agreed*, it is time to move into the closure phase, without further unnecessary dialogue. If the customer sounds *indifferent* (e.g., "That's impressive, but I'm not sure I really need it"), an experienced salesperson will start asking a few more questions to see if the customer has left some important need unspoken, which can then be addressed. If the customer raises *objections* (e.g., "It's impressive, but it will take a lot of work"), the good salesperson will try to correct the objections with facts—not opinions—or put them into the proper context (e.g., "We help a lot with the first steps and, once you've tried it once or twice, you'll find it's not time-consuming"). If the customer responds with skepticism (e.g., "I'm not sure that wellness programs will really lower sick time."), a good salesperson will try to offer factual proof (e.g., "Control Data found that it did with its workforce"). With a response that sounds indifferent, objecting, or skeptical, however, the good salesperson sets a personal limit on the time that he or she will invest in this further dialogue.

Following either an early indication of agreement, or one that seems to have been secured after further dialogue, an experienced salesperson will move quickly into the closure phase, to get an agreement to try the service. It is important to preplan how this will be accomplished. Can the salesperson schedule an appointment, commit to a date, leave a contract for signature, etc.?

Reportedly, as many as 30% of hospitals now have sales teams, and many include nurses. They may be selling laboratory services to physicians and companies, wellness programs to industry, screening programs to government agencies, childbirth education classes to mothers, nursing education to nurses at other hospitals and so on. Many of these efforts are handicapped by hospital administrations that require the representative to consult with them before closing deals, rather than predefining what they can sell on the spot. This approach almost certainly reduces the number of deals that the representatives secure by as much as 50%, by failing to allow them to follow through instantly with a client who is ready to commit.

One common technique used by experienced salespersons is the presumptive close. Once the customer appears to have agreed that the service meets his needs, the salesperson starts the closure phase by presuming that the client is already committed (e.g., "Let me look at my calendar—we can have our first session on August 23rd at noon"). The alternative—of asking a question (e.g., "Would you like us to schedule your first session?")—affords another opportunity for an apparently convinced customer to defer his decision. If the customer is not yet ready to commit, he or she will say so. Why, therefore, ask?

Nurses are involved increasingly in acting as agents, representatives, or salespersons for health services. This role brings them into direct contact with potential customers who are in the information search phase of the service selection process. The techniques of good salespersonship developed in other fields, and as described briefly here, can be employed to structure these relations productively. The contact between a customer and a salesperson is intrinsically different from that between a nurse and a patient, or an educator and a student. It should be approached with different techniques of structuring and concluding the dialogue.

How Health Customers Make Decisions

Once customers conclude their information search, they arrive at the third stage of the service selection process. They make decisions on the services that they will use. How do they actually make such decisions?

Jeremy Bentham and John Stuart Mill, who were among the Victorian economists and social philosophers who first pondered this question, believed in the idea of a *rational customer*. Their answer was "the theory of utility." They realized that people select products or services that satisfy bundles of benefits. How, they wondered, did they weigh different benefits against each other? If someone wanted a doctor who was both able and accessible, but found one who was very able but not very accessible, while another was not so highly regarded for his ability but was very accessible, how did the customer make a rational selection? Their theory of utility stated that people make such decisions by adding the value of different units of utility, which they called "utiles."

Thus, the person evaluating the two doctors might conclude that the first doctor offers 7 utiles of ability plus 2 utiles of accessibility, while the second doctor offers 4 utiles of ability plus 7 utiles of accessibility. The second doctor would be preferred, so long as the customer saw one utile of ability as equal to one utile of accessibility. If the customer placed twice as much value on ability as upon accessibility, he or she would prefer the first doctor — $(7 \times 2) + 2 = 16$ — while the second doctor scores $(4 \times 2) + 7 = 15$. The first doctor is thus more "utilitarian," which is what this group of thinkers were termed.

The growth of Freudian psychology in the 20th century and in the number of social theorists who employed psychological ideas led to the rejection of this notion of decision making. Instead, customers were seen as making purchase decisions primarily on an emotional basis. The notion of the rational customer gave way to the idea of the *emotional customer*, in whom purchase decisions resulted from a power struggle among ego, id, and superego, each a product of childhood experiences.

Some of the early applications of scientific processes to marketing seemed to produce strong evidence for this emotional theory. Major manufacturers discovered the power of *test marketing*. If a new product was to be launched and its success of failure rested on obscure psychological forces, it made sense to test out possibly important variants before committing to them on a large scale. For instance, the product could be tried in Phoenix in a red box and in Boston in a blue box. Often, such test marketing did show that such variants could be very important; the red box version might outsell the blue box version by 2 to 1—hardly evidence of a rational customer.

Gradually, however, marketing scientists came to see that, even though many emotional factors entered into purchase decisions, there were patterns to be discerned in them. A new field of research emerged in the 1970s. Known as *psychographics*, it is dedicated to identifying such patterns of behavior. Aided by psychographics, marketing managers can still seek to influence the ways in which customers recognize needs, conduct information searches, and reach decisions about the products or services they will use.

Abraham Maslow's theory of the hierarchy of needs (Maslow 1954) helped to reconcile these two notions of the rational and emotional customer. It showed that once people have satisfied basic psychological needs, they seek to fulfill other needs—for security, esteem, or self-actualization—that are rooted in emotions, but are just as important to the customer.

How rational customers are in their information searches and product decisions depends upon three major factors:

1. What type of need they are seeking to satisfy

2. How important they deem the decision

3. Their different personalities

There are people who approximate the Victorian social theorists' model of the rational customer. They try to conduct a systematic and logical search when the decision seems important to them. Earlier in this book a patient was described who adopted such an approach to screening hospitals for her childbirth until she found one that satisfied her personal criteria. By contrast, other people place a high level of trust in their "intuition" and "sense of judgment" and make quick decisions. The color of the box may influence the choice of a brand of tea but play a lesser role in buying a microwave oven. Despite differences in personality, however, people tend to approach market decisions that they judge to be important more rationally than those that they consider trivial.

Influence of Marketing

Can marketing influence the decision phase of the service selection process? As discussed earlier, marketing can clearly influence the information search that precedes purchase decision. Active market guidance can help to clarify the customer's options, narrow choices and lead to one choice emerging as preferable. Many marketing textbooks, however, do not identify any direct means of influencing the decision phase itself. They tend to treat it like the jury deliberations in a trial. A lawyer can argue his or her best case in court, but once the jury adjourns to consider its verdict, the attorney is isolated from their decision process. Similarly, the customer is often viewed as reaching the point of decision and retreating into some cerebral choice process, detached from further influence.

However, many customer decisions are accompanied by the act of accessing the product or service. Marketing can influence the decision itself, as Figure 3-2 suggested, by ensuring the *fulfillment* of the accessibility of the product or service.

Consider a common example of such fulfillment. A customer decides to purchase a carton of fresh orange juice as part of his or her next stop in the local supermarket. The customer has a particular brand in mind — for instance, Tropicana. The supermarket must fulfill that expectation by having Tropicana in stock, and by having it in a place where the customer can easily find it. If the customer has to search too much for the product, he or she may opt for a substitute, or worse for the supermarket, decide to buy that item elsewhere, or, worse yet, get angry with the supermarket and vow never to return. Where, however, should the Tropicana be displayed? Where does the customer expect fresh juice to be — in the dairy aisle with the milk or in the drink aisle with the sodas and frozen juices?

Salespersons for food distributors go to great lengths to advise stores on where and how to display their products, because they know that accessibility is vital at the point of sale. Major food companies invest heavily in test marketing to establish on which shelves, where on those shelves, and where in the store their various products sell best. Their salespersons compete with those of other producers to see who can persuade store managers to give them the most preferential shelf footage and shelf locations.

Many services depend upon potential customers coming in person to a point of service — such as a bank, a hair salon, or even an emergency room. If the point of service is not organized to expedite fulfillment of the customer's decision, he or she may revise the decision and go elsewhere. One reason, for example, why banks have invested so heavily in automatic teller machines is to extend their access to customers. The machines can be in more locations than the banks themselves, can function when the banks are closed, and can relieve peak-time lines at the counter by providing an alternative point of service. One reason why a very successful hair styling salon may franchise another one to use its name is to extend its access to more people who want their hair styled under that name.

Consider, by contrast, the case of the hospital that was always closed. A hospital chief executive officer (CEO) was stopped in the lobby by a medical staff member who was obviously angry. Since the doctor accounted for several hundred admissions a year, the CEO decided to listen carefully. The doctor said that six times in the last month, he had been called in the middle of the night by patients with emergencies. He had told them to get to the hospital emergency room (ER), where the staff on duty would see them and, if necessary, admit them. He would see them in the morning at the hospital. On each occasion, he could not find the patient in the hospital, and the ER had no record of having seen them. When he checked with the patients, each had been told by the local ambulance squad that the hospital was full. Each had been taken to another hospital where the doctor did not have privileges and which he regarded as a very inferior facility.

The CEO promised to look into the problem immediately. He found that his hospital frequently ran out of critical care beds, causing it to notify local squads of this status. In fact, this occurred more than 100 nights in the last year. He called together a group of nurses, administrators, and the physicians in charge of the ER and the intensive and critical care units and asked them what it would take to run a hospital that never closed to ambulance squads. Several ingenious ideas surfaced, including designating "add-on" beds to be used and staffed only when no other solution existed. He was convinced in the end, however, that there was no way of always staying open to critical cases without compromising standards of care.

He, therefore, posed another question. What would it take to assure the 50 or so major admitters to the hospital that their patients would never be turned away in an emergency? It was estimated that, among them, these doctors might have some 200 such cases annually. About 60 might arise on nights when the hospital was "closed" — or less than 1, on average, on each such night.

The result of this discussion was the installation of a dedicated hot line into the ER, known only to these doctors, who could thus call to alert the ER of an incoming patient. It was made clear that a bed might not be available in every case, but the best effort would be made. For instance, suitable cases might be admitted to an intermediate unit and assigned extra nursing until an ICU or CCU bed opened. Most of the doctors agreed that a patient would be better off in such a bed than in the ICU of a less well resourced hospital.

This solution did not, therefore, keep the hospital always open to any patient. It did, however, keep it open most of the time to the patients of these loyal physicians. A year later it was estimated that the hospital had received 60 such admissions that, under the previous policy, it would have sent elsewhere. Effectively, what the hospital had done was to increase *access at the point of service.*

Many other health services do not operate on an emergency basis. Patients consummate their purchase decision by calling and making an appointment. Although a certain percentage turn into "no shows" — by not keeping their appointment — the call to make the appointment is the effective decision point. The practice's telephone thus constitutes a major point of service.

Consider all the things that can possibly inhibit customer access in calling a health service for an appointment: The line may be repetitively busy; it is not staffed 24 hours; if an answering service covers, it usually cannot schedule appointments; the caller may not call back if advised to do so; if the caller leaves a number, it may take the office several attempts before it can return the call; an appointment early enough and at a convenient enough time to satisfy the caller may not be available.

Consider the case of the missing coordinator. A hospital ran an ad for its childbirth education classes. The ad had been several months in development and, unfortunately, no one thought to check back with the childbirth education department before scheduling the ad in the local paper. The department, for its part, had never thought to assign a second person to handle calls when the nurse educator was unavailable. The ad ran just as the educator went on vacation for 2 weeks. On her return, she learned that the ad had run and asked how the calls had been handled. She was told that over 40 calls had come in and that each person had been told about her vacation and was asked to call back in 2 weeks. No one had asked for callers' names and numbers. Not one of those 40 callers ever called back.

Staff managing health services can make a major impact on customers in the decision phase of service selection by making service as accessible as possible at the point of service. This point of service might be the telephones that customers call for appointments or the places to which unscheduled customers are likely to come. Many services, supported by otherwise excellent marketing strategies, lose large numbers of potential customers by not being sufficiently accessible at the decision stage.

Remember that, in certain situations, several people may share in the decision-making role of the customer. If a doctor decides that a patient should be admitted to a hospital, both the doctor and the patient may well be involved in the choice of facility. Doctors themselves are consumers of the hospital's services when their patients are admitted: the services enable doctors to achieve their own goals of practicing their profession, caring for their patients, and earning their fees.

About 16% of the employed population also now have health insurance that requires precertification of hospital admission (Medical Benefits, 1987). An even larger percentage of the population is covered by Medicare or Medicaid, which has similar requirements. Although not strictly a customer of the hospital, these third parties do act as gatekeeper in a hospital admissions. They may approve or disapprove of the doctor's and the patient's decision.

Recall also the earlier discussion of the role of surrogates who may make decisions on behalf of customers. For instance, in 24% of cases of elderly persons moving into a "senior living community," an adult child also participated in the final decision (Laventhol and Horwath 1986). Some probably did so as surrogates, effectively making the decision on behalf of the parent. The others shared the role of customer, and shared the decision, with the parent. In another 69% of cases, an adult child was not involved in the final decision, but had visited the facility previously with the parent and was an influencer of the decision. Indeed, one common challenge to salespersons for both nursing homes and retirement communities is trying to mediate between the resident and an adult child, who seem to have different opinions, to reach a shared decision.

The role of the customer as a decision maker may be shared among several people. It may also in health care require the concurrent approval of others, including doctors and insurers. To influence the decision, a supplier may, therefore, have to influence several parties.

References

American Board of Family Practice. 1987. *Rights and responsibilities, Part 2: The changing health consumer and patient/doctor partnership.* Lexington, KY: American Board of Family Practice.

American Medical Association. 1987. *The socioeconomic characteristics of medical practice.* Chicago: American Medical Association.

Anderson, R.M., G. Fleming, and C. Aday. 1981. Study points out medical manpower needs. *American Medical News* 24:29-31.

Berki, S.E., and M. Ashcroft. 1984. HMO enrollment: Who joins what and why. *Millbank Quarterly* (Fall): 588-632.

Brown, S. 1980. Comparing attitudes and opinions of Arizona physicians and consumers. *Arizona Medicine* 17(3): 174-179.

Dove, R. 1986. Exploring the selection of a nursing home: Who, what, and how. *Journal of Health Care Marketing* 6 (2): 63-66.

Fisk, T. 1987. Perceptual Mapping: Hospitals' competitive images. Paper presented at College of Health Care Marketing Annual Symposium, February 16-18, Orlando, FL.

Fisk, T., and E. Somers. 1987. HMO's: A negotiating strategy for university hospitals. *Journal of Health Care Marketing* 7 (3): 60-70.

Gochman, D.S., G. Stukenborg, and A. Feler. 1986. The ideal physician: Implications for contemporary hospital marketing. *Journal of Health Care Marketing* 6(2): 17-25.

Hall, J., D. Roter, and C. Rand. 1981. The communication of affect between patient and physician. *Journal of Health and Social Behavior* 22(1): 18-30.

Halpern, K., T. Fisk, and C. Brown. 1983.

Cooper data: The doctors people want. Camden, NJ: Cooper Hospital/University Medical Center.

Halpern, K., T. Fisk, and J. Sobel, M.D. 1984. Consumer preference: The overlooked element in health planning. In *Health care: An international perspective.* ed. J.M. Virgo, pp. 267-278. Edwardsville, IL: International Health Economics and Management Institute.

Hugstad, P., J. Taylor, and G. Bruce. 1987. The effects of social class and perceived risk on consumer information search. *Journal of Consumer Marketing* (Spring): 41-46.

Laventhol and Horwath. 1986. The senior living industry: 1986. Philadelphia: Laventhol and Horwath.

Maslow, A. 1954. Motivation and personality. New York: Harper and Brothers.

Medical Benefits. 1987. Employee benefits in medium and large firms. *Medical Benefits (July 30): 5.*

Medical Economics. 1985. June.

Newman, J.W., and R. Staelin. 1972. Pre-purchase information seeking for new cars and major household appliances. *Journal of Marketing Research* (August): 249-257.

Robinson, P., and T. Fisk. 1988. The role of perceptual mapping in image management and strategic positioning. Paper presented to the Academy of Health Care Marketing Conference on Market Research Innovations, May 6-7, Chicago.

Scotti, D.J., G. Bonner, and A. Wiman. 1986. An analysis of the determinants of HMO re-enrollment behavior. *Journal of Health Care Marketing* 6(2): 7-16.

Smith, H.L., and R. Rogers. 1986. Factors influencing consumer selection of health insurance carriers. *Journal of Health Care Marketing* 6(4): 6-14.

Review Questions

1. From what sources do patients get the information they need to make choices about health care?

2. What are the four main factors that determine whether a patient will form a loyalty to his or her health care providers?

3. "All that people think about in choosing their health insurance is what it costs." Comment.

4. "What patients want most from nurses, doctors, and hospitals may differ." Discuss.

Chapter 5

Using and Assessing Health Services

Service Usage

Once a customer has decided upon a product or service, he or she reaches the fourth stage of the buying process—actual usage. Purchase and usage are not necessarily simultaneous events. Many products are bought for later consumption. Appointments are made, or contracts signed for many services that are actually performed later.

Chapter 3 noted that *customers* are not necessarily *consumers*. A customer may purchase a product or initiate arrangements for a service on behalf of someone else who will actually consume it. This chapter focuses on the consumer who, as stated, may or may not be the customer.

Some marketing experts argue that there is a basic difference between the usage of a product and the usage of a service. They hold that, unlike products, services are intangible and perishable, that the supply of a service and its consumption occur simultaneously, and that services are "heterogeneous," meaning that their performance varies (Zeithmal, Parasuraman, and Berry 1985). However, this idea does not stand up to scrutiny. Certain services are tangible—they can be sensed in advance. Plastic and oral surgeons, for instance, can now use various devices, from photographs to computer graphics, to show a patient what he or she will look like postsurgery. It may not be possible for the patient literally to sense the surgeon's skill in advance, but that is not the service. The service being bought in plastic surgery is its outcome, a changed appearance. The customer no more views the surgery itself as the service than someone buying an automobile views the dealership as the

97

product. By the same token, many products are not capable of being sensed in advance. A shopper cannot taste the soup before buying the can; a person buying a car cannot test how it will perform 24 months and 40,000 miles later; yet he or she assumes a certain minimum performance time frame.

Services are perishable only if they involve a supplier's personal time and cannot be rescheduled. Automatic tellers are services, but they are by no means perishable. Indeed, the whole logic behind them is that they are nearly always accessible. Many products are perishable (as anyone who has ever eaten a stale pretzel can testify).

Production and consumption of services do not necessarily occur coincidentally. A physician ordering a computed tomography (CT) scan for a patient may wait several hours or days to "consume" the results in his professional care of his patient. By contrast, production and consumption of some products (like cotton candy) occur almost simultaneously.

Many services are indeed heterogeneous; they vary each time they are performed. Many others, however, are standardized. The service supplied by automatic tellers is an example, and so are many medical procedures where quality is assured in part by following standard protocols and treatment regimens. By contrast, many products are deliberately nonstandard, such as made-to-measure suits or personalized license plates, as are some health care services, such as options in childbirth or the rights of patients with some forms of health insurance to refer themselves either to a primary physician or directly to a specialist.

To claim that all products are distributed to consumers, while consumers must come to a center for service, is furthermore not a valid distinction between products and services. Home care, physician answering services, information hot lines, and air conditioning maintenance are all services that move to the customer, or involve no movement at all. Similarly, a bumper sticker saying "I Love NY" or that "Virginia is for Lovers" is a product, but you may have to travel a long way to obtain one.

When people say that they "work in a service organization," they usually mean that they have a close and multifaceted relationship with their customers. Increasingly, however, all types of manufacturing companies are adding a wide range of customer services to their narrower task of manufacturing. Repair services, trouble-shooting hot lines, ensuring the accessibility of parts and accessories, calls to check upon consumer satisfaction, training programs for users, "no-hassle" return policies, and so on are all examples of service supplements to products. At the same time, some service organizations, like many banks, are limiting hours of personal access, are relying more on telephone service, and are still in the process of developing easy ways for customers to pursue complaints.

The only real difference between a product and a service is, therefore, in the philosophy of the supplier. The "service mentality" can be found just as much among manufacturers as in suppliers of a personal service. The "production mentality"—that responsibility is limited to delivering the direct benefit of the product and does not extend to any broader interaction with the consumer—can be found in some so-called service organizations as much as among producers of consumer goods.

The most important question for any supplier to consider when consumers actually reach the point of using their products or services is not, therefore, "Are we in a service business?" but "What does the customer expect?"

The supplier's objective should be consumer satisfaction. According to the marketing philosophy stated earlier in this book, individuals and enterprises achieve their own goals by satisfying the goals of consumers. Because the typical consumer has recognized the need to obtain a bundle of benefits, a supplier who interprets those consumer needs too narrowly, and concentrates only upon the central and most obvious benefit of the service, runs a high risk of creating a dissatisfied consumer. The supplier who sees consumer needs as multifaceted is more likely to secure the customer's satisfaction.

Consumers are satisfied when services fully meet their expectations. They are dissatisfied when a service fails to meet their expectations in some important component of their desired benefit bundle.

How do consumers form their expectations? How are those expectations met (or not met) in service usage? Figure 5-1 summarizes the process. The lefthand column of this patient satisfaction model shows the most common sources of patient expectations for health services. The righthand column shows the major components of the service encounter through which those expectations are either confirmed or denied. Note that two of the righthand boxes are shaded.

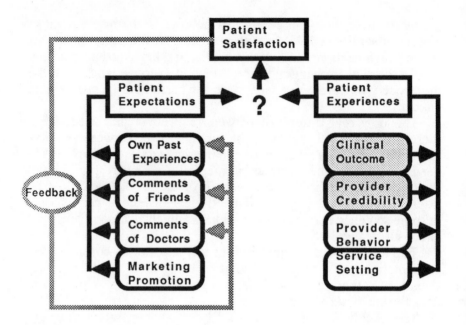

Figure 5-1 Patient satisfaction model.

The marketing theorists who developed the original concept upon which this model is based (Parasuraman, Zeithmal, and Berry 1986) argued that in practice it is difficult for a service supplier to confirm or deny the credibility image that a consumer has already formed by the time of service. Based on personal interviews with large numbers of recent users of various services, Parasuraman et al. found that, through the information search process, most consumers attach a high credibility to the supplier that they have chosen. By the time of service itself, they have come to "believe" in the supplier's competence. The supplier can destroy that credibility by an obvious error, but, otherwise, it is taken for granted.

Parasuraman et al. (1986) also argued that consumers find it difficult to assess the technical outcome of a service like health care. This idea is debatable. While patients cannot assess the outcome of their care with clinical accuracy, the patient surveys conducted at Thomas Jefferson University Hospital show that most people are able, without effort, to express an opinion on whether their problem is "cured," "substantially better," "about the same but easier to cope with," "about the same," or "worse" following an episode of care.

The two unshaded boxes on the right of Figure 5-1 deal with behavioral and environmental aspects of the service. Parasuraman et al. (1986) argue that these aspects are the most crucial to consumers' evaluation of whether their expectations have been met or not. Again, this claim is debatable, but it is undoubtedly true that behavioral and environmental service aspects play a critical role in consumers' health care satisfaction. But specifically which behavioral and environmental factors? The answer to this question can be both difficult and misleading. "Patients want us to smile." "The reading material in the waiting room should be up-to-date." "In-patients want TVs off by 10 PM so they can sleep." "Nursing home residents like eating in groups." "Home care patients like you to talk to them a lot." Opinions such as these may or may not be valid. Even if they are based upon experience, they may not be true of all patients.

At Thomas Jefferson University Hospital, in Philadelphia, large samples of inpatients are regularly interviewed regarding more than 80 different aspects of their care and service. Many hospitals now follow similar practices to see how patients rate different attributes of their stays. At Jefferson Hospital, however, the results are also analyzed to see how important different aspects are to patients' overall first impressions of the hospital. Complex analytical software developed at Jefferson is used to study the relationship between patient ratings of individual features of their stay and their overall satisfaction. Each of the 80 or so aspects is categorized as "very important," "somewhat important," "less important," or "not important" to the patients' overall feeling that his or her expectations are being fulfilled. This process has shown that behavioral and environmental issues rank with clinical issues as among the most important to patients. It also shows, however, that only some such issues are "very" or "somewhat" important. These studies thus provide nursing and other hospital services with both an indication of how patients rate different aspects of their work and of how important each aspect is to patients, allowing the hospital and staff to assign priority to specific activities to improve patient satisfaction. At one point, for instance, it was found that noise was among the 10 or so most negative factors in patients' reactions to the hospital. The survey was detailed enough to ascertain that it was not noise from other patients that was the problem—which might have been the erroneous assumption—but noise among the hospital personnel themselves. A concerted awareness program was initiated, resulting, 12 months later, in substantially higher patient ratings on this service feature.

This approach to researching patient reactions has been extended at Jefferson to different types of outpatients and to patients visiting some of the physician practices on the campus. The results have also been reanalyzed in various formats to identify *segments* of patients with different personal priorities. The results from Jefferson may not be a guide to other health care providers, as both patient preferences and actual circumstances can differ.

Both these and other studies, however, show that nursing is among the most important factors contributing to patients' reactions to health care encounters. Table 5-1 provides a sample of the type of data yielded by the method developed at Jefferson Hospital. For simplicity, it includes only eight service attributes, arranged in descending order of importance to overall patient satisfaction. The righthand column shows how a group of patients rated the performance of the nurses. The actual questions asked at Jefferson use a method known as "semantic differential scaling," which lowers the risk of "positive bias,"—that is, respondents tending to rate services higher because of the tenor of the questions. Most importantly, respondents see negative descriptions as much as positive descriptions and are asked to grade services between two extremes (e.g., "nurses friendly" versus "nurses not friendly"). Each pair of opposites is formally tested before being used in the surveys, to ensure that its intended meaning is understood. In the preceding example, for instance, it was found that the best opposite for "friendly" was "not friendly," rather than "unfriendly." To most people "unfriendly" means "hostile," rather than "aloof" or "cold."

The software developed at Jefferson converts the scores obtained by semantic differentiation into ratings out of 100 points, to make them easier to read than a scatter of readings on a scale. It also calculates the statistical accuracy of the data, taking into account the number of responses upon which they were based. In Table 5-1, the scores are accurate to within 4%. A score of 80 may, therefore, actually be a score of between 76 and 84. (These calculations are made at a 95% level of confidence.)

Clearly, the breakdown of these factor scores enables health care professionals to evaluate the importance of each factor in relationship to the others and to patients' overall satisfaction. Of course,

Table 5-1 Patient Satisfaction Scores

Service Feature	Score (out of 100)
Overall satisfaction	85
Very important to overall satisfaction	
Overall nursing	87
Nurses friendly	93
Somewhat important to overall satisfaction	
Nurses seem experienced	80
Nurses come quickly when I call	75
Nurses explain things well	77
Less important to overall satisfaction	
Nurses helpful to my visitors	69
Not important to overall satisfaction	
Nurses introduce themselves	94

Source: Based on patient sampling method developed at Thomas Jefferson University Hospital, Philadelphia (see text).

none of the features listed is a priority if the overall satisfaction score is acceptable. However, in this instance, it is not. The target score for total satisfaction in this system is 90 or higher. If it is significantly below 90, large numbers of patients are likely to criticize their experience in discussions with friends and resolve not to use this health service again.

This simplified example of satisfaction testing dealt only with the responses from patients as a whole. Jefferson Hospital's thorough version also subdivides respondents into segments of patients with varying expectations of nurses and other health professionals. Some patients, for instance, seem to attach most importance to how experienced nurses seem to be. Other patients, aware of the talk of a nursing shortage, are most concerned with how well staffed units seem to be. Because this group cannot assess nurse staffing levels directly, they use a *proxy* measure—how attentive the nurses seem to be personally and how quickly they respond to calls for help.

Consumer satisfaction occurs when the individual's expectations are matched by his or her actual experience in using a product or service. Some of the assessment of a health service starts while it is being received. These "first impressions" are important to consumer satisfaction. Since so many aspects of a health service may potentially influence patient satisfaction, it is important to identify those that matter most.

Postcare Evaluation

After consumers have used a product or service, they enter the fifth phase of the service selection process, that of evaluating their experience with the product or service. They assess the extent to which the product or service met their expectations of it. This assessment may be limited and cursory, or it may be thorough and extensive. It tends to be most thorough when one or more of the following conditions applies:

1. The benefits sought from the product or service were regarded as important. (For instance, a consumer is likely to conduct a more thorough assessment of his or her experience in buying formal evening attire than in buying a pair of jeans for routine wear.)

2. The consequences of the purchase will last for some time. (For instance, a clothes dryer may be used for years, while a vacation, although often as expensive, is of short-term consequence.)

3. The purchase was "expensive" in either dollars spent, time involved, or disruption to normal activities. (For instance, a microwave oven costs more than a hair dryer. A weekend away requires more time commitment than a dinner in a restaurant.)

4. The consumption of the product or service was shared with others to whom the consumer feels responsible or whose opinions the consumer values. (For example, a gift for a relative or close friend may matter more than the identical item bought for yourself.)

5. Other people are likely to notice the product or service and to ask questions about it, so that the consumer has

to "explain" or even "defend" his or her decision. (Redecorating the living room has more visible consequences than repainting a basement.)

Nearly all health services have these attributes, which tend to stimulate the consumer to make a thorough postusage assessment. Not only are the consequences of these services often long-lasting, but the program of treatment and of billing may be spread over a prolonged time. Many health services are seen as expensive in both cost and personal time commitment. Often, a health service directly involves other people important to the consumer, such as family and friends visiting an inpatient, or a possibly reluctant spouse participating in marital therapy. Finally, the use of a health service will often be inquired about by friends interested in the consumer's health or who want to expand their own information about available services for possible personal use.

Cognitive Dissonance

Health consumers tend to make thorough postusage assessments of health services, particularly if a serious disease and a greater personal commitment of time and expense were involved, and if the experience involved others or was visible to them. What does such a postusage assessment entail? First, the consumer compares his or her expectations for the service with the actual experience. If a gap exists between the two, the consumer undergoes what marketing scientists call *cognitive dissonance*. Cognitive dissonance happens when two mental images do not fit together, therefore producing a state of psychological discomfort or confusion. If the service experience fails to meet the consumer's expectations, he or she forms doubts about the wisdom of the service selection made. If the service decision was important, of lasting impact, expensive, involved others, and led to questions from others, this cognitive dissonance may be magnified.

Studies among patients at Jefferson Hospital, for instance, have been paralleled by further surveys some 3 months postdischarge. These studies have tended to show not only that consumers' ratings of service features change slightly as reflected in their postusage assessment, but also that the relative importance of some service features to consumers' overall satisfaction is altered. For instance, patients who perceived their medical problems to be quite serious usually attached less importance during their hospitalization to the quality of hospital food than in their postusage assessment. Two major factors probably explain this shift. First, the patient, when recovered, slightly revises his or her priorities. Second, patients after discharge are subjected to questioning by friends. It is more difficult to describe to friends the less tangible aspects of a hospital stay, such as nursing care or attentiveness, than to comment upon readily understandable matters like food or amenities. Indeed, friends may inquire specifically about such service features, because of widespread public impressions about standards of hospital food and accommodations. It should not be assumed that these service features come to dominate the postusage assessment of patients; the available data only show that the features play a larger role in consumers' lasting impressions about hospital stays.

It is also possible that patient expectations are partly modified during the experience itself. This area of consumer behavior is still being researched and debated among marketing scientists. Indeed, the idea of *informed consent* rests upon a belief that patient expectations can be modified by dialogue with health professionals. There is, as yet, an imperfect understanding of the extent to which this effect is possible, of how precisely it can best occur, and of what impact it has on postusage assessment, given that patients may well have firmly established expectations before they reach the point of actual service usage.

Consider, as an example the case of a woman who required surgery to remove a bowel obstruction confirmed by magnetic resonance imaging (MRI) and colonoscopy. The day before surgery, she asked her surgeon two questions of concern to her — the amount of permanent scarring that would result and the level and extent of any postoperative pain. The surgeon considered three answers to her questions about scarring:

"There will be some permanent scarring. Its extent may well depend on what I find when I go in. I assure you I will do my best to keep it to a minimum."

"I have done this procedure hundreds of times and most patients find the scars that result not to be a big issue to them."

"I really cannot give you a precise answer. I depends upon so many things."

He considered three possible answers to her question about postoperative pain:

"This is major surgery and there is always postoperative discomfort. We have some of the best anesthesiologists around and they are up-to-date with all the latest approaches to limiting postoperative pain."

"There's no easy answer to that. Recovery from major surgery does involve some pain, but people vary a lot in their reaction to it. You'll be on some standard medications that we use to limit pain, but if you're having a problem, call your nurse and we'll see what else we might do."

"Since it's an issue for you, I could enroll you in a clinical trial that our anesthesiologists are conducting with a new approach. It's very promising and has worked well with some patients, but it is experimental."

This patient has clearly included minimal scarring and minimal postoperative discomfort in the benefit bundle that she wants from her surgery. Consider whether any of the three possible answers just described to these two questions is likely to confirm the patient's expectation of minimal scarring and pain. If the patient's expectations are firmly established, she may heed none of these answers and simply maintain those expectations. Each of the possible answers quoted is a legitimate response, yet each may have very different consequences for patient expectations.

The expectations that patients bring to health care service encounters are largely formed during the needs recognition and information search stages of the service selection process. At the beginning of their service usage, patients often have a further opportunity to ask questions and to participate in a formal informed consent process. It is uncertain to what degree their expectations are modified by these opportunities. The answers and explanations that they receive may confirm, lower, or raise their expectations, or have no impact on them.

Some authorities argue that cognitive dissonance either occurs or does not occur (in the latter case, the consumer's expectations are met in full or largely in full and the consumer is considered satisfied with the experience). Other marketing experts argue that cognitive dissonance always occurs to some degree, because the consumer's image of a product or service never coincides completely with its reality.

If cognitive dissonance occurs or, in terms of the other school of thought, it occurs and is substantial, three important practical consequences result:

1. Patients determine not to use the service again; they do not form *brand loyalty*.

2. They do not recommend the service to friends. Instead, they criticize the service.

3. Patients may well blame others who shared in the service selection process, including friends who were influencers, a doctor or health insurer who shared in the role of customer, or anyone to whom they delegated the decision as a surrogate.

Brand Loyalty. Much research has been conducted into consumer brand loyalty. Satisfaction with past usage of a product or service; frequency of usage; products or services perceived as "routine" and "easy to find" or, at the other extreme, as "important" and "hard to find"; and products or services whose outcomes are easily predicted in satisfying needs are all factors that shape brand loyalty in general (Engel and Blackwell 1982; Nicosia 1966).

Most health care services are needed infrequently by consumers. Even a visit three or four time a year to a primary caregiver is not a frequent event in comparison with many consumer activities. The growing supply of doctors and the falling occupancy rates in hospitals have made health services seem relatively easy to find. Increasing public health awareness also seems to be widening the realization that the quality, and hence the outcome, of different health services vary. As a result, more health consumers are engaging in *brand switching*. A recent survey (*Medical Economics* 1985) reports that a majority of adults have switched primary care providers in recent years, and also indicates that the percentage of this population of "switchers" is now much higher than at any time over the last 20 years.

In terms of brand loyalty to hospitals, two reported surveys of patients, discharged several months previously from 30 different hospitals, showed that only about 50% names the hospital in which they were recently as their preferred hospital for any future care (Fisk 1986). Sixty percent of female respondents and 40% of male respondents named another hospital. Although the number of patients surveyed for each hospital was too small to draw valid conclusions about specific hospitals, patient loyalty did seem to differ by hospital. Thus, it appears that some hospitals do a better job than others at generating brand loyalty.

In the health care area, patient satisfaction is not the only factor that leads patients to form brand loyalty, but it is a major factor. Available evidence suggests that many patients of both doctors and hospitals do not form brand loyalty as a result of their postusage assessments. Instead, they become brand switchers who intend to go elsewhere for future care.

Many products and services depend most for their marketing effectiveness upon word-of-mouth communication from satisfied consumers. Even large-scale advertising may not succeed at countering a negative image spread by word-of-mouth. For instance, consider the case of the disliked hospital (a true example). Some 30% of adults in the town where it is located state that they would refuse to go to it under any circumstances. Only some 25% of people who have been inpatients there name it as the hospital to which they would prefer to be admitted for any future care. The local community is rife with jokes and anecdotes about it. The hospital has tried many approaches to living down this negative image, but so far has been unable to beat word-of-mouth communication.

Criticizing the Service. One consequence of significant cognitive dissonance is that patients are likely to spread negative comments about a health service to others. How far does word-of-mouth testimony by consumers spread?

One detailed study (TARP 1986) suggests that satisfied American consumers of products and services, on average, praise a service to three acquaintances. By contrast, dissatisfied consumers share their negative impressions with between 12 and 21 other people. Women share information on their dissatisfaction with products or services more widely than do men. Female consumers, if dissatisfied, tend to tell up to 21 other people, while dissatisfied male consumers tell closer to 12. This finding underscores the practical importance of patient satisfaction to health care providers. Not only is any patient dissatisfaction potentially harmful, but, because negative comments travel up to seven time farther than positive comments, the percentage of dissatisfied patients must be kept very low. Organizations that take consumer satisfaction seriously therefore aim to achieve high scores when they survey consumers. Table 5-2 shows the net effect of several different levels of patient satisfaction on the information about a service that circulates by word-of-mouth communication.

As shown in the table, even with only 3% of consumers dissatisfied, almost 1 in every 5 people who hear about the service from a patient will hear negative comments. With 6% of patients dissatisfied, almost one-third of the information circulated about the service by word-of-mouth is negative. The percentage of dissatisfied patients has only to exceed 12% before most of the word-of-mouth comment about the service is negative.

Blaming Others Who Participated in Service Selection. The other potential consequence of patient dissatisfaction is that the patient may attribute part of the blame for poor selection of service to those who influenced or who shared in his or her decision. This result may increase tension within a family; it may lead to a patient's changing health insurance; to the patient blaming any physician who influenced the selection; and if dissatisfaction is strong enough, to the patient actually switching doctors. At the least, many patients will share their dissatisfaction with a referring doctor or agency. One survey (SRI Gallup 1987) shows that the single most important factor mentioned by physicians as influencing their referral decisions is the satisfaction of previous patients referred to particular services. Another study (Halpern, Fisk, and Brown 1983) shows that a large percentage of patients dissatisfied with hospitals stays blame their physicians for that service selection.

What actions by a health professional are most likely to provoke patient dissatisfaction? As earlier comments in this volume have indicated, patients are highly segmented in the benefit bundles which they seek from health services and in the priorities they attach to various aspects of these bundles. Therefore, any general observations must be carefully interpreted. Nevertheless, it appears that the most likely causes of patient dissatisfaction with a primary care

Table 5-2 Effect of Word-of-Mouth Communication on Patient Satisfaction

% satisfied	Positive comments per 100 patients (@ 3 per patient)	% dissatisfied	Negative comments per 100 patients (@ 21 per patient)	% Negative comments
97	291	3	63	18
94	282	6	126	31
91	273	9	189	41
88	264	12	252	49
85	255	15	315	55
82	246	18	378	61

physician are that the doctor does not spend enough time with them and that the doctor is not good at listening to or explaining things to patients. One study (American Board of Family Practice 1987) found that 75% of patients complained that the doctor did not give them enough time. Interestingly, the same study also interviewed doctors, and 69% agreed that this was a problem in contemporary primary care. Fifty-six percent of patients complained about their doctors' listening and communications skills. Forty percent of doctors admitted to this problem, a surprisingly high percentage. Other studies have reported analogous results (Brown 1980). Remember, however, that among any group of patients, varying aspects of the health provider's ability, availability, articulateness, and accessibility will be significant factors in satisfaction.

In terms of outpatient visits to hospital services, emergency room visits, and hospital stays, the patient surveys at Thomas Jefferson University show a broad list of service attributes to be either "very important" or "somewhat important" to patient satisfaction. In the perceived outcome of the care, the behavior of nurses, the behavior of physicians, and a few selected aspects of the amenities and environment are among these more important features. In practice, however, any health service needs to investigate what matters most for its particular patients and how patients rate its current performance. Acting on the basis of general findings may mean missing the mark in what specific patients most want, and might lead to allocating effort to service features that are already well regarded, while neglecting others that are problems.

*Patient dissatisfaction can lead to negative feedback to referral
sources. It can thus have a "multiplier effect" by discouraging
future referrals. Although certain aspects of health services
seem most likely to cause dissatisfaction, any health service
should ideally investigate the priorities and reactions of its own
patients, as these may not reflect general findings from elsewhere.*

Influencing Health Consumers'
Assessments of Services

How can nurses and other health professionals influence the assessment that patients make of their services, and thereby patients'
future interest in using the service again and recommending it to
friends?

1. The best opportunity that nurses and other health
   professionals have to influence patients' final assessments of services is during those services, by trying to
   fulfill each patient's expectations as completely as possible.

2. There may be more opportunity than is currently being
   realized to obtain input on particular patient concerns,
   preferences, and benefits sought through the initial nursing assessment, or nursing diagnosis process.

3. Through an early discussion with patients, there may be
   opportunities, otherwise missed, to modify unrealistic
   patient expectations.

4. The last day, or last few hours, of an inpatient stay and
   the last few minutes of an office visit or an outpatient
   service, provide an opportunity to leave the patient with
   a strong positive impression, and even, possibly, to compensate for any negative impressions created earlier. In
   many health services, by contrast, attention to the
   patient diminishes in these last critical minutes or hours
   of service. For instance, an inpatient about to be discharged is a lower nursing priority than patients being
   admitted, or others at critical points in their care.

5. Many service organizations deliberately contact consumers within a few days of service, both to catch any problems that may lead to dissatisfaction and to show the consumer that their interest in him or her still continues. Some health services do routinely engage in such follow-up calls, but they are still the exception rather than the rule.

6. Many service organizations routinely survey recent customers, both to obtain feedback and to express their interest in their views. This practice is growing in health care.

7. The billing process may also influence the lasting impression that patients form of health services. Again, many organizations have reviewed their billing procedures to ensure that they result in payment but maintain their "message" of consumer orientation.

8. The relationship that a patient develops with nurses as professional caregivers is, in certain situations, a close and strong one. Thought must be given to how best to manage the end of the relationship, such as when an inpatient is discharged, to convey a continuing interest in the patient's health and well-being and to avoid a feeling of an abrupt loss of interest.

Summary of the Health Service Selection Process

The previous chapters have described the five steps that health customers undergo in the service selection process—need recognition, information search, decision, actual service usage, and post-usage assessment. It has been shown that other people are often involved, along with the actual consumer of the service, in this selection process.

It has furthermore been seen that circumstances differ among patients. They may perceive different bundles of needs or benefits; they may conduct their information searches in slightly different ways; and their approaches to making final decisions about services can differ, as can their reactions during and after service usage. Nevertheless, they do follow certain common patterns, which are possible to research, understand, and attempt to influence. Even where people differ in their approaches, often it is possible, with the aid of computer-assisted analysis, to categorize the major differences into market segments. Strategies to address different segments can then be developed.

To summarize the key aspects of this entire process, consider the diagram in Figure 5-2, based on an original concept applied to other types of services (Solomon 1986). The figure depicts the five steps of the process and the ways in which formal marketing efforts can influence each of them, similar to Figure 3-2. This more complicated version, however, also depicts the role of various people other than the customer personally. Note that Figure 5-2 only applies to some instances of health service selection. Other customers' interactions would have to be depicted differently.

As a helpful exercise, you might try to describe a typical health services selection case that fits the diagram in Figure 5-2. One such version is contained in the following Case Example #3, but, clearly, the diagram could apply to several different case histories. Alternatively, read the case history provided here and then try to develop a parallel version depicting a case known to you (possibly involving a friend, relative, or yourself personally).

The following case history accompanies Figure 5-2.

A 17-year old boy (*customer*) felt pain in his side at school and went to the school nurse (*surrogate*). She was concerned and called the boy's mother (*surrogate*). The boy's mother called the family's physician (*doctor*), who told her to bring him at once to his office. The boy's discomfort increased on the journey to the office, and the doctor diagnosed appendicitis. This completed the need recognition.

The doctor recommended hospital admission, as the symptoms suggested that the problem was worsening and the appendix needed surgical attention. The doctor had admitting privileges at three hospitals and offered them as choices to the mother. The mother called her husband at work (*surrogate*), brought him up-to-date on the situation, and consulted him on the choice of hospitals. This step completed the information search. Because of the emergent nature of the son's condition, the parents did not feel they had time for a more comprehensive search.

Together the parents decided on one of the doctor's hospitals. The doctor confirmed their choice by calling the hospital to alert

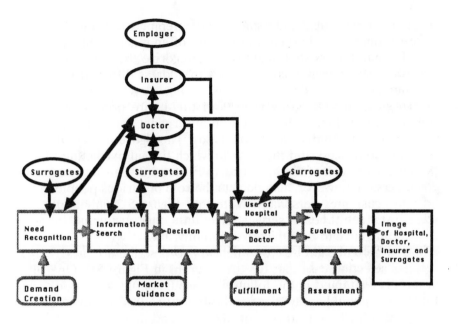

Figure 5-2 Roles of various people in a sample service selection process.

them to the emergency admission. The hospital asked what insurance the family had. The parents responded that it was a health
maintenance organization (*insurer*). The father had selected that
HMO from the health insurance options offered at his company
(*employer*). Fortunately, the hospital selected by the parents was a
participating provider for that HMO. Otherwise, the parents might
have had to select another hospital. These steps completed the
decision.

The boy was taken to the hospital and admitted. Several hours
later he underwent emergency surgery, performed by a surgeon
selected by the primary physician. The patient stayed in the hospital
several days. The parents (*surrogates*) visited him regularly. On two
occasions, they took along an old friend (*surrogate*) who was a nurse
at another hospital. She was very concerned at the apparent short
staffing on the nursing unit where the boy received his postsurgical
care. She also did not feel that the dieticians had given enough
thought to the boy's diet during recovery from his operation. She
shared these views with the parents. Together, they tried to address

these concerns with the nursing staff, but were unhappy at the level of response. The boy stayed in the hospital for two days longer than expected. The primary doctor hinted at "one or two complications," but was not specific. The friend with nursing experience said that his postsurgical nursing care was to blame. The boy's discharge ended the usage step.

The boy's condition after discharge was excellent and remained so. The parents, however, remembered their anxieties over his postsurgical care and the apparent lack of response when they had voiced them. They reached the conclusion that the hospital was inadequate and also blamed the primary physician for agreeing to admit their son there for surgery. The father also blamed his HMO. That hospital was one of its participants, but other hospitals that might in retrospect have been preferable were not. The father resolved to change his health coverage when the opportunity next arose. He also felt slightly resentful toward his employer for offering this HMO, and told several colleagues at work about his feelings.

References

American Board of Family Practice. 1987. *Rights and responsibilities, Part 2: The changing health consumer and patient/doctor partnership.* Lexington, KY: American Board of Family Practice.

Brown, S. 1970. Comparing attitudes and opinions of Arizona physicians and consumers. *Arizona Medicine* 17(3): 174-179.

Engel, J.F., and R. Blackwell. 1982. *Consumer behavior.* 4th ed. Chicago: Dryden Press.

Fisk, T. 1986. *Positioning: projecting your services as different.* Paper presented to the Health Services Marketing Symposium, October 8-9, Houston, TX.

Halpern, K., T. Fisk, and C. Brown. 1983. *Cooper data: The doctors people want.* Camden, NJ: Cooper Hospital/University Medical Center.

Medical Economics. 1985 (June):

Nicosia, F. 1966. *Consumer decision processes.* New York: Prentice Hall.

Parasuraman, A., V. Zeithmal, and L. Berry. 1986. *A conceptual model of service quality and its implications for further research.* Report # 84-108. Cambridge, MA: Marketing Science Institute.

Solomon, M.R. 1986. The missing link: Surrogate consumers in the marketing chain. *Journal of Marketing* 50(4): 208-218.

TARP (Technical Assistance Research Programs Institute). 1986. *Consumer complaint handling in America: An update study.* Consumer Affairs Council of the U.S. Office of Consumer Affairs. Washington, DC: U.S. Department of Health and Human Services.

Zeithmal, V.A., A. Parasuraman, and L. Berry. 1985. Problems and strategies in services marketing. *Journal of Marketing* 49(4): 41-50.

Review Questions

1. "Patients are satisfied when health services meet their expectations." Comment.

2. "We need to know what is really important to patients as well as how they rate our performance." Why?

3. Why do some satisfied patients still not become loyal patients?

4. "Dissatisfied patients talk about their experiences more than satisfied patients." What are the implications for nurses?

Chapter 6

Families and Doctors as Nurses' Customers

Families and Friends as Customers of Nursing

The previous chapters' discussion of the service selection process frequently referred to the role of patients' families and friends as either influencers or surrogates. It was also noted that at times influencers and surrogates may share with the patient in one or more aspect of the role of customer: in initiating demand for a service, deciding which service to select, and paying for it.

When coming into direct contact with nurses or other health professionals, families and friends may act in one of these roles. This fact implies that their impact upon a patient's decisions and upon his or her postusage assessment of services can be significant. They cannot, therefore, be treated as having a lesser relationship with the service without risking that they will negatively influence the patient's eventual assessment of the service. Prior to service, families and friends may be an important part of the "network" that assists the patient in his or her service selection. And during and after the service, they may be part of the network that shapes how the patient will assess the service, influencing whether he or she will develop brand loyalty toward it and recommend it to others.

Family members and friends may also, however, be *customers* in their own right. They are not currently customers for clinical care, but they may have distinct personal needs in their role as close associates of the patient. Depending on the circumstances, these necessities may include need for information (to enable them to better discharge the role they perceive with the patient and to prepare for any special postcare needs the patient may have), *assurance* (to cope with their own anxieties about the patient's health), *access* (to

119

enable them to discharge what they see as their obligations to help and comfort the patient), and *pastoral support* (to adjust to the likely or actual death or serious disability of the patient). Even though these benefits lie outside the narrow technical definition of clinical care, some family members and friends may well expect these services to be available from a caring institution.

Influencers and surrogates may, therefore, have their own service expectations and, like patients themselves, assess whether they are fulfilled by the health professionals they encounter. As with patients, however, any two family members or friends will often place different emphases upon the same two benefits. The best approach to providing some services, therefore, may be simply offers of assistance. For example, "Can I answer any questions that you have about Jane's illness?" might be preferable to "I want to tell you about Jane's problem." "Would you like to stay after visiting hours are over?" may be better than "I'm sure you'd like to stay after visiting hours." "Would you like me to see if the chaplain can come up?" might be preferable to "I'm sure you'd like to see the chaplain."

The approach of asking questions to identify the benefits that matter to a particular person, rather than assuming that you know resembles a fundamental aspect of selling mentioned earlier in this book—how good salespersons start person-to-person sales encounters. They do not know what the customer wants, so they try to find out. Only after they know do they present their products or services as solutions. The same technique can help to customize the help given to family members and friends.

Family members and friends are also *potential customers* themselves. Because they do not recognize a current need for health care themselves, they may not be engaged in an active information search on their own behalf. Their focus may well be on what the nurse is doing to assist the patient, and on what they can do to help the patient. As a result, they may be quite tolerant of personal inconvenience. Most family members or friends of a patient know and accept that they are not the center of attention for the nurse or other health professional. Nevertheless, their health care experiences in assisting the patient may well be recalled at a later date when they do have a personal health need. In one study of inpatients at Thomas Jefferson University Hospital in Philadelphia, 1 in every 10 patients reported that they had been to the hospital before to visit a family member or friend. If family and friends are impressed by their experiences, they may become future customers of the service themselves. If they are not impressed by their experiences, the reverse is likely to apply.

Even if a family member or friend is unlikely to need the health service that he or she witnessed personally, he or she may become an active proponent of it to others. In one focus group study conducted by one of the authors, for instance, a woman admitted that she always recommended one particular hospital to friends for childbirth, even though she had had two children elsewhere and was returning to the same hospital shortly for her third. She explained that she was committed to her obstetrician and also now felt familiar with her hospital. However, she had visited two friends who had had babies at the other hospital and thought it much better, so she always recommended it when asked for her opinion.

Family members and friends visiting patients may be customers for nursing and other health professionals in four different ways:

1. *Family members or friends may be major influencers of the patient's choices and subsequent assessment; they may have acted as surrogates in selecting the service; or they may share some part of the customer role with the patient. In this capacity, they perceive themselves as having a stake in the patient's care.*

2. *Family members and friends may be customers in their own right, with perceived needs that the patient does not share, and which they expect nurses to help provide, ranging from needs for information to support in bereavement.*

3. *Family members and friends are potential future customers of the health service. Their experience now, even though focused upon the care and help given to the patient, will influence whether they may choose to use the services personally.*

4. *Family members and friends may positively, or negatively, recommend a health service, even if they have no likely personal need of it, because of what they observe when visiting or accompanying the patient.*

As emphasized here, nurses can influence family members and friends in each of these roles by the way in which they treat them.

Doctors as Customers of Nursing

Doctors too, as customers of nursing services, hospitals, health agencies, or other physicians to whom they refer, follow the broad model of customer behavior as discussed in detail in the foregoing sections.

Need Recognition Phase

Like the patient as a customer, doctors also *recognize needs,* undertake an *information search* into methods of achieving those needs, reach a *decision,* experience *usage* of services, and, finally, conduct a *postusage assessment* of those services. However, there are important differences between doctors as customers and patients as customers.

Previously in this book, it was stated that in the need recognition phase of the service selection process, patients formulate personal benefit bundles, or groups of needs that they seek to fulfill through a health service. For instance, in the case of the patient with a bowel obstruction mentioned in Chapter 5, the patient recognized a need for surgery but also placed high personal priority on both minimal permanent scarring from the procedure and minimal postoperative pain. The patient's needs were not necessarily limited to these three benefits, but they were uppermost in her thinking. Similarly, the discussion earlier in this volume of why people join health maintenance organizations (HMOs) showed that price and quality both matter, but that different patients attach varying importance to these two features.

What benefits do doctors typically assign priority to when engaging in service selection decisions? Several studies of why doctors with multihospital affiliations choose particular hospitals for specific patients tend to show that the most important considerations are the quality of nursing at the hospital, the availability of specialists and equipment that may be needed, the hospital's public reputation, and the convenience of that hospital for the physician personally (IEC Marketing Group 1981).

Another study of the characteristics sought in the specialists to whom physicians refer their patients listed the top six factors as satisfaction of previous patients with the consulting physician, ease and promptness of communication with the consulting physician, personal knowledge of the consulting physician, the range of services available, the ease of getting patients appointments, and the helpfulness of the consulting physician's staff (SRI Gallup 1987).

Taken together, these findings suggest that referral and hospital selection decisions by doctors are relatively complex. That is not surprising. Most customers needs recognition processes are complex, as was demonstrated in the discussion earlier in this book of patients as customers.

Overall, four main types of needs seem to enter into most physician service selections (Fisk and Brown 1987):

1. Professional needs (Where will a doctor get the best care for his or her patients?)

2. Practice needs (Where will a doctor get the most help with his or her own practice's goals — such as ease of referral for his or her staff, return of the patient to his or her continuing care, quick test results, etc.?)

3. Patient needs (for an early appointment, personal and family satisfaction, etc.)

4. Personal needs (for convenience, familiarity with a hospital, etc.)

Just as patients have multiple roles in seeking health services (as a patient, a person with family responsibilities, a person with career obligations, a human being with psychological as well as physiological concerns), so do doctors as customers of health services to which they bring or refer patients. A doctor, considering the needs entailed in a patient referral, or patient admission, has four roles: he is a health professional with clinical responsibilities, a practice manager with concerns for the efficient use of his or her time and staff, a marketing manager with concern for satisfying his or her patient and any family members closely involved, and a customer himself with an interest in personally convenient and supportive service.

For nurses and other health professionals who deal with doctors as their customers, it is important to recognize these four types of needs that may combine in the benefit bundle the physician seeks. It is easy to treat doctors as though they were one-dimensional customers with professional needs only, rather than recognizing these other roles. A surgeon, for instance, whose operating room schedule gets delayed by an overrun on a prior case may not suffer any consequences in terms of his professional needs. The delay may well, however, affect his practice by making him late for subsequent office hours; it may generate patient and family dissatisfaction; and it may cause personal inconvenience by requiring him to cancel the birthday lunch he had promised his wife. The OR delay thus frustrates his practice, his patient, and his personal needs.

Doctors, like patients, differ in the weight they attribute to different parts of their benefit bundles. The relative importance of these four types of need may vary with physician personality, physician familiarity with the service, changing personal circumstances, and specific features of a referral. Regarding personality, some physicians, for instance, attach more importance to personal convenience than others. They may also differ in their attitudes about the variability of professional quality. Two studies (Mason 1985; SRI Gallup 1987), for instance, seem to show sizable minorities of physicians who do not select quality issues, such as "leading specialists" or "good nursing," as among the major needs in their referral decisions. Instead, these doctors seem to refer almost exclusively to the medical staffs of one or at most two hospitals with which they are principally affiliated. One major factor behind their selection is, "I tend to refer to physicians who refer, in turn, to me." These findings do not necessarily imply that these doctors totally ignore quality concerns. Rather, they may not see professional quality as sufficiently variable to justify referral beyond the institutions with which they are most involved. Even so, this attitude makes them different from other doctors who seem to refer to specialists at a number of institutions whom they regard as professionally outstanding.

Regarding familiarity, physicians' needs are likely to be more extensive if referring to a resource or admitting to a facility with which they are less familiar. Again, it is a common consumer trait to view the less familiar as more risky, and, therefore, to formulate more precise and extensive needs, than in contemplating a more familiar resource. Hospitals that have expanded the number of their operating rooms have often found an initial hurdle to overcome in persuading surgeons to try an unfamiliar working environment, even though the staffing, design, and procedures duplicate existing suites. A physician making a first-time referral, such as to a home care agency, is likely to formulate a wider set of needs than one already familiar with such referrals. The new referrer will need to become more informed about the practice, patient, and personal implications than one who has already developed a familiarity with the service.

Changing personal circumstances can also alter the relative importance of different needs for a physician. Consider, for example, the obstetrician who not only maintains a private practice, but, as a member of the voluntary faculty of a medical school, is required to contribute several hours a week to supervising residents in the obstetrics clinic. He enjoys this regular commitment, as it provides him an opportunity to help in the development of the house staff and brings him into contact with a wider variety of interesting cases. He is regarded as a willing workhorse, who never hurries the patients or residents, often stays late and picks up extra patients if someone else is absent or sick. In one afternoon session, however, he is booked with an unusually heavy load of patients because two of the residents are out sick. Rather than being his usual self, he hurries through the cases and is abrupt with everyone. Finally, a senior nurse summons the courage to ask him what is bothering him. He replies that he had promised to take his two sons camping that night and realized early into the session that he will be 2 or so hours later than he had expected. The nurse asks him why he had not explained the situation. He replies that he always put his professional commitments first. She replies that he obviously was not doing so this afternoon — his professional and personal needs were in conflict. Now that she knows his problem, she will talk to the other doctors present to rearrange things so he can leave.

The relative importance that a doctor attaches to professional, practice, patient, and personal needs also varies with the specific referral situation. For instance, the following are six types of referral that a physician may make to a radiology service (Fisk and Brown 1987):

1. Referral within a hospital of an inpatient by his or her attending doctor for a diagnostic study.

2. Referral of an inpatient by his or her attending physician to an offsite radiology service (at another hospital or free-standing center) for a diagnostic test not available at the hospital itself.

3. Transfer of an inpatient by his or her attending physician from one hospital to another for inpatient radiation oncology not available at the first hospital.

4. Referral of an outpatient from a doctor's office for a diagnostic test, with the expectation that any treatment shown as necessary can be provided by the referring doctor at his or her office.

5. Referral of an outpatient from a doctor's office for a test, with the expectation that the patient may then need to be admitted to a hospital by the referring doctor.

6. Referral of an outpatient from a doctor's office for a test, with the expectation that the patient may have to be referred to another doctor for treatment on either an inpatient or an outpatient basis.

Which type of physician need is likely to be uppermost in the physician's mind in each of these situations?

1. A doctor referring an inpatient within a hospital for a radiology study is mainly motivated by a professional need. The doctor is not even making an active choice of supplier. The choice that he made was to admit the patient to that hospital. Even though professional needs predominate, the doctor may still have practice (quick results reporting), patient (a good experience while in radiology), and personal (again, quick results reporting) needs at stake. If such needs are not well met, the doctor may admit fewer patients to the hospital in the future.

2. A doctor referring an inpatient off-site for a test not available at the hospital is probably motivated exclusively by a professional need. It would serve the doctor's practice, patient and personal needs better if a comparable test were available at the hospital.

3. In transferring an inpatient to another hospital for advanced inpatient care, a doctor may well have several choices of suitable hospitals available to him. All four types of need probably play some role. The most important may well be practice needs. Will the patient be returned to the physician's care?

4. In referring an outpatient for a test, with the expectation that any subsequent treatment can be provided at his or her office, a doctor almost certainly has several radiology services to choose from that are nearly equal so far as his professional and personal needs are concerned. His thoughts, therefore, are more likely to be dominated by practice needs (e.g., ease of scheduling, speed of results reporting) and by patient needs (location, convenience, satisfaction, possibly price).

5. In referring a patient from the doctor's office for a test, in the expectation that the patient may then need hospital admission, all four needs play some role. However, for most routine tests, patient needs may well dominate. The doctor will be concerned about the first impressions that a patient may form of the hospital to which he or she then may have to admit the patient. Many hospitals fail to realize their full potential for outpatient tests because otherwise loyal doctors are concerned that the patient will receive a poor first impression from the hospital's diagnostic services. Doctors often send patients to free-standing diagnostic centers to keep them from experiencing a part of a hospital that may be less service oriented.

6. In referring office patients for diagnostic tests, in the expectation that the patient may then need referral to a specialist, a doctor probably focuses on professional, practice, and patient needs. The doctor's personal needs in this situation are limited. His professional inclination will be to refer to the location where the specialist is also located. This preference may receive more scrutiny, however, if practice needs (e.g., for an early appointment and quick reporting) or patient needs (e.g., for friendly staff, a reasonable waiting period) may be better served elsewhere.

The needs of doctors in referring or admitting patients are complex. Oversimplifying them leads to ineffective marketing efforts. Nurses or other health professionals cannot meet the needs of doctors by concentrating upon professional quality issues alone, or practice support alone, or patient satisfaction alone, or doctors' personal needs alone. Doctors seek fulfillment of a complex benefit bundle from the health professionals with whom they work.

Information Search Phase

The information search that a doctor undertakes will vary in intensity and duration, depending upon the doctor's familiarity with the type of needs that a patient presents. Some marketing scientists distinguish three types of information search behavior (Hawkins, Best, and Coney, 1983). In situations with which a customer has become familiar, the information search is often so cursory as to amount to an automatic response. In less familiar situations, a customer may have a preference from prior experience, but may nevertheless compare it with a few other known options, in a search that consists of limited problem solving. In situations not experienced before, or only experienced rarely, a customer may engage in a much more thorough consideration of alternatives, based upon extensive problem solving.

Some doctors encountered in the authors' work clearly engage in all three types of information search behavior. An example would be a pediatrician in private practice, with admitting privileges at three community hospitals, who admits patients with common problems routinely to one of those hospitals; he refers patients with less frequently encountered problems to specialists at one of the two other hospitals; and for the infrequent but most serious conditions, such as musculoskeletal tumors or neurological impairment, he refers patients away to one of several university hospitals based upon careful consideration of the complexities of each case.

It should also be noted that, as all doctors encounter more patients with firm views and preferences about different hospitals, and as satisfying patient expectations grows in importance to their own practices, physicians may be forced into more extensive problem-solving approaches to hospital and specialist selection. One physician known to the authors has reported that only 60% of his patients will now accept referral or admission to the hospital with which he is affiliated. He has been forced to develop a list of acceptable alternatives to offer to the other 40%.

One survey of doctors (Jensen and Larson 1987) reported that 50% of responding practices have designed and implemented new strategies to improve patient satisfaction in the past 12 months. This level of innovation in patient relations strategies rises to 70% among group, as opposed to solo, practices. This trend is almost certainly influencing the approach that many doctors are taking to searching for acceptable referral options for their patients.

Decision Phase

As noted earlier in this book, doctors' decisions about referrals and admissions are also increasingly involving more consultation with patients regarding the choices available to them. A growing minority of patients see the choice as exclusively theirs. Between 20% and 25% do not even mention a doctor as a source of influence in hospital selection. The American Board of Family Practice now speaks of a "patient/doctor partnership" in such decisions (American Board of Family Practice 1987).

Despite this growth of patient involvement in service selection, however, it would be unwise to discount the role of physicians, who still represent the major source of influence on patient choices. The American Board of Family Practice (1987) estimates that 45% of patients are "decision sharers," while 55% remain "decision delegators." Dividing patients into two such rigid categories may, however, be slightly misleading. In reality, there seem to be more than two segments, with subtle but significant differences in the degrees to which patients defer to doctors, are guided by them, debate with them, overrule them, or, lastly, ignore their advice. Even so, the doctor remains, with the patient, the major determinant in referrals and admissions.

Usage Phase

In their usage of health services, doctors, like patients, form impressions and arrive at assessments based on how well their set of expectations is fulfilled by nurses, other health professionals, and health enterprises. Just as it is crucial to identify with patients what service attributes are most important to them, so it is with doctors.

Postusage Assessment

In their postusage assessment of health services, doctors again follow the same general model described earlier in this book for patients. Often, however, a doctor is a much more frequent user of a service than any individual patient, and is therefore more familiar with it. However, the doctor is less dramatically affected by the outcome of a patient's care than the patient and family. For the doctor, it is not a personal matter of life and death, relief from pain, improved self-esteem, or whatever other major need initiated the patient's search for a solution.

Frequent usage, low perceived risk, and high familiarity with products or services are among those circumstances mentioned in Chapter 5 as tending to generate brand loyalty. The typical doctor is thus, according to marketing science, likely to be more loyal to health services that he uses regularly. The doctor may voice criticisms more directly, because of ongoing access to the nurse, or others involved, but he or she usually does so from a foundation of brand loyalty. The exceptions are those physicians who try a service for the first time, or are infrequent users of it. They cannot be expected to have yet developed any inherent brand loyalty.

The best methods for obtaining information on what matters to doctors differ, however, from those discussed earlier for researching patient reactions during or after service. The ideal methods vary for two major reasons:

1. Doctors are *repetitive customers* for health services. Whereas some patients are also repetitive users, they are the exception, and often there is a long gap between episodes of service. As repetitive customers, doctors' opinions are important for what they reveal about that doctor individually, not for what they reveal about how other similar, but different customers might react to the service.

2. The patient population of even a medium-size hospital or health agency can consist of many thousands of customers each year. The number of doctors who are important and repetitive customers is probably quite small. One basic law of statistical inference — of sampling opinions and drawing conclusions from the sample — is that drawing inferences about a large population calls for a different approach than drawing inferences about a small population. When sampling a few hundred patients drawn from a population of many thousands, conclusions can be drawn that are *generally* true for

patients as a whole. With advanced computer-aided analysis, a hospital or agency can even differentiate the opinions of varying *segments*. There is a margin of error to the sampling, but so long as this margin is taken into account, the service can cope with it. This is because the service is not trying to draw conclusions that apply to *every* patient; it is only looking for guidance on what to do to increase the percentage of satisfied patients. When sampling a small population, on the other hand, responses are needed from a much larger percentage in order to be representative of the whole, because each respondent may be very important to the hospital or agency. It may be much more damaging to a hospital's service for 2% of doctors to be dissatisfied with it than 2% of patients. Even though 2% of a hospital's patients are many more people than 2% of its doctors, the patients can probably do it much less harm.

Because the doctors who are crucial to many health services are repetitive customers and relatively small in number, the best way to gather their input may not be by survey. Such surveys may occasionally have a use, but more frequently what you want to know is what Dr. A. or Dr. B. expect personally, not what "87% of our most active doctors" expect.

The way then, to learn the individual needs, expectations, and reactions of a small number of influential customers is not by market research methods such as surveys, but by salespersonship techniques, such as those discussed earlier. Those techniques involve face-to-face discussion of doctors' needs and reactions to the service. In marketing terms, the patient is an individual customer whose needs at the time of service should be met by consumer satisfaction. The doctor is a "repetitive account" who calls for ongoing customer service. That customer service is best performed directly and person-to-person.

What can nurses and other health professionals do, therefore, to serve doctors most effectively as customers of their services? Following are several suggestions and points to keep in mind.

> *1. Although doctors' "needs" in relation to health services may be more articulated than those of patients, because doctors' use of services is often repetitive, the*

concept of active steps to generate demand still applies. Nurses, other health professionals, and health enterprises can help to share doctors' needs by keeping them informed about services, changes, and developments. It is unwise to assume that a doctor is always fully informed about a service. Even if the doctor is in close contact with the service, it is usually on a case-by-case basis, from which he or she may not discern a broad knowledge of the service.

2. *Remember that doctors are professional clinicians, practice managers, patient satisfiers, and people themselves. They have "needs" of a health service in each of these roles, not just as clinicians.*

3. *These needs change in relative importance in different circumstances. Different types of referral, for instance, bring different needs to the fore.*

4. *Surveys are useful to assess the needs of a large population of people, how they seek information about satisfying those needs, and their knowledge and opinions of your services. In some circumstances, surveys are useful among doctors, such as when a health center has a large and diverse referral base.*

5. *For relatively small numbers of customers, such as the most active doctors, surveys can be misleading. It is better to maintain a "sales dialogue" with these physicians, exploring their individual needs and reactions to your services.*

6. *Informal conversations with doctors can contribute to the effectiveness of a service. So can formally arranged meetings, even scheduled visits to doctors' offices. Remember, however, to maintain the formalized structure of a sales call. Person-to-person dialogue requires a systematic approach in order to obtain valuable information.*

References

American Board of Family Practice. 1987. *Rights and responsibilities, Part 2: The changing health consumer and patient/doctor partnership.* Lexington, KY: American Board of Family Practice.

Fisk, T., and C. Brown. 1987. *Marketing the Radiology Practice,* pp. 10-12. Reston, VA: American College of Radiology.

Hawkins, D., R. Best, and K. Coney. 1983. *Consumer behavior: implications for marketing strategy.* Plano, TX.: Business Publications.

IEC Marketing Group. 1981. *Snowmass Advisory,* Spring.

Jensen, J., and S. Larson. 1987. *Survey of physicians.* Lincoln, NE: National Research Corporation.

Mason, D. 1985. Referral relationships between New Jersey physicians and university hospitals. Master's thesis, Wharton School of Business Administration, University of Pennsylvania, Philadelphia.

SRI Gallup. 1987. Admitting/referral behaviors. *Hospital Marketing Monitor* (Spring):

Review Questions

1. What are the four distinct ways in which members of patient's families may be customers for nursing?

2. "Family members watch what nurses do for patients even more than patients do themselves." Discuss.

3. "It is dangerous to oversimplify about how and why doctors make referrals." Comment.

4. "The concept of the service selection process applies to doctors, too." How?

Part III

Strategic Marketing Issues

Chapter 7

Identifying Market Opportunities

Every field of human enterprise is full of opportunity for new initiatives, programs, products, and services. Yet about 50% of all new ideas brought to the marketplace fail. How can these two facts be reconciled?

The answer is that many new products and services are poorly conceived, poorly considered, inadequately studied, insufficiently developed, not well tested, and not properly launched. It only takes one serious mistake in any of these six critical steps (see Figure 7-1) to create a "lemon."

Also, that 50% average failure rate for new products or services is itself misleading. The failure rate for products is closer to 40% (Nielsen, Marketing Services 1980). The failure rate among services, by comparison, is almost certainly greater than 50%. The difference is not that service development is inherently more difficult, but that the service sector is dominated by quite small businesses often serving local markets, whereas the goods sector contains many giant enterprises. The very large enterprise can afford more sophisticated approaches to market opportunity assessment. They do not always take advantage of this ability, but many do. They conceive, consider, study, develop, test, and launch new products more carefully. These larger enterprises can also subsidize new products for longer periods to give them a chance to succeed. Companies like Xerox and IBM have advanced systems staff developing product ideas that will not be launched for 7 to 10 years, and even then only if they pass various rigorous steps of internal review. One major company lost money for 11 years on a major new product before it became a success (Quinn 1979). In contrast, many service enterprises are small in scale and cannot subsidize a new idea for a long time with profits

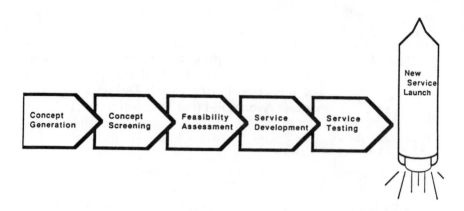

Figure 7-1 The service innovation process.

earned from old ideas. Indeed, many service businesses only have one idea — the one that they are presently offering.

The development of a product also creates physical assets, such as a factory and stocks of finished products, while the development of a service idea only creates goodwill among clients. A lender will often tolerate losses in product development for a longer period, safe in the knowledge that, if the business fails, some money will be recoverable from sale of the assets. In contrast, many small service companies go out of business quickly because the bank withdraws its support. What is the value of a failing service?

Consider the case of a home care agency that was put up for sale. Founded by two nurses, this small agency quickly developed a good reputation with two major referral sources. For three years, it offered a good service to a small number of clients. It actually made a small profit on its clinical activities, but it needed an office, a phone service, and several staffpersons just like a home care agency handling twice its volume. These overheads turned its profits into a loss. After three years, it owed the bank about $150,000, and the bank said enough. It looked for a buyer who would repay the bank loan and help the nurses cut the overhead to a more affordable level. It was lucky and did find one, but the buyer knew that he was gambling on the two major referral sources remaining loyal, or on the agency finding some other, equally large referrer. The only real value in the agency was the dedication of the two nurses who founded it and the goodwill of the two referral sources.

The other advantage that large producers have is that they can afford some failures. Even with their methodical assessment procedures, they can make mistakes. Ford's Edsel, DuPont's artificial leather, RCA's videodisk, Avon's ill-fated acquisition of Tiffany's and Citibank's loans to Brazil are just a few examples of expensive mistakes by major corporations. They can, however, afford them. Indeed, they expect to make some mistakes if they are pursuing a broad and aggressive approach to product innovation (Peters and Waterman 1983).

There are, of course, some quite large health services organizations that can at least partly imitate these major businesses. They can afford some sophisticated planning, a long time horizon for some investments to pay off, and some mistakes. If they are not-for-profit entities, as many hospitals are, they may even be able to afford to subsidize some unprofitable activities for a very long time, as part of their social mission, as long as those that are profitable exceed those that are not by enough to keep the organization viable.

The small, one-idea enterprise has a much more difficult task. The odds are against its success. How much so can be seen in the *64-32-12-6-2-1 rule*. Studies (Cadbury 1975; Booz Allen and Hamilton 1982) of companies with a long history of success at innovation suggest that:

1. It takes 64 product concepts ("bright ideas") to find:

2. 32 product concepts that pass an initial screening to find:

3. 12 product concepts that survive project analysis to find:

4. 6 product concepts that can be made to work in product development to find

5. 2 products that are successful in test marketing to find:

6. 1 product that is successful.

Two clear conclusions emerge from these data. First, a one-idea enterprise that does not think through the viability of its idea carefully is almost certain to fail. Successful products or services are rarely born of intuition. Second, beating the odds calls for:

1. A lot of bright ideas

2. An ability to discard half of those ideas rapidly as not even worth the effort of detailed study

3. An intellectually honest method of business analysis that fails as many candidate ideas as it passes

4. A rigorous approach to product or service development that avoids taking incomplete ideas to market

5. Some method of testing new products or services on a small scale before committing to them on a large scale

6. Expertise at launching new products and services in the market

7. A tolerance of failure and an ability to survive it.

These are easy attributes to summarize but much more difficult to achieve. The following sections review in detail the first of these steps in the service innovation process. The next two chapters discuss the remaining steps.

Generating Service Innovation Ideas

Where do innovative organizations obtain their ideas? The obvious answer is that they get them from innovative people, but that is not the whole truth. As one analyst of product planning noted, "Most companies are formed on the basis of one good idea. But the second and third ideas, which are essential if the company is to be truly successful . . . are engendered by thorough analysis of markets and technologies" (Zarecor 1975).

Those innovations that do arise from individuals also come from a much more diverse group than is often assumed. The dominant image of the innovator is that of one person so consumed by an idea that he forms his own company to pursue it and leads it on to growth and fame. There are, indeed, many examples of that process. Ford, Polaroid, Apple Computer, Walt Disney, and Hospital Corporation of America are just a few. However, there are just as many examples of people who came to leadership roles in companies that already existed and made them grow by applying new ideas to what the company was already doing. IBM, General Motors, Citibank, and Baxter Travenol are some cases in point.

The majority of innovative ideas do not in any case come from one dominant corporate leader. Salespersons, dealers, assembly-line workers, outside inventors, competitors, and — most overlooked of all — customers are often the original source of innovative concepts (Von Hippel 1978). The challenge in most organizations, large and small, is not to generate bright ideas. Where there are people there are ideas. The challenge is to create a climate that encourages those ideas to surface (Von Oech 1983; Roberts 1987).

The more ideas that surface, however, the more ideas there are that will not be pursued. Some of the 63 out of every 64 ideas that are rejected along the way are just bad ideas, yet many good ideas are not pursued for a whole range of reasons of which their originator could not have been aware. A creative climate, therefore, does more than just encourage ideas to surface. It also entails rejecting many bright ideas without turning their originators off from thinking up and suggesting more.

Formal "suggestions schemes" that only reward people whose ideas are adopted tend to fall into disrepute because they choke off further suggestions from many people whose ideas are rejected. Schemes that provide at least a token aware for any suggestion, except the obviously flippant, are a step forward. A further improvement would be to reward all suggestions, provide a greater reward for those that are adopted, but provide an explanation to those whose ideas are not pursued to encourage them to think of other ideas that overcome the objections.

Can nurses and other health professionals genuinely innovate? Do present circumstances permit and encourage them to do so?

The health care industry is clearly, in the late 20th century, among the most innovative fields of all human enterprise. Perhaps the only other field in which innovation is occurring at an equivalent pace is that of electronic communications, data storage, retrieval, and analysis. Most people associate the current prolonged period of medical innovation with M.D.s and Ph.Ds in the biological sciences, working at universities and in the research laboratories of pharmaceutical companies and medical equipment enterprises. Just as many innovations, however, are occurring in clinical nursing, in organizational methods in health care, and in the structure of the health care delivery system. "Innovation thus refers to the process of bringing any new, problem-solving or opportunity-addressing idea into use" (Kanter 1984).

There has been an encouraging growth in nursing research, as well as in the number of specialized publications in which nurses, pharmacists, medical technologists, physical therapists, and other health professionals, publish their own innovative ideas. Just as important, however, as the academic model of innovation of research, trials, peer review, and publication is the organizational one, which involves advocating, justifying and being allowed to try out new methods of organizing care and responding to new opportunities.

As an example, in late 1987 nurses in several hospitals were actively involved in trials in the advanced application of bar coding. This technology has been around for some years, most visibly in the form of check-out scanners in supermarkets. The same concept applied to unit doses, checked with a wand against a bar-coded patient bracelet and automatically recorded in a minicomputer, promises to both reduce nursing paperwork and cut down the number of medication errors. This development may not receive much publicity for some time in the professional literature, but by 1990 or soon after, the practice will be widespread in hospitals. People may not even remember where the first innovative work was done. The effort may well, however, have as broad and positive an impact on patient care as at least half of the research reported in the medical journals. What started it? Very simply, no more than four people in a hospital who thought it was an idea whose time had come.

To take another example, in the late 1970s, an emergency room physician in Rhode Island got into an argument with his hospital's CEO about his contract and staffing patterns in the emergency room. He had some fixed ideas about how emergency rooms should run. His ideas would take more money and require some radical changes to traditional ER staffing models, but, he was convinced, would also bring in much more volume and provide a better service. The doctor and the CEO could not agree, and so the physician resigned and announced that he would build his own ER across the street. Thus was born the first American free-standing urgicenter. By 1983, there were more than 2,000 imitations of this idea in operation across the nation (Witt 1983). Some have been failures, for reasons that will be discussed later, but many have been successes.

Many innovative concepts in health care start with one person with a bright idea. That person may be anywhere in the organization, or may be a customer. Mechanisms to encourage and reward staff suggestions and to solicit patient feedback are thus invaluable. Not every good idea, however, is in the right place or at the right time. Explaining to staff why their ideas are not adopted is therefore vital to maintaining a further flow of ideas.

As valuable as individuals inside and outside an enterprise are as sources of new service concepts, most such ideas come from a much more formalized *service development process.* Large enterprises often have special staffs dedicated to using standard approaches to sifting out possible innovations. Estee Lauder developed its Clinique brand, for instance, because a formal and continuous internal process geared to spotting new markets reported a rising number of women wanting cosmetics without the health risks possibly associated with more traditional formulas.

These formal approaches look for their service innovation concepts chiefly in five areas:

1. Technology
2. The economy
3. Public policy
4. Competition
5. Social trends.

Each of those areas will be reviewed shortly, but there is another important concept that precedes them.

Successful innovative enterprises have a well-developed sense of themselves — of the business they are in, what they know and can do well, what they don't know and may be unable to do, and the geography of their market.

One of the most famous of all marketing texts spelled out the danger of *marketing myopia* (Levitt 1960). In that essay, Theodore Levitt documented the failures of many enterprises that had defined their field of interest too narrowly. The horse-and-buggy industry was eclipsed by the rise of the automobile. It need not have been, if it had seen itself more broadly as being in the personal transportation business. Indeed, the early auto makers used exactly the same carriage construction techniques as were pioneered in the buggy business. (That is why, to this day, some upscale cars have names dating back to the heyday of the carriage industry, like "sedan" and "brougham.") The horse-and-buggy makers had mastered one of the two technologies needed to build an automobile. The early auto pioneers had the other — the internal combustion engine. They went out and learned how to build carriages. If, instead, the established and rich buggy companies had seen the writing on the wall, and acquired know-how in auto engines, the car industry today would be dominated by an entirely different set of names.

Levitt's article helped to change the way in which many organizations thought of themselves. It became the vogue throughout the 1960s and 1970s for companies to redefine their mission. Some took the concept to an extreme. They defined their mission as "managing things well," and developed into conglomerates with activities spread from chemicals to rental cars, from hotels to aerospace components. Levitt never intended his idea of marketing myopia to be pushed that far. He recognized that organizations have fields of competence, beyond which they may have no special expertise to offer. His one point was that it is short-sighted to define that field of competence too narrowly and to assume that changing circumstances will not impact it.

Clinically, the opposite of myopia is presbyopia — the farsightedness that comes with hardening of the lens of the eye. By the late 1970s, some authorities were beginning to see that *marketing presbyopia* was also dangerous. A myopic person sees clearly the path one or two steps ahead, but does not spot in time the oncoming truck. A presbyopic person can see where he is heading, but does not notice that he is already standing on the edge of a cliff. As various major corporations, from Penn Central to Chrysler, with excellent reputations for their long-range diversification plans, ran into unforeseen immediate and dire problems, the risks of marketing presbyopia became as apparent as those of marketing myopia. By the early 1980s, the successful companies seemed to be those that "stuck to their knitting" (Peters and Waterman 1983). They know how to change, but they do not stray far from their basic areas of expertise (Hrebiniak and Joyce 1986).

Many of these organizations try to codify that philosophy of change but within their scope of competence in what is often called a *mission statement*. Often very short — no more than one or two paragraphs — a mission statement says what business the organization is in. It heeds Levitt's warning by not defining it too narrowly. The "hospital business" may well, for instance, be too narrow a concept in an era when medical advances and other forces are reducing the need for inpatient care.

An example of the importance of mission definition is the tuberculosis sanitoria of the 19th century. Throughout the 1800s and into the 1940s, the best defined treatment for tuberculosis was to move to a location with a mild climate without air pollution. For instance, one of the best-known centers of medical care in the U.S. was Saranac Lake, New York, Even the Scottish novelist and poet Robert Louis Stevenson relocated across the Atlantic to take care of his tuberculosis at a center in this small Adirondacks town. There were scores of similar centers across the United States. Then, suddenly, between the late 1940s and the mid-1950s, advances in immunology eliminated an estimated 300,000 tuberculosis beds. In less than ten years, an industry that had thrived for nearly a century was wiped out. A few of these institutions managed to convert to new roles. Deborah Hospital, for instance, in the New Jersey town of Browns Mills, originally founded as such a "lung hospital," had well before 1950 also developed as a cardiac hospital and survived the collapse of its tuberculosis caseload. Many sanitoria, however, with a more myopic sense of mission, just closed their doors.

A good, brief mission statement, therefore, states the organization's sense of purpose, but not in terms that are too constricting. Just as importantly, however, a good mission statement should state what the organization will not do. It should define the boundaries of its field of competence. First, because all organizations and people do have limitations. Why should a hospital, for instance, believe itself competent to run commercial restaurants and gas stations, as at least one hospital has tried to do. Second, a too broadly defined mission can easily dilute attention from the organization's core area of expertise. Even if it feels that it cannot continue in the long run to depend on its traditional activities, because the need for them is warning, it will almost certainly need to keep them intact and well managed in the short run to give it time to broaden its scope of activities.

In the early 1950s, a company that was then the major maker and distributor of household cleansers in the northeastern United States noticed that several giant consumer product companies, such as Procter & Gamble and Lever Brothers, were developing their own cleanser products. These rivals were new to household cleansers but had tremendous competence at marketing and distributing consumer products from soaps and detergents to cereals. They had defined their own missions not in terms of a product but in terms of shipping and distributing products to supermarkets and stores around the United States.

The cleanser company made three important decisions. First, it reached a conclusion very difficult for any organization. It decided that it had no choice but to exit the cleanser business. Second, it estimated that it had 5 more years in that business before the sky fell in on it. Third, it immediately increased both production and marketing, even though it foresaw only a limited future in that field. This expansion earned the company more money over those 5 remaining years than it would have earned otherwise. At the end of that time, because of this expansion, it was able to sell its factory for a high price to one of the new rivals. Now with no cleanser business but a lot of cash, the firm implemented a strategy it had been developing in secret through those 5 years. It changed its mission and injected the cash into an entirely new field.

This case exemplifies a major danger of having too broad a mission statement. If an organization that has to change becomes to preoccupied with its new ventures, its traditional ventures, upon which it depends during that transition, may collapse even faster. The cleanser company saw that danger and responded with two missions, one for now and one for later, and gave the more immediate one priority. It avoided marketing presbyopia.

The other reason why a good mission statement puts limits on the organization's scope of endeavor is that it helps to focus the process of looking for new opportunities. As it scans the five areas of possible opportunity mentioned earlier, it is looking at them through a particular set of lenses. It rapidly sets aside opportunities that do not fit its mission and concentrates more on those that do. Even a quick look, for instance, at social trends would reveal that the number of working mothers and of single-parent households is increasing. One result is greater demand for low-priced family restaurants and ready-to-cook meals. Fewer households have someone with the time to prepare an evening meal from basic ingredients. That is a very useful piece of information if an organization's mission places it in the fast-food or prepackaged food business, but it can be rapidly passed over by one with a mission in casual clothing and footwear or in time-shared data processing services.

Hospitals that respond to changes in their environment by expanding in an unplanned manner into many new ventures may find themselves in the situation of the old woman in the nursery rhyme. If the old woman's mission was to have a lot of children, she should not have chosen to live in a shoe. If her mission was to live in the shoe, she should have practiced family planning.

One small community hospital was among the first to conclude that small hospitals could not easily survive alone in the future unless they were geographically isolated from serious competition. This hospital was not isolated, but was in the suburbs of a large city, with at least 20 competitors within as many miles. It decided to revise its mission and was one of the first hospitals anywhere to elect to become a "health system" rather than just a hospital. As a health system it would try to combine several hospitals and other allied types of health services.

For several years, the hospital pursued this mission very effectively. It acquired two other hospitals from a for-profit chain that had decided to concentrate its own activities in another part of the United States. It developed a home care agency and obtained licensure to operate an emergency medical system in its county. Then it began to deviate from that health system mission. Its successful administration began to see other business opportunities, not strictly allied to health care, to which it thought it could extend its managerial talents. Within another 2 years, the hospital had eight other subsidiaries, engaged in services from hiring out temporary secretaries, to catering, to word processing, to printing, to handling billing and collection for doctors.

It was, of course, as a hospital, already involved in all these activities for itself, so it seemed an easy matter to do the same things for businesses not related to health care. What it did not see, however, was that, as a hospital, it was only into these activities as an incidental part of providing health services. Once the hospital started selling them outside of health care, it had no special expertise to offer. Indeed, it had less expertise than companies that specialized in these activities. One important dimension in which it lacked expertise was customer relations. Its dietary department did not have to worry about whether the hospital would use its services again tomorrow. It had a monopoly within the hospital. So did the billing department, the print shop, and the other services.

Almost two years after these new ventures were started, the hospital trustees called for an audit of their financial performance.

Collectively, in 2 years they had yielded about $200,000 of profit on total sales of about $1.5 million. They had, however, required almost that sum in legal and accountants' fees to set up in the first place. They had also consumed about 50% of the time and attention of the top four or five administrators in the hospital through those 2 years. The hospitals and other health services that represented their core mission, in contrast, yielded a surplus of some $5.0 million over those 2 years on total revenues of some $125.0 million. The top administrators were thus, as the trustees saw, spending half their time on activities not related to health care and that amounted to just over 1% of the size of the health activities. They told the administration to close the companies down.

This hospital thus initially avoided marketing myopia by realizing that the demand for hospital inpatient programs is declining and by moving into a more comprehensive array of health services. As its sense of vision expanded, however, it fell victim to marketing presbyopia, and strayed well beyond its field of competence.

A brief mission statement helps an enterprise to look at its environment with a clear perspective. It makes it easier to spot relevant opportunities from environmental analysis, because it keeps the enterprise from wasting time on irrelevancies. A good mission statement should be broad enough to allow the organization to change if the environment changes, but narrow enough to keep it within its fields of competence.

Opportunities and Threats in the Technological Environment

The Changing Health Care Environment

As already noted, health care has been changing more rapidly and dramatically over the past two or three decades than in all prior human history. Between 1945 and the early 1970s, inpatient use of hospitals in the United States expanded at a rate of between 3% and 6% annually. No other industry in the history of the American economy has seen such high growth sustained for a period in excess of 25 years. The main reason for this growth was technology. There were many more good reasons for people to be in hospital beds in 1975 than there were in 1945. Many diseases previously regarded as incurable or chronic were now treatable in an acute care setting. For example, it was not possible prior to 1953 to operate on an open heart to bypass coronary blockages; it was not possible before the mid-1950s to maintain very premature babies with immature lung function on a monitored respirator in an intensive care nursery; it was not possible before the 1970s to fit a patient with an artificial larynx, or an artificial tendon, or an ear implant for deafness.

Hospital inpatient occupancy rates have fallen sharply, however, since the mid-1970s. The reason is not that medical advances have stopped. They are, indeed, more profuse and more rapid than ever. The pace of technological advance in health care has speeded up, not slowed down.

The fall in hospital occupancy rates is the result of a common phenomenon in marketing. The same technological advances that propelled the growth of inpatient care between 1945 and the early 1970s also caused the decline of inpatient care after 1975 (Fisk 1986). Medical techniques became so efficient that they could achieve the same results with shorter lengths of stay. As one example, an acute myocardial infarction led, in the 1960s, to an average hospital stay in excess of 25 days. By 1980, the average heart attack patient stayed in hospital under 15 days. That means that for every 100 hospital beds dedicated to myocardial infarction patients in 1960, only 60 were needed by 1980 to treat the same number of people. As a result, the total daily census of U.S. hospitals started to fall.

Some medical techniques became so efficient that they could now be safely performed without a hospital admission at all. In 1960, about 15% of all surgery, for instance, was performed on an outpatient basis. By 1980, the figure was over 30%. Such trends have caused the total admission rate to fall. In 1960, well over 200 people in every thousand were hospitalized each year. In the mid-1980s, that figure has fallen below 150 per thousand. That decline in hospitalization rates eliminates the need for about 25% of all hospital beds.

The combined impact of these two two trends has been dramatic. In 1975, one 200-bed hospital had 7,300 admissions, with an average length of stay of 9 days. Consequently, its average occupancy was 90%. Because of fewer elective admissions on weekends and seasonal variations in the incidence of some diseases, a hospital that runs at 90% occupancy is virtually at full capacity.

Since 1975, admissions to this hospital have fallen by 18% — less than the average fall in hospital admissions since 1975, but still a loss of 1,300 annual admissions. The average length of stay also fell, from 9 days in 1975 to 6 days in 1985. Again, that level of reduction was not exceptional.

In 1985, therefore, the hospital had 6,000 admissions, with a 6-day average stay. As a result, its average occupancy for that year was 49%. Ten years after operating at virtually full occupancy, the hospital was now half-empty. Almost all of that reduction could be attributed to improved medical methods, requiring fewer admissions and shorter stays.

The technological impact that hospitals have been experiencing since the early 1970s is not over. There is every reason to believe that the pace of improvement in medical technologies will continue through at least the next 40 or 50 years, and may well speed up. Clinical advances are always preceded by breakthroughs in basic science. The advances in clinical care of the last few decades were made possible by advances in basic microbiology, in computers and solid-state electronics, and in other fields. In many cases, there was quite a long lag between the basic research discoveries and the consequent medical advances. For instance, magnetic resonance imaging is still in its infancy as a clinical tool, but the discoverer of magnetic resonance won the Nobel Prize for Physics for his basic research into the field in 1950. There will continue to be a rapid and accelerating rate of medical advances because all the basic science work to fuel it has already been done, and yet more is in process (Galton 1985).

With the possible exception of computers and telecommunications, no other sector of the U.S. economy is experiencing such prolonged and far-reaching technological change as health care. That, in part, is what makes the application of marketing science to health care such a special challenge. The marketing of these new technologies raises special issues. In Chapter 3, it was seen that an important task of marketing is to influence how customers identify needs and benefits. The benefits of established products, like detergent or automobiles, are well understood, making the marketer's task more one of explaining why one version is superior to another. The benefits of new technologies, by contrast, have to be explained. What, for instance, is the benefit of radioactive implants at the time of breast tumor surgery? What reason might there be to travel 100 miles to a center offering this new technology, when there may be 20 centers closer to home treating breast cancers by other means? What is the advantage of a home care agency with the expertise to administer intravenous chemotherapy outside of a hospital, and is it safe?

The next few decades will therefore continue to be characterized by rapid and wide-ranging innovations in clinical techniques. Even though they may continue to depress hospital admissions, they will in fact lead to a larger health care industry. The growth will be away from the hospital inpatient setting, but it will be substantial as yet other diseases still regarded as incurable or chronic become treatable, and as better methods are devised for presently treatable diseases.

These changes will have a profound impact on the health care delivery system. They may well create opportunities for new modes and settings of health care. They will certainly create new and different opportunities for nurses and other health professionals.

Technology, Needs, and Opportunities

Those organizations that seek out new opportunities systematically are regularly scanning their own technological environment for new opportunities. Those might be:

1. Customer needs for which an emerging technology offers a better solution. For instance, cling foil grew out of research to find a better way to insulate railroad boxcars. It did not work for that purpose, and so the company asked itself if there was something else that it could do.

2. Technologies that are going to produce a need for new delivery systems. Bar coding, for instance, gave birth to a new type of supermarket cash register.

3. Technologies that are going to create a need for new and complementary products. The microwave oven, for instance, created a demand for frozen microwaveable meals.

4. Technologies that are going to require new support services. The personal computer has, for instance, created a demand for computer stores, adult video games, specialized software, books, training courses, and even a new

design of bedroom furniture to house terminals and peripherals.

5. Technologies that are going to require new skills. Cable television has created a need for electricians with special training in installing and repairing cable systems.

The following case describes a development in health care that had all five of these types of effect. By the mid-1960s, the Beatles' income was so great that they hired professional investment advisers to manage it for them. One of their investments gave them a large stake in a British electronics firm, EMI. Some time later, unimpressed with the company's dividends, the Beatles' money managers started pushing for a shake-up at EMI. As one concession, EMI brought in an American consultant in research and development.

Like all large electronics firms, EMI was investing heavily in research and development of new products. The consultant saw, however, that it had too many small and under-funded research programs under way. The company needed to review them, pick the most likely winners and fund them better, while dropping the losers. One candidate to be dropped was a project that a small team had been working on for about 10 years, but had yet to make work well enough to consider producing and selling it.

The consultant met with that research group and asked them what the invention was intended to do. They explained that it could, in theory, produce images of slices of the human body much more precise than conventional radiology and using lower doses of radiation. The consultant immediately saw the U.S. market potential, and asked them how much money it would take to perfect a prototype within 15 months. After a decade of underfunding, the research team saw its chance and gave him an estimate. Finally, he asked what they called this thing and was told, "computerized axial tomography," or CAT scanning.

The early work on CAT, or CT, scanning was not pursued with health care in mind at all. Its probable use was thought to be in manufacturing processes that required looking inside a substance. It was only later that the EMI group saw that this technology could provide a new solution to an old problem in health care, that of imaging soft tissue. The technology has fostered new delivery systems, right through to mobile CT units in trucks rotating around hospitals too small to afford or justify a dedicated scanner. It has generated complementary products, including additional computer peripherals to enhance the image and store and compare images. It has generated new support services, including preventive maintenance programs. It has created a need for new skills among physicians, radiological technicians, biomedical engineers, and others.

A look at the technological environment may, of course, show up threats to the existing activities of an enterprise, as well as opportunities. The trends that halved occupancy at the hospital discussed above are a case in point. Many hospitals have broadened their activities in recent years in response to such trends, by expanding outpatient surgery, developing home care agencies, and so on. The example of the tuberculosis showed how the impact of technological change can even render specialized health care institutions obsolete.

What is technology? Although the term is most associated with tangible, physical equipment, much technology consists more in know-how (Nelson, Peck and Kalachek 1967). Indeed, most industrialized nations, such as the United States, are shifting from a labor- or capital-intensive economy to one in which know-how is a primary commodity in itself (Porat 1976).

Technology can therefore be subdivided into know-how and equipment, or people-based and hardware-based technologies. Indeed, some enterprises have compiled formal know-how inventories, seeking to identify and catalog what it is that their people know that gives them a unique competitive advantage, and reviewing what it will take to convert that know-how into marketable products or services.

A certain university medical school has been for many decades among the most productive in basic medical research and in publication of the results. Its faculty, however, predominantly defines its mission as ending there — at the discovery and transmission of new knowledge. The task of converting that know-how into actual clinical protocols or into new equipment and pharmaceuticals has often been left to doctors elsewhere, or to commercial companies. There is nothing wrong with that mission, as long as there are sufficient funding sources to sustain it. If there are not, it must begin to consider one of three alternatives: It could start selling parts of that know-how instead of giving it away. It could become more directly involved in joint ventures with commercial companies in the translation of that know-how into saleable products. It could put more effort into converting that know-how into clinical protocols first in its own university hospital, to give it more of a competitive advantage. The additional patient care revenues generated could help to sustain further research. This university hospital, despite the major research innovations of its faculty, has been for several years experiencing declining admissions and financial deficits. It has a reputation among both referring doctors and the public of being a leader in research but not a particularly distinctive hospital. Any of those three options, however, calls for a redefinition of the university's mission, which to many of the faculty would be a perversion of its role and its ethics.

A contrasting example is that of a major national computer software vendor that developed a comprehensive internal employee wellness program. It also kept careful track of the reduced health care costs that resulted. During the course of compiling a know-how inventory, the company saw that it could combine its successful track record in corporate wellness with its know-how in documenting complex programs, to create a new product: selling its corporate wellness expertise to other companies. The firm also had know-how in on-site training for companies that bought its software products, and it had a large and successful sales force. What it sold was a substantial documented guide to the program, plus on-site training of its own wellness managers, plus computer software that generated fitness profiles and exercise prescriptions for individual employees.

Types of Technological Change

The contrast between these two organizations illustrates another key point about technology. There are three areas of technology (Capon and Glazer 1987).

1. Product technology (the know-how embodied in the product or service)

2. Process technology (the know-how required to deliver the product or service)

3. Management technology (the know-how to sell, finance, control delivery, and collect revenue from the product).

The university in the case above possessed only product technology. The software company possessed all three technologies. In fact, its product was not particularly distinctive. There are many comparable corporate wellness programs and some that are probably even better. Its management technology was not particularly distinctive, as many companies have good corporate sales forces. Its critical strength lay in its ability to apply its process technology to this new product.

Figure 7-2 shows how the two types of technology relate to these three areas of technology. In each cell is one example of a non-health care enterprise and one example of a health service that has its main competitive advantage in this field of technology. Coca-Cola's ability to package and market its product is probably equalled by many other soft drink makers. Its distinctive technological advantage lies in its syrup formula. It remains the leading soft drink worldwide largely because people like it most. Likewise, genetic testing is one of the most advanced and fastest growing medical technologies, yet it requires no complex equipment and is relatively easy to process and manage. Its unique technological edge lies in the know-how of the people doing it.

Automated tellers require no major banking skills and are easy to maintain and easy to market. Their unique technological strength lies in their hardware and what it does. In the same way, positron

Area of Technology :	Type of Technology :	
	Know-How	Hardware
Product / Service	Coca-Cola Genetic testing	MAC machines PET scans
Process	Exxon Nursing	Japanese radios Radiation therapy
Management	American Express Surgi-centers	ADP Shared Medical Systems

Figure 7-2 The technological advantage matrix.

emission tomography (PET) although it does require know-how, processing, and management, has its distinctive competitive advantage in the equipment itself. It is expensive, and there are not, as yet, many PET scanners.

Exxon is not particularly noted either for its inventiveness or for its marketing or general management skills. It uses a great deal of hardware, but it is not particularly different from that of many lesser oil companies. Exxon's competitive strength lies in its ability to manage a very complex technological process of extracting oil, shipping, refining, and distributing it.

Nursing, too, is largely a process technology. Doctors may see patients on rounds, write orders, and operate, but it is nursing that takes direct and face-to-face charge of shepherding patients through the complex array of actions that together comprise their care, and ensuring the coordinated delivery of services. The frequent preoccupation in medicine with product technology and with hardware often leads to nursing being regarded as an inferior technology. It is, however, just as vital to the overall technological chain of service delivery as any other component. Nursing thus shares this technological focus upon managing process with some of the world's largest and most successful companies.

The Japanese radio manufacturers are particularly strong neither at product innovation nor at management. They have come to dominate American and other competitors by being much better at managing the process of radio manufacturing. Radiation therapy, an innovative and complex technology, may not seem to be a process technology. Unlike PET scanning, however, linear accelerators have now proliferated to such an extent that most doctors and patients have several rival centers among which to select in their region. The distinguishing advantage of one center over another has become less a matter of what hardware it has than of how well its physicians and technicians can plan, simulate, and manage the use of the equipment. Just as radiation oncology hardware is becoming more commonplace, new advances in combining radiation and medical or surgical therapies make the field even more one in which process technology matters most.

American Express has neither a unique product nor a unique process. It continues to lead the credit card industry mainly by its superior management and marketing know-how. Surgicenters, similarly, have no unique hardware, services, or processes. They succeed or fail solely on their ability to manage an operating suite more efficiently and with greater convenience for both surgeons and patients than hospital-based outpatient surgery. If hospitals can learn to match their management know-how, surgicenters will lose any technological advantage they have.

ADP has grown into one of the largest vendors of payroll management services. In principle, there is no reason why any reasonably sized organization should not be able to manage its own computerized payroll system. Many do, but many others try and fail and decide to contract this task out to companies like ADP that have superior ability at managing payroll programs. Shared Medical Systems (SMS) is one of the largest vendors of computerized hospital accounting systems. Most of its clients do their accounting through local terminals connected to SMS headquarters outside Philadelphia, although SMS now also offers to install completely self-contained systems. SMS's product is not unique. There are a number of competitors in the market, and the process of time-shared data processing from remote sites to a common mainframe computer is now widely applied in airline reservation systems, car rental systems, computerized tills in department stores, and the equipment used in many stores to obtain authorization for credit card purchases. The competitive edge of SMS lies in its ability to manage such a complex system and ensure effective service to multiple client organizations.

One use of the matrix in Figure 7-2 is to determine in what areas your service has an edge over competitors, and where competitors may have the edge.

A second use is to consider where, if anywhere, the service needs to add new skills to withstand a competitive threat. As an example, a nurse who had developed a small but quite successful home health agency saw her strength as being in process technology know-how (Figure 7-3).

She attempted to analyze her major competitive threats. She was hearing a lot about medical equipment distributors diversifying into home health services. It was a logical strategy for them. Medical equipment sales and rentals to the home care market were growing and were very profitable. Direct control of home health agencies would give such companies direct control over a larger part of their own markets. The main competitive advantage that such companies had over her own lay in their knowledge of hardware management technology (they knew the equipment rental business) and their

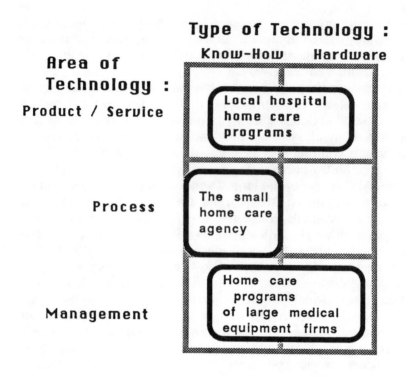

Figure 7-3 The technological advantage matrix facing a home health care agency.

general management technology know-how (many of these companies were large, with good financial and marketing management).

The nurse also noticed that several local hospitals who had been customers of hers had started their own home care agencies. Again, this seemed a sensible strategy, enabling them to provide more services through a longer period to their inpatients who needed home care after discharge. She did not see them as rivaling her in process technology know-how. She had been in home care for several years and knew that it required special skills to coordinate that hospitals usually lacked.

She was convinced, however, that in the future more and more services would be delivered in the home. The growth would be most pronounced in fields such as home chemotherapy, intravenous feeding, and cardiac monitoring. Such services called for a much broader range of professional skills—in respiratory and physical therapy, biomedical maintenance, and specialty nursing—than a small home health agency could afford itself. For a hospital, with all these resources already in place, expanding them into the home would be easier. A hospital's competitive edge in home care thus lay in product technology know-how and hardware.

The nurse's agency was strong today because of its process technology know-how, but threatened from above by hospitals with stronger product technology know-how and hardware, and from below by medical equipment companies with stronger management technology know-how and hardware. After careful thought, she concluded that she could not meet either threat alone. She lacked the experience, size, or resources to move into more advanced home care modalities or to upgrade her management technology. She had to seek a partner.

She saw three options. She could sell out to a medical equipment company seeking to expand into home health services. One might let her stay in charge of the clinical program, but as its employee. She could seek to merge with a hospital on similar terms. Finally, she could seek to merge with other similar home care agencies. Perhaps together they could also get into medical equipment rental and even acquire more management technology, such as a computerized staff scheduling, patient record, and billing system.

She had heard of visiting nurse associations in some areas combining together into quite powerful and well-managed home care agencies. Her first preference was to merge with like agencies. Six months and a lot of meetings later, however, this strategy was getting nowhere. Several similar agencies were enthusiastic in principle, but saw major problems in practice. She fell back on her second best option—merger with a hospital, which she felt would be more compatible with her personal mission of service than a commercial medical equipment company. She did find a hospital partner. In fact, it not only added more product technology to the agency, but also helped to upgrade its management technology. The hospital was one of her own customers but, she later discovered, was about to go into home care for itself, and would have cut her out of its referrals had she not come up with the merger proposal.

A third application of the matrix in Figure 7-2 is to spot possible gaps in some other organization's strengths which you can fill as a vendor to it. That is what ADP did, by realizing that many otherwise sophisticated companies still could not run an internal payroll system that gave its workforce checks that were both accurate and on time. Many health care consultants thrive by identifying know-how that they themselves possess, but that some organizations lack. It may be a missing product technology know-how, such as how to create an effective women's health center. It may be a missing process technology know-how, such as how to increase laboratory efficiency or how to introduce a successful guest relations program. It may be a missing management technology know-how, such as an effective operating room scheduling system or quality assurance program.

While the role of a consultant is to help an organization fill a gap in its know-how, service organizations also exist that will take over that missing role on a continuing basis. Again, they may focus on missing product technology. One commercial enterprise now runs ambulatory clinics on some naval bases, under contract to the Department of Defense. Others may focus on some missing process technology, such as contract nursing agencies. Still others may focus on some missing management technology, such as nurse recruitment or biomedical repairs.

Some 25% of hospitals now have sales teams that visit the offices of potential referring physicians or of companies to sell wellness, industrial medicine, and other services. Most of these hospitals have identified a common dilemma: The ideal person to sell such services—a health professional experienced in selling, or a professional salesperson knowledgeable about clinical medicine—is very rare, is often happy with his or her present job, and is dubious about swapping it for a role in a first-time hospital excursion into the untested field of direct selling of its services.

A number of consultants have seen this dilemma as an opportunity to offer either advice on setting up such efforts, sales training for health professionals, or an introduction to clinical medicine for people with other sales backgrounds. Several service companies have seen this opportunity also but offer a different solution: They offer to do the hospital's selling under contract. They see their competitive edge as their ability, while serving several client hospitals, to hire both experienced salespersons and health professionals to work with and learn from each other. Few hospitals are willing to staff a large enough team to contain both sets of know-how for what is still an experimental concept.

*Enterprises that formally scan their technological environment
do so to identify emerging technologies that offer new opportunities to them, to provide a better solution for their existing
customers, to serve as the delivery system for the new technology, or to make complementary products, run new support services, or provide new skills that the technology may require.
They also look for threats to their existing activities in emerging
technology to see how they should best respond. They look at
both technological know-how and technological hardware opportunities and threats. They look at product technology,
process technology, and management technology, since an effective enterprise must have competence in all these areas and
a distinctive competitive edge in at least one of them.*

Opportunities and Threats in the Economic Environment

National and International Economic Conditions

The economic environment surrounding an organization can
also offer new opportunities and pose new threats. Although it may
not be relevant to many health care enterprises, for others even the
international economic climate can make a critical difference.
Several major U.S. medical centers, particularly those close to the
Mexican and Canadian borders, draw at least some patients from
foreign countries. There is demand for American health care among
some of the rich of such countries, primarily because their own
economies have not been able to afford the same rate of proliferation of new medical methods. For certain types of service, consequently, they have to travel to the United States. There are, at least,
small flows of such patients from countries further afield, for instance of Irish patients in need of liver transplants.

The size of the flow, however, is critically dependent upon
another international economic variable: exchange rates. The sharp
decline in the value of the Mexican peso in the mid-1980s, to cite
one example, reduced the flow of patients into the United States.
Conversely, it increased the flow of American patients to Mexico.
Across the California-Mexico border, around Tijuana, a quite strong
"offshore" U.S. health network has developed, consisting of some
services not approved by the Food and Drug Administration, such

as certain unorthodox treatments for cancer, but also of health spas which, by virtue of the weak peso, offered bargain prices for luxury fitness courses.

The flow of foreign patients to the United States remains quite small and is usually the result of special circumstances, such as an immigrant family bringing a relative here for care, or a foreign U.S. trained doctor referring some patients to his American alma mater. Some medical centers have launched more formalized international marketing programs to attract target groups from other countries. Whether these efforts have so far shown a profit is open to question. It is entirely possible that some will, but it is not an effort worth mounting without a lot of careful thought and planning, as the costs can be high and the returns uncertain.

By contrast, the state of the national economy can provide major marketing opportunities. Times of higher-than-average inflation, for instance, increase demand for various types of bank services, such as floating-interest loans, and decrease demand for fixed-interest loans. Such times also tend to depress consumer demand for high-priced products and to favor less expensive alternatives and discount stores.

The impact of the state of the national economy on demand for health services does not appear to have been well researched. It was believed for a long time that, because health care is a necessity, it is largely immune to cyclical economic changes. That may, however, have been a false assumption. Overall demand for health services grew so strongly over past decades, basically for technological reasons discussed above, that this long-term growth may well have masked short-term cyclical fluctuations. The fact is that many modern health care services are not necessities — matters of life and death — but are discretionary elective services. Some at least of these needs can be postponed. There are also now more options available than ever before for many health needs, and these options vary in price. It is, therefore, entirely likely that demand for certain services varies with consumers' perceptions of how much discretionary income they have available. Cosmetic surgery is a case in point. It is even more likely that times of higher inflation favor lower cost health suppliers, and that, by comparison, when consumers perceive their disposable incomes to be rising they are more likely to base health services selection on quality considerations.

It would certainly seem that the prolonged high inflation of the mid-1970s and early 1980s played a part in the growth of HMOs and of such health services as urgicenters, chiropractic, and free-standing imaging and therapy centers. That does not mean that they will disappear in a subsequent era of low inflation and higher growth, because each now has some established consumer loyalty. It does mean, however, that they might well have found it much more difficult to grow as much as they have but for the economic climate of that period.

Times of low economic growth, higher-than-average unemployment, and high inflation favor health services that meet essential customer needs and those that are lower priced. Conversely, times of high economic growth, moderate unemployment, and low inflation are good periods for higher priced and more discretionary health services. Since any new enterprise faces a special challenge in its start-up phase, timing the launch of a service to coincide with the most favorable economic climate strengthens its chances of success.

Local Economic Conditions

Whatever the status of the national economy as a whole, there are often profound regional and local variations. Even if, for instance, the national economy is in a period of growth and low inflation, increasing as one of its consequences the growth of cosmetic surgery or more expensive types of fitness centers, new ventures in those fields will face a much less certain market in a service area that is not following the national trend. Even in periods of high overall economic growth there are still older industries that are on the decline, and towns and regions where such older industries are concentrated.

Thus, the danger in trying to steal new opportunities from other enterprises is that they may be operating in a very different economic climate. As one example, in the early and mid-1980s Manhattan saw the successful launch of quite a number of higher priced executive fitness centers. Various entrepreneurs tried to imitate that innovation in other locations that lacked the vital factor present in Manhattan. That factor was a very high concentration of affluent executives, who perceived themselves as having income available for luxury spending, within a very short distance of such fitness centers. In fact, the key to the most successful of those centers has been that they are accessible on foot and in under 10 minutes in the middle of clusters of skyscrapers with high numbers of executives working in them. Very few cities in the United States have such a high density of affluent executives within walking distance of a given location.

One of the most dramatic illustrations of the impact of the local economy on opportunities in health care is that of Texas in the mid-1980s. Sustained growth of the local economy through several decades encouraged the emergence in Houston of the Texas Medical Center, a campus of over 30 hospitals, health institutes, and health-related schools. This growth helped to generate a number of opportunistic health-related ventures whose prospects would have been highly questionable elsewhere. They included a very large fitness center, the Richardson Institute of Preventive Medicine, a gourmet restaurant — Chez Eddy — dedicated to low-calorie and low-cholesterol dishes, an "international hospital" dedicated to foreign patients, and several large hotels to accommodate outpatients and campus visitors.

The slump in the Texas oil industry in the mid-1980s had a major impact upon such opportunities. It had a quadruple impact upon the local health care industry. First, the number of unemployed people in Houston, with more limited health insurance coverage, rose. Second, those local residents with jobs found many companies tightening their belts by being less generous with improvements to their health benefits than they had been previously. Third, the flow of charitable donations from oil companies to not-for-profit health organizations fell, giving them fewer dollars to invest in new ventures. Fourth, banks and other lending sources became more nervous about the growth prospects for health care in the city, and so borrowing money for new projects became more difficult.

It is probable that the Houston economy will again see better days and that the local health care industry will respond to its new challenges. This change in the local economy, however, certainly put some brakes on the development of health-related innovations.

Local economic conditions can vary substantially from national trends. An area might be experiencing strong economic growth while the overall national economy is not, or vice versa. Unique opportunities may, therefore, exist in an area — for lower cost services in a poor local economic climate, or for more discretionary types of health services in a strong local economy. For this reason, it can be dangerous to look for opportunities in what similar health suppliers are doing successfully in other parts of the country. The economic circumstances that made a particular innovation effective for them may not exist in other areas.

Opportunities and Threats in Public Policy

The past training of hospital and nursing administrators has often placed more emphasis on the role of public policy in shaping new opportunities and threats for health providers than it has on the other sources of new challenges discussed in this chapter — technology, economics, competitive forces, and social trends. The potential impact of public policy changes can, indeed, be considerable. For instance, the introduction of Medicare opened up new opportunities for medical practices and hospitals that had previously treated large numbers of elderly people, but without recouping their costs for doing so. These providers had been subsidizing the care of senior citizens out of what they could charge to younger patients and their insurers. Once they started recovering their costs under Medicare, many of them could use that income from younger patients to pursue new opportunities. The advent of Medicaid had a similar impact upon providers caring for large numbers of poor patients. However, the scope and generosity of Medicaid vary among the states and still leave, in most states, many uncovered poor people whose care must be paid for out of higher charges to other patients.

The public policy that generated these extensions of health insurance coverage in the 1960s and early 1970s was called the *doctrine of entitlement.* It held that no one should be deprived of access to needed health care on the grounds of age, sex, race, or income. In the late 1970s and the 1980s the priority in public policy toward health care has shifted toward a policy of *cost containment.*

Perhaps the most far-reaching manifestation of that new priority was the federal introduction of case rate payments (the prospective payment system), rather than daily payments, to hospitals for Medicare patients. This change too has had a major impact. It essentially seeks to determine the average cost of treating a particular diagnostic group (e.g., myocardial infarction without surgery) and calculates a case rate based upon that average. Various other allowed costs are added on, based on particular hospital circumstances.

As an example, consider three hospitals A, B, and C. To treat a particular diagnosis, hospital A keeps patients for an average of 15 days and incurs costs of $10,000 per case. It is the average hospital in this case. Hospital B keeps such patients 18 days and incurs costs of $12,000 per case. It is the high-cost hospital of the three. Hospital C keeps such patients only 12 days and incurs costs of $8,000 per case. Each hospital has the same daily costs of $667. They vary only in how long each keeps patients with this disease. When they were paid on a daily rate basis, each hospital received that $667 per patient day. (In reality, they usually got slightly more than cost.) Under that payment method, hospital B received the most money for these patients. In fact, it received half as much again as hospital C.

The new system pays not by the day but by the case. The average cost for this type of patient is hospital A's $10,000. If that price is paid to all three hospitals, hospital A notices no difference. Hospital B, however, now loses $2,000 on each case, while hospital C makes $2,000 on each case. Hospital B will find it increasingly difficult to cope with losing money on each of these cases, while hospital C will have a surplus to invest in new equipment, buildings, or more people. The system thus rewards the efficient and punishes the inefficient. That is, in part, its intent.

How does hospital C treat these patients more efficiently? One possible answer is that it is cutting corners and not giving good care, but there are, in reality, other checks exercised on hospitals to try to prevent that occurrence. Another possible answer is that patients with this diagnosis who go to hospital C are less sick on average than patients with the same diagnosis at the other two hospitals. Perhaps, for instance, hospital C has fewer elderly patients who have a range of chronic conditions which exacerbate this disease and make their treatment longer and more costly. There are, indeed, cases where this payment system may fail to allow sufficiently for such variations in patient mix. The other possible explanation, however, is that hospital C may have done the best job of introducing new methods of health care that allow these cases to be treated more quickly, while hospital A has been an average innovator and hospital B a slow innovator. If that is true, the system is fair in penalizing those hospitals that perpetuate older clinical approaches, and in allowing innovative ones to make a surplus to fund even more innovation.

Marketing science uses the term *technology diffusion* to describe the process by which new methods in any field spread until they become standard practice. An important innovation starts with one innovative enterprise. If it works, others start to imitate it. By such imitation, the innovation diffuses to other enterprises until it becomes standard practice.

In health care, technology diffusion has usually been quite rapid, because the medical profession's ethics are not to protect better ways of treating people from imitation, but to teach others how to imitate them. However, as was noted earlier, the rate and scope of medical advances in the late 20th century are proving to be significant. A fast rate of technological innovation when combined with a fast rate of technology diffusion poses a special public policy problem. It is extremely costly. Not only are the major medical centers, where much of the innovation originates, constantly introducing new and better methods, but each doctor and hospital away from those centers is continually trying to absorb the latest wave of innovations. The process is being aided by pharmaceutical companies and medical equipment manufacturers. They do not want to see innovations, which have been costly for them to develop, restricted to a limited number of doctors and centers. It is in their marketing interests to see any new medical technology diffused quickly and broadly.

Nor have federal and state agencies tried to block the rate of medical innovation. Consistently through recent decades, the federal government has, indeed, sought to encourage clinical innovation. Through the National Institutes of Health, it is one of the largest funders of the basic and clinical research that fuels medical innovation. Through the Food and Drug Administration, it is one of the final arbiters of whether a particular technology is sufficiently proven to allow it to diffuse and become standard practice.

Through those same decades, however, public policy has sought to place some limits on the extent of that diffusion. Federal health planning acts and individual state certificate-of-need laws and regulations have required providers to obtain approval before engaging in the most costly types of technological innovation, such as installing MRI units or running open heart surgery programs. The problem that these certification processes have encountered is that the majority of medical innovations are not associated with expensive items of equipment. More often innovation is implemented through substituting one improved drug for another, or by doctors acquiring new knowledge and skills. Often, also, it takes the form of new equipment that is relatively inexpensive, like many surgical lasers, but which amounts to a major cost if many thousands are installed across the United States over just a few years.

Consequently, public policy toward health care in the 1980s and 1990s is faced with a major dilemma: how to reconcile technological advance, technology diffusion, and cost containment. That is why part of the purpose behind the change in systems of public payment to hospitals and health professionals is not only to contain cost, but also to try to concentrate the more expensive forms of health care delivery in fewer locations.

The former issue of entitlement has not disappeared from the public policy agenda, even if it has been joined by these other priorities. A considerable amount of effort and funding by official agencies is still expended to seek better and more cost-effective methods of health care delivery to those who depend upon the public purse to pay for it. The latest issue to arise in entitlement policy is, of course, that of AIDS patients. It is recognized that they need care and cannot be denied it, but who will pay for it and how?

Federal, state, and municipal administrations are also quite significant direct providers of health care through the Veterans' Administration, the armed services, state and municipal hospitals, and a wide range of public nonhospital health agencies and centers. In the 1980s, however, a new agenda item has begun to enter into public policy: *privatization.* Serious consideration is being given to a smaller governmental role as a direct provider of health care, and the subcontracting of responsibilities for these services to enterprises whose mission and field of competence lie in health care.

Public policy can be a major source of both opportunities and threats to health care providers. It cannot, however, be divorced from the other factors considered in this chapter. Public policy toward health care is not created in a vacuum. Technological, economic, competitive, and social trends all shape governmental policy.

The relatively simple public policy priority of the 1960s, namely, entitlement, has given way to a new public agenda with several component priorities. Each may represent an area of opportunity or an area of threat for a health provider, depending upon the provider's specific mission and circumstances. This new public policy agenda of the 1980s and 1990s will favor:

1. *Innovations that promote improved health, particularly if they are also less costly than previous standard practice*

2. *Innovations that promote cost containment without lowering quality*

3. *Innovations that facilitate the more rapid diffusion of new, less costly technologies*

4. *Innovations that limit excessive diffusion of the more expensive technologies, by sharing them or by merging several health providers and limiting the duplication of these technologies among them*

5. *Innovations that offer more cost-effective methods of meeting entitlement needs among the elderly and the poor*

6. *Innovations that allow government agencies to privatize some health services they currently provide directly*

7. *Innovations that improve treatment of certain high-visibility diseases (e.g., cancer, AIDS, trauma) but that limit the number of centers involved in such care.*

Opportunities and Threats in the Competitive Environment

Monitoring the Competition

Successfully innovative companies also systematically study the actions of their competitors. They look for opportunities they might imitate, and for threats they might have to counter. Such companies tend to study the behavior of five different types of enterprise (Porter 1985):

1. Most obviously, they watch other enterprises selling similar goods or services.

2. They also keep a watch on possible new entrants into their business. These new entrants may be organizations like their own, or they may be companies that previously concentrated in other fields, but have decided to diversify. RCA, for instance, was not a competitive threat for Avis until it decided to take over Hertz. Campbell Soup was not a competitor of Hershey's until it brought out Godiva Chocolates. Coca-Cola was not a rival of Levi Strauss until it decided to promote Coca-Cola casual wear. Marriott was not a rival of Hospital Corporation of America (HCA), until Marriott decided to offer hospital contract management services.

3. Companies also watch sellers of substitute products. Steel is used in many manufactured goods that can also use concrete, aluminum, fiberglass, or metal alloys as substitutes. Cloth is used for hospital gowns, but paper is now a common substitute. Sutures may be made of thread, but can also be made of other materials. The steak that was once the mainstay of many American diets has lost ground to fish.

4. Companies watch their suppliers. Many companies grow by *forward integration*. They decide to take a step closer to the final consumer of their product, by eliminating the enterprise in the middle. U.S. Steel developed a bridge construction division. Some shoe and clothing makers, like Florsheim and Benetton, have franchised their own stores. Many hospitals now operate primary care satellites, staffed by their own salaried doctors, rather than depend upon a self-employed doctor in private practice to refer patients to them.

5. Companies watch their customers. Sometimes retail firms decide to expand by *backward integration*, by taking direct control over the source of some of their own supplies. They may even start selling those supplies to others as a new product line. Some automobile makers, for instance, have expanded into direct production of some components that they previously brought in from

outside. One large chain of furniture stores has its own advertising agency, its own direct mail company to handle mailing of its catalog, and even its own restaurant near its corporate headquarters. Some physicians in fields such as neurology, obstetrics, and cardiology now perform in their own offices laboratory or radiological studies that they previously referred out to pathologists or radiologists. The largest hospital company in the United States, HCA, tried, unsuccessfully, to merge with the largest hospital supplies distributor, AHS.

To monitor all these potential competitors, enterprises must gather competitive intelligence. The term conjures up thoughts of industrial espionage, of bribing insiders and of hiring away key personnel from competitors. Such actions are, however, very rare and are often acts of desperation by companies who have failed to pursue more ethical, legal, and effective means. Organizations that are good at collecting and analyzing information on their competition rely, for the most part, on published material. They obtain their information from newspapers, magazines, the trade press, and data shared among competitors through their trade associations. They supplement that information with intelligence gathered by their own salespersons, dealers, and distributors. If a key customer is buying from a competitor, a representative who discovers that information in the normal course of his work reports it to a competitive analyst in the company.

How do such enterprises convert thousands of snippets of published or reported data into useful competitive information? They do two relatively simple but time-consuming things:

1. They define what they are looking for

2. They file any pertinent information systematically

Companies that have a well-defined mission statement for their own business can define clearly what information they are looking for. From that definition they can develop a list of key competitive variables that are worth monitoring, and pay attention only to those issues that really matter to them. Any competitor is likely to take many actions that are totally irrelevant, because it has a different mission.

One large medical center decided several years ago upon a strategy of seeking contracts to manage hospitals in Third World countries. It saw this move as a way of earning large profits that could be repatriated to support its own growth. It has had some minor success in acquiring such contracts, and the total effort has probably been worthwhile.

Various nearby hospitals watched this plan unfold with awe. Their concern was misdirected, however. The medical center's international expansion posed them a competitive threat only if they had similar plans. Even then the threat would have been trivial. There remain many thousands of hospitals and more than 50 countries in the Third World that this effort had not touched. As it happened, none of these competitive hospitals shared that goal of seeking Third World contracts.

The main reason the other hospitals wasted time analyzing their competitor's action was that they themselves lacked a defined mission. Had they possessed one, they would have seen this action as an irrelevance, or even as an advantage to them. The more energy the medical center put into this endeavor, the less time it would have to undertake activities that might be truly threatening to its local competitors' missions.

The more crowded and competitive any industry becomes, the more likely it is that major competitors will pursue divergent missions. Each is likely to prosper more by trying to get out of the others' way, rather than fighting head to head. One good approach to limiting the competitive challenge is to define a somewhat different mission. Macy's and Sears, Roebuck have very similar missions, but they are carefully differentiated. Each tries to position itself in a slightly different segment of the market. They have also pursued very distinct growth strategies in recent years.

An organization with a clear mission, therefore, studies its competitors with a focus. It looks most at actions that seem a challenge to its own mission. It may also take a quick look at other actions of its competitors to see if they represent an overlooked opportunity. There is a real danger, if the technological, economic, regulatory, or social environment is changing rapidly, of missing the boat (Dickson and Giglierano 1986). Texas Instruments failed to see the potential of the LCD watch until Casio and Seiko had entrenched themselves in this market. The U.S. Postal Service failed to see the demand for guaranteed overnight delivery until Federal Express had established itself as the market leader.

However, a competitor's actions should not be imitated merely in retaliation. They have to make sense in terms of some other environmental opportunity. Federal Express should have worried the Postal Service not because it had come into existence, but because the whole speed of business communication has accelerated, with computer links, Telex and FAX systems, and enhanced telephone features like teleconferencing. There was a clear demand for a more rapid means than the normal mails could provide of transporting documents too bulky or requiring too high a standard of reproduction to transmit by electronic mail. The Postal Service should have "followed the herd" in this instance, because in doing so it would have strengthened its ability to fulfill its own mission. Usually, however, it does not make sense to follow the herd (Peters and Waterman 1983). The herd may be heading in a different direction than your organization wants to go, or it may just be running around in circles.

The federal government started, in the mid-1980s, to seek out HMOs willing to enroll large numbers of senior citizens. Its goal was to test whether the HMO mechanism could provide a means of cost containment for the Medicare trust fund. Some HMOs saw this as an attractive new product line, but realized that contracting with the federal government is very different from contracting with a large number of employers. Despite supplemental insurance and private pay, so much of the medical care of the elderly is financed by the federal government that it is a virtual monopsonist (sole buyer) of health services for this population. An organization that sells to a sole buyer has less freedom of action than one with multiple customers. If one of many buyers starts making unreasonable demands, a seller can refuse to do business with that buyer without destroying his or her business. An enterprise with only one customer and no other potential customers can only withdraw from that contract if it is willing to close down that entire product line.

Those HMOs that realized that dealing with Washington was different, but wanted the extra business, took steps to limit their risk, such as setting a ceiling on the percentage of their total revenue that they would allow to become dependent on this product line. Most of these HMOs have coped reasonably well with Medicare contracting. Some other HMOs, however, were concerned that they might miss the boat, and so they followed the herd into accepting Medicare contracts. Exercising less prudence than the competitors that they were imitating, many of these prepaid plans have fared very poorly, and even lost large sums of money, on Medicare contracting. Still other HMOs watched where the herd was going and decided that federal contracting was not part of their mission. They elected to ignore this opportunity. Most of them remain happy with that decision.

Those organizations that perform effective competitive analysis not only look at competitors' behavior with a defined focus, but also file what they discover systematically. One isolated fact about a competitor may mean nothing, but three or four items of intelligence pointing in a common direction may mean a lot. By filing information about competitors as they come across it, companies can analyze it periodically to look for patterns of behavior. Relying on memory to pull random facts together is much less certain, particularly in large organizations, where different people may come across different pieces of a puzzle, but no one person is assigned the task of putting them together into a picture.

For example, a doctor associated with one hospital heard from a realtor friend that a rival hospital was about to lease a large building some 20 miles away, in an area from which the doctor derived a number of referrals. The doctor was worried enough to share this information with the hospital's planner, who made a note of it. Three months later, the rival hospital announced the opening of a radiology satellite at that location. The doctor and the planner both relaxed; their hospital was not strongly interested in that specialty. Another 3 months passed before a senior nurse at the first hospital learned from a friend who worked at the rival hospital that she was studying a possible radiation therapy satellite. The nurse also shared this comment with the hospital's planner, who now understood why the rival hospital had leased so large a building.

Either piece of intelligence—that the rival hospital had leased too much space for an imaging center, and that the rival hospital was considering a radiation therapy satellite—was inconclusive in itself. The extra space might have been planned for anything. The radiation therapy satellite might have been anywhere. Together, these two clues pointed to a reasonable assumption that the rival hospital might place a linear accelerator in the large vacant space.

The hospital planner and the doctor saw that as a much bigger threat than the initial imaging center. Their hospital took various actions to minimize the potential damage, including calling on all the oncologists in the area and announcing a free bus service for patients to its radiation oncology unit. The rival hospital opened its center 15 months later. It proved reasonably successful, but by taking patients away from other hospitals, not from the one that got advanced warning of the threat and took some steps to contain it.

Successfully innovative organizations invest in gathering and analyzing information about their competitors. They do so, however, with a focus derived from their mission statement. They look for specific trends that threaten that mission. They may also look at competitors' actions to check that they are not missing the boat themselves with a new market opportunity. Most of the time, however, they rapidly discard those actions as "right for them but wrong for us." They do not follow the herd unless it definitely furthers their own mission.

Competitive Geography

Successful innovative organizations also seem to have a well-developed sense of the *competitive geography* of their markets. They realize that their ability to sell diminishes with their distance from the customer, unless they can develop an effective distribution system in-between.

When Gallo launched Bartles & Jaymes wine coolers, it took almost 2 years before the product was available nationwide, because a distribution system of trucking, warehouses, and local dealers had to be built first. Some 10 years earlier it took Coors Beer even longer to do the same; in the interim a thriving black market for the product developed on the eastern seaboard.

Despite the high visibility of the major nationwide sellers of products and services, the vast majority of U.S. businesses thrive by restricting themselves to regional or local markets. Some do so because they lack the ambition or drive to expand their sales territories, but others have examined the idea and concluded that, in their field, the extra costs of a larger service area are greater than the extra revenues obtainable.

For example, there have been several attempts to organize national networks of hospitals in order to seek direct contracts with major national corporations. The hospitals' goal is forward integration: trying to cut out the insurance companies that stand between them and the corporations whose employees they serve. Some of these efforts may eventually prove successful, but they confront one major geographical obstacle. Any one of the Fortune 100 companies tends to have its major concentration of employees in a different locality from any of the others. A network of hospitals that could serve General Motors well would have major gaps in trying to serve any of the other 99 companies in the top 100. A network with reasonable national contracting ability would have to be very large, with very high overhead, and would yet only be able to deliver quite minor advantages to many of its member institutions.

The majority of organizations that serve small regional or local markets still need a strong sense of market geography to be successful. One of the fields in which this concept is best developed is retailing. The locations of shopping malls are seldom chosen randomly. They result from very careful study of population distribution and tolerable travel times. These studies also look very carefully at the locations of existing and competitive retail stores (Applebaum and Cohen 1961). To do so, they use various sophisticated computer models. One relatively simple version that illustrates the principles involved is the *gravity model*. Although now used for such decisions as store or urgicenter location, this model originated with Isaac Newton's study of the planets.

In Figure 7-4, A is the intended location of a new shopping mall, B is the location of an existing mall, and C is a town 2 miles from B and 4 miles from A. At the moment, mall B gets all the shoppers from town C who want to shop in a mall, because there is no other mall nearby. The percentage of those shoppers that the new mall A will draw away obviously depends on which is the better shopping mall. The gravity model recognizes, however, that distance is by far the most important determinant of where people shop. (It is also by

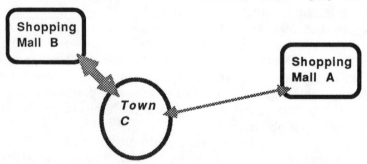

thickness of arrows show Mall B's attraction to Town C is four times greater than Mall A's, while Mall A is only twice as distant from the town as Mall B.

Figure 7-4 Sample gravity model.

far the most important determinant of where people will go for health services. As long as the nearby hospital offers all the services available at the farther hospital, most people will opt for the nearer facility).

One might suppose that, because it is twice as far away, mall A will draw half as many shoppers as mall B. However, gravity model states that "the relative pull of two locations upon a third location is proportional to the ratio between the inverse of the square of the distance of each to that location." That sounds complicated but is in fact quite simple. Mall A will be 4 miles from the town. The square of 4 is 16. Mall B is 2 miles from the town. The square of 2 is 4. Four is one-quarter of 16. Therefore, the new mall will only draw away one-quarter of the shoppers from the old mall, even though it is only 2 miles further from the town.

Stated simply, the gravity model says that the number of people that a service location will draw diminishes very quickly with distance. Consider the case of a group of doctors who were planning a breast imaging center, to be located at the middle of three concentric rings of population (Figure 7-5). The rings extend out 5, 10, and 15 miles from the planned center. Each ring has the same population: 20,000 people. From the inner ring the medical service expects to draw 1,000 patients each year. How many will it draw from the middle and outer rings?

Starting with the middle ring, 10 squared is 100, while 5 squared is 25. One hundred is four times 25. Therefore, the center will only draw one-quarter as many patients from the middle ring, or 250. Now looking at the outer ring, 15 squared is 225, while 5 squared is 25. Because 225 is 9 times 25, the service will only draw one-ninth as many patients from the outer ring as it does from the inner ring, or 111. The total of the three rings is 1,361. Thus, if this center needs 1,500 patients to cover the costs, the gravity model predicts that the center will have difficulty attracting enough patients to be viable.

In reality, of course, the gravity model gets more complicated. The density of population may well differ from ring to ring. Also, distance is less important than actual travel time, and it may be quicker to get to the center from some places 10 miles away than from others only 5 miles away. A proper gravity model, therefore, uses real population data and estimated travel times, but the underlying concept is the same.

For some services walking time is more relevant than driving or public transport time. Another practical example of the gravity

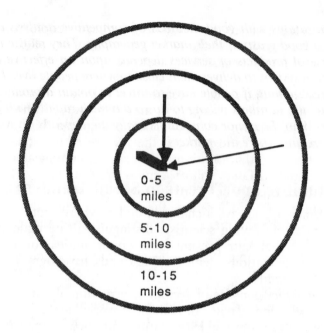

Figure 7-5 Gravity model for a proposed breast imaging center.

model is that of a hospital in a declining inner city area that decided that it should try to attract other businesses to its immediate neighborhood. These businesses would draw more people to the area, who would then become familiar with the hospital. The one business that did express interest was McDonald's, a company that studies its locations very carefully using concepts such as the gravity model. About 8 blocks north of the hospital was the only other still-thriving part of the old downtown area, around the city hall and courthouse. About 4,000 people worked in that area, compared to 2,000 at the hospital. McDonald's did open a restaurant, 4 blocks from the city hall and 4 blocks from the hospital. It brought nobody near the hospital, but the hospital's own cafeteria, which had been profitable, went into the red as some employees took a walk to McDonald's on pleasant days. Because many of them were nurses on hurried meal breaks, the hospital also had to invest in more trash receptacles for all the McDonald's containers that ended up back in the hospital. The nurses also had to keep a closer eye on visitors sneaking in a McDonald's snack for patients on restricted diets.

Organizations with good methods of competitive analysis also have a good grasp of their market geography. They realize that the use of products or services depends upon an effective distribution system to deliver them close to where people live. They also realize that, if people have to travel to obtain a product or service, the numbers willing to do so diminish rapidly with distance. Who the major competitors really are depends on where they are and where the market is.

Opportunities and Threats in Social Trends

The times are always a-changin', and nowhere more so than in social trends. Marketing scientists distinguish three main types of social trends that can present new opportunities, or pose new threats, to organizations: demographic trends, psychographic trends, and life-style trends.

Demographics consists of factual information about who people are: their age, gender, place of residence, workplace, education, ethnic background, income, marital status, household composition, and so on.

Psychographics consists of what people think, believe, like, and dislike, and how they behave in approaching decisions.

Life-style consists of what people spend their time doing, what activities they value, and how they choose to live. Life-style stems from demographics and psychographics. For example, affluent people who like travel and sun may take winter vacations in the Sun Belt or the Caribbean. Lifestyle, however, is observable. It is the behavioral result of a population's demographics and psychographics.

For many industries, there is one social issue so critical to their success that it needs special attention. The fortunes of the automobile industry, for instance, are critically dependent on people's travel patterns. These are a result of their demographics, psychographics, and life-style, but they are so central to an auto maker's viability that they are worth monitoring and analyzing in their own right. For AT&T, that fourth issue is communications behavior. For the clothing industry it is the changing shapes and sizes of people (a demographic fact), changing preferences for clothing (a psychographic fact), and changing life-style (work hours, leisure pursuits, etc.). For health services, that critical social variable is *epidemiology*, or changes in the incidence of disease, length of life, accident rate, and other factors.

Other chapters of this book have described some of the most important general trends in demographics, psychographics, life-style, and epidemiology that are impacting health care in the 1980s and will do so in the 1990s. The following comments, therefore, focus on how to analyze them from a strategic perspective.

As mentioned earlier, all environmental analysis should be performed with a focus provided by the service's mission statement. The only social trends worth studying are those relevant to the success or failure of that mission.

Demographics

To make effective use of demographics, it is first essential to define who constitutes the *target audience* for the service or organization. The next step is to compile a *demographic profile* of that target audience, outlining who and where they are, their gender, education, income, and so forth. Official U.S. Census data are now published in software as well as book form. As a result, it is now possible to analyze local, regional, and national demographics with more precision than ever before. In the past, for instance, it was difficult to access demographics for areas smaller than the official census tracts. With computerized census data, it is relatively easy to break out a demographic profile of individual city blocks.

If, for instance, a health care organization is planning some special program for senior citizens, it is worth mapping in detail where they live in the service area. As the gravity model suggests, a medical center or practice ideally located for the population under 40 may be very poorly located to attract a critical mass of senior citizens.

The mass media and the health care press are a rich source of demographic trends that may represent new market opportunities (e.g., the graying of the population) or threats (e.g., the falling birthrate). However, it is vital to check these overall national trends out against the local demographics of an organization's service area and its sense of its competitive geography. For instance, central areas in many cities are undergoing gentrification and the average age of the population is actually falling, despite the graying of the population as a whole. In other areas both the elderly and the young adult population are growing, but the number of adults in their middle years has declined. Still other areas have large concentrations of young adults or of ethnic minorities; here births are likely to continue to rise for some time.

It is also vital to realize that demographics change, whereas many health care services are planned with permanence in mind. HCA prospered in the 1970s by building small, well-managed hospitals in many new suburban areas being populated by young families. The main health needs of these families were for routine childbirth, pediatrics, and the more common conditions of young adulthood such as asthma. These small, attractive suburban hospitals did well catering to these needs.

By the mid-1980s, however, this population had entered its 40s. Many had remained in those suburbs, which had, therefore aged along with them. These families were now out of their childbearing years, and their children had grown up or were now in their teens. The hospital needs of these families began to tilt more toward more serious medical, surgical, and gynecological needs, for which a small community hospital now seemed less appropriate. Demographic change has not been the only change affecting HCA's profitability, but it has played an important role.

It is just as important to avoid jumping to conclusions based on demographic comments in the media. Often, the real truth is more complicated. The demographic truisms of the day need study to verify their accuracy before they become the basis for strategic decisions.

Consider the case of a hospital located in an ethnic neighborhood in the center of a major American city. With declining average length of stay and rates of hospitalization, it saw its financial strength erode over a period of some 5 years. It decided to "start marketing" in a attempt to boost admissions. First it analyzed where its current patients were coming from. Nearly 80% came from the immediate neighborhood, where the local public rated it by far the best hospital. Another 15% of its patients came from a variety of adjoining neighborhoods, just as the gravity model would predict. However, 5% of the hospital's patients came from two suburbs some 20 miles distant.

This fact excited one board member. He pointed out that these suburbs had been settled 20 to 30 years earlier by outward migration from the hospital's neighborhood. These suburbs were full of families of the same ethnic background. Many even spoke in the distinctive accent of the old neighborhood. Once or twice a year many of them came back to the old neighborhood to reestablish their roots. He himself lived in one of these suburbs and had always been annoyed at how few of his neighbors used the hospital, despite the ethnic ties. The hospital decided to start an advertising campaign targeted at those suburbs and playing on the ethnic connection. It was completely ineffective.

The hospital's analysis contained four major demographic misunderstandings. First, it is a commonly heard but totally erroneous belief that most American suburbanites grew up in the inner cities. Their grandparents or their parents might have, but most American suburbanites alive today grew up in American suburbs (Newitt 1984). Second, many of today's suburbanites grew up in the suburbs of other cities. It is understandable that some, when relocating for work, gravitate toward suburbs with an ethnic flavor similar to their own. These migrants do not necessarily adopt the consumer preferences of their new neighborhood. Third, even though many of these suburbanites do revisit the old neighborhood once or twice a year to enjoy its ethnic flavor, they do not go there for services. Their service orientation is largely within the suburbs. If they do travel elsewhere for health care, it is to a specialized or tertiary center, not to another community hospital. Fourth, it turned out that the 5% of admissions that this hospital was getting from those suburbs was entirely attributable to one physician on its staff who had an office in those suburbs. Most of his patients accepted his recommendation of the hospital out of belief in him, not because of any affinity with the hospital or its neighborhood.

The graying of the population is another often-overstated demographic myth. It is happening, but at a much slower pace than the media headlines and the flurry of health care activity in geriatric programs justify (Kiplinger 1986). It is true that the fastest growing age group in America from now through 2005 will be the population over 85, which will more than double in size. However, it will still only represent 3% of the total population, compared to about 2% today. It will remain a quite small market segment.

The population aged 75 to 85 will grow about 25% between 1985 and 2005, but will remain a constant 4% of the total population. People aged 65 to 75 will also increase about 25% by 2005, but will, in fact, decline as a percentage of the total population, from 7% to 6%. In terms of absolute numbers, the greatest increases through 1995 will be in the 35-to-45 age group and the 45-to-55 age group. Between 1995 and 2005 the greatest increase in numbers of people will be in the 45-to-55 and the 55-to-65 age groups. The percentage of the population aged 65 or over will in fact remain static, at 13%, through 2005. There will be more "very elderly," but a larger percentage of those under 75 will be the "well elderly," without major health care needs. The true graying of the population will start to be seen beyond 2005 and will not be very significant until after 2015.

The underlying reasons for this strange phenomenon date back to the 1930s. During the Depression the birth rate fell dramatically. World War II prolonged this situation. Consequently, an unusually small number of people will turn 65 between 1995 and 2010. Those that do will, on average, live longer, producing a growth in the over-75 population. World War II was followed by the baby boom, as many couples started the families they had deferred in the Depression and the war. As a result, an abnormally large number of people were aged 25 to 35 in 1985, will be aged 35 to 45 in 1995, and so on.

Beyond 2015, it is likely that an even larger percentage of those aged 65 to 75 will be the "well elderly," and many may remain in employment until 70 or beyond. Because of increased life span, by about 2025 there may be quite large numbers of people over 75, and indeed over 85.

However, taking major steps in the late 1980s in anticipation of a situation some 30 to 40 years distant would be like having made decisions in 1950 about needs in 1990. These statistics should not imply that all efforts to develop health services around the growing number of senior citizens and of "frail elderly" are misguided. That market is growing. For a long time ahead, however, it will be much smaller than implied by many comments in the media, which have been assumed by many health care providers to be more significant and more immediate than they really are.

Another oversimplified demographic myth is that the typical American household (a married couple with two or three children) is breaking down. Yet this typical household never was universal. For several decades, many households have consisted of couples whose children have left home, widows, and young people living alone. These groups have increased in size because of increased general affluence, allowing people to leave home early in larger numbers, and because of the higher divorce rate and increased longevity producing more widows and widowers. The prototype American family now constitutes a smaller percentage of households, but it is still alive and plentiful.

Demographic changes can create new market opportunities. The rising number of fit and affluent retirees has increased the demand for air travel. The growth in the percentage of women working outside the home has increased the demand for female business attire, quick-to-cook meals, day care centers and kindergartens. The increased numbers of young people leaving the parental home has created more demand for low-cost but fashionable furniture. The growth of the suburbs has increased auto sales and lawn services. The growth of population in the Sun Belt has helped to make air conditioning a standard feature of the American home.

In health care, the growth of the elderly population has increased the demand for nursing homes. The arrival of the baby boom into its childbearing years has increased the demand for obstetrics and pediatrics. Increased personal incomes have led to a higher demand for cosmetic surgery. A longer life span has increased the demand for prostate surgery in men and breast cancer surgery in women. The growth of the Hispanic population in some areas has increased the demand for bilingual health personnel. Rising affluence and population movements have increased total automobile miles driven and thus the number of major trauma cases.

Demographic changes can also pose new threats. Levi Strauss & Co. found sales stagnating as the baby boom aged, until it introduced fuller cut jeans. The growth in white-collar jobs actually hurt custom tailoring, as middle managers made off-the-rack suits commonplace corporate attire. The movement of population out of the old center cities destroyed many small stores, just as the gentrification of some inner cities has now created demand for others.

In health services, the aging of the baby boom is now lowering the birth rate and the demand for childbirth services. The larger percentage of well elderly has reduced the appeal of retirement communities with finance plans that assumed people would move into them in their early 60s. The depopulation of some areas has forced hospitals to close and reduced the profitability of some medical practices.

Demographic changes occur continually. They can create new or expanded market opportunities for health services, or they can threaten existing services by lowering the demand for them. It is vital, however, to look behind superficial demographic trends. They may not apply to a specific service area, and their impact may be much more complex than it appears at first sight.

Psychographics

The same risks are inherent in looking for opportunities and threats in psychographic trends. Superficial findings can be very misleading. It takes careful thought and some experience in interpreting market research to draw meaningful conclusions about customers' values, preferences, dislikes, and expectations.

A number of hospitals in one area agreed to contribute to the costs of a shared large-scale public survey. They decided that they had more to gain from using the shared data intelligently than from concealing the data from each other. They jointly hired a survey company, and 2 months later, they all received the same 100 pages of tables. The survey asked people which local hospital was best for a wide variety of services. Table 7-1 lists some of the items surveyed and the percentage of "don't knows."

What excited several hospitals was the large number of "don't knows" in response to questions about which hospital was best for specific services. Each hospital saw these data as indicating that hospital advertising about specific services would pay off. A hospital that emphasized its women's services might capture a large number of the 50% who did not know which was best; so might a hospital that focused on advertising cancer care, and so on.

Table 7-1 Results of Hospital Preference Survey

Which Hospital:	% Don't Know
Are you most aware of ?	1
Do you most prefer for your own care?	1
Has the best nursing?	5
Has the best overall quality?	5
Has most concern for its patients?	10
Is best for cancer ?	35
Is best for cardiac care?	40
Is best for trauma care?	40
Is best for women's care?	50
Is best for ear, nose, and throat care?	60

A flurry of product line ads appeared in the local media — at least $4 million worth of such advertising over the next 12 months. Then, a follow-up survey showed that very little had changed.

What had gone wrong? Had the hospitals misinterpreted the data? All the clues that they needed to act more wisely are in the table above, and in one or two of the comments already made in Chapter 4.

First, the hospitals only paid attention to the last several questions in the table. The first few percentages show that almost everyone is well aware of hospitals, has a preference, and has an opinion about which hospital is best for important overall qualities. The other questions show that large numbers are uncertain about which is best for specific services. These two findings seem contradictory.

The paradox may be resolved if you think of your own behavior as a customer in other fields — for instance, buying jeans or shoes. Many customers have a firm opinion about the best place to go to buy jeans or shoes, but "don't know" where is the best place to look for "blue dress shoes to match that new dress," or "white jeans with a slim fit." That is a level of detail that many customers do not think it reasonable to know or want to know. If they want "blue dress shoes to match that new dress," many of them will go to their "best" shoe store, and only look elsewhere if it cannot help them. Even if a rival shoe store advertises "blue shoes to match your new fall dress," those people who see or hear the ad may not pay much attention to it, unless they are currently confronted with the need for blue shoes. Even then, many will still try in their "best" shoe shop first.

Second, this table alone does not say much about the "don't knows." They may not be at all like the "knows." Perhaps, for instance, they are mainly from that segment of the population described in Chapter 4 who align themselves with a primary physician and let him or her recommend hospitals as they need them. Perhaps the other segment that likes to make its own hospital selections, and may shop around to see which is best for different services, already have their minds made up and are unlikely to be swayed by product-specific ads.

In fact, elsewhere in the survey, the interviewers had asked a number of questions about the extent to which people had regular doctors and relied on them in hospital selection. If the hospitals had spent a little more to have the market research company run further analysis about the "don't knows," they would have learned more about this group's approach to hospital selection. Perhaps that information would have confirmed that product ads were the right strategy. If it had, it would have given the hospitals some valuable additional data about those people in order to better target their advertising to them.

This case does not prove that product ads are a waste of time. In many circumstances they are a good strategy. What the case does show is the risk of oversimplifying data about customer psychographics. The information available to these hospitals about those "don't knows" was inadequate as a basis for such a major and costly decision.

Conducting and interpreting market research in a way that minimizes these risks takes a little knowledge of statistics. It also takes quite a lot of knowledge about techniques of market research. Both subjects are beyond the scope of this book, but if you intend to conduct or to interpret market research findings, it would pay to take a course or read a basic text in statistical methods (e.g., Hamburg 1974; Mendenhall and Reinmuth 1974) and to take a course or read a basic text in practical market research methods (e.g., Chase and Barasch 1977; Vichas 1982).

However, reports of market research studies conducted by other people are appearing with increasing frequency in health care periodicals. Health care enterprises are also increasingly commissioning or conducting their own surveys, and health professionals will become more involved in reviewing and reacting to them. Unfortunately, some of these studies, like the example quoted above, lead to oversimplified conclusions. Even in some of those that reach the health care journals, the headline or major conclusions are at times not supported by the data. For instance, there are quite frequent reports about the "increasing number of adult Americans who regularly exercise." Other reports from the Surgeon General and other sources seem to call that finding into question, by reporting that the number of overweight and sedentary adults is stable or growing.

More probing studies of exercise habits seem to suggest that, although the majority of adults now take some regular exercise, for most it consists of "short walks." Others may exaggerate their exercise programs to interviewers, because they know that exercise is good for their health and that they should be more active. Similar studies of smokers and drinkers, for instance, show that they tend to understate their consumption of tobacco or alcohol. They also do so more in oral interviews (face-to-face or by phone) than in anonymous and written surveys.

It seems that the percentage of American adults who exercise regularly enough, vigorously enough, and for long enough to make any appreciable difference to their cardiovascular fitness may be growing, but it is still only a minority. Yet many health professionals and others have launched exercise programs or fitness centers based upon a superficial interpretation of the available data.

A hospital in the Chicago suburbs commissioned a study of local exercise patterns. As in the surveys mentioned above, a high percentage of respondents claimed to exercise regularly. The survey did probe a little into the types of exercise that people preferred. Again, it showed that walking predominated. Even among the minority who exercised more strenuously, it showed that their main exercise interests varied widely, from tennis to basketball, from aerobics to jogging, from weightlifting to cycling.

Despite this information, the hospital launched a fitness center with a very restricted range of options, largely Nautilus and aerobics. It proved to be a major money-loser. A large number of those regular exercisers preferred solo exercise programs, like jogging and cycling, which gave them relief from being around other people. Others belonged to one-sport clubs for swimming or tennis and were disinterested in Nautilus or aerobics. Still others saw their regular exercise as a social opportunity to be with family or friends, playing basketball or softball or touch football. Even among those interested in Nautilus or aerobics, many already belonged to clubs nearer their home, or to their commute to and from work, than the hospital. Some of these individuals had taken out lifetime or multi-year memberships in those clubs and were unlikely to switch, even to a club that might appear better, because they had not yet gotten their money's worth out of those memberships.

If you become involved in reviewing and reacting to market research reports, you should check the conclusions that their authors draw against the data they present. Ask yourself whether the data really support the findings. What may be an opportunity for others may not be an opportunity for your enterprise.

Even if you do not wish to become an expert statistician, it is worthwhile to understand a few essentials of statistics. There are, in fact, many forms of statistical analysis. In Chapters 3, 4, and 5, reference was made to some important conclusions drawn from studies that used complex statistical techniques such as multivariate analysis, varimax rotation, and various complicated correlation methods, to achieve such goals as describing psychographic segments and imputed attribute ranking. Many worthwhile studies depend, however, on more basic types of statistical inference. Common to many of them are a few concepts.

The first basic concept is that of the normal distribution. It asserts that many natural phenomena are "normally distributed," as in Figure 7-6, with most observations grouped around the average and only a few observations found at either extreme. Consider a simple example: the height of adult U.S. men. If the average height of adult men is 5'10'', one would expect most men to be close to that average, say, between 5'6'' and 6'2''. One would expect only a few men to be shorter than 5'6'' or taller than 6'2''. One would expect very few indeed to be less than 5'0'' or more than 6'8'' in height.

It may seem a stretch of the imagination to state that the same normal distribution applies to people's attitudes and beliefs, how satisfied they are with their doctors, which of two presidential candidates they favor, and whether they prefer their coffee strong or weak. The process of statistical inference, however, starts with that assumption or hypothesis.

Returning to the height of adult men, what would you conclude if you gathered the actual heights of the 250 male house staff at a university hospital and found that their average height was not 5'10'' but 6'0''? Suppose you also found that, rather than being grouped

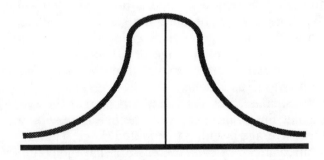

Figure 7-6 The normal distribution.

around that average, as the normal distribution predicts, only 100 of the doctors are below that average, while 150 are above it, and 10 of the doctors are actually over 6'8''.

Your obvious inference from these data would be that "Doctors at this hospital are not typical of the population at large with respect to their height. Or you might draw another conclusion: "If doctors at this hospital are typical of the population at large, then the average height of the population has increased since someone calculated it at 5'10'' for adult males."

Both conclusions *seem* to be supported by the data. Are they? Statisticians have devised calculations to help test such conclusions. One type of statistical test tries to answer the question, "If we know this is true of the population at large, but we get a different result looking at 250 people, is there something special about this group of people, or is it just a random fluke that our sample seems different?" A statistician may, in this example, come back with the answer that, if the average height of adult men is 5'10'', there is quite a reasonable probability that the average height of any sample of 250 men will be 2 inches, or 3%, different. There is nothing special about your group. Another type of statistical test tries to draw conclusions about the population at large from sample data. In fact, a *statistic* is a piece of data about a sample, such as its average height. A piece of data like this for the population at large is called a *parameter*. In this example, therefore, the question becomes "If the statistic of a sample of 250 adult men is that their average height is 6'0'', what is the average height parameter for the entire population of adult men?"

A statistician might come back with the answer that, based on the sample size and the sample statistic, the average height of the population of adult males at large is between 5'9'' and 6'3''. One cannot be more certain, because the statistician has only a small sample to work from. Rather than giving a precise answer, therefore, the statistician gives a range or a *confidence interval*. Rather than stating the range as 5'9'' to 6'3'', the statistician may express it as 6 feet plus or minus 3 inches.

The statistician is not absolutely certain that the average height of adult males lies in this range, but he or she may be 95% certain that the true average is within the quoted range. That degree of certainty is called a *level of confidence*. Note that the confidence interval is always a *range*, while the level of confidence is always a percentage probability.

What if a 95% level of confidence is not precise enough? After all, it leaves a 1 in 20 chance that the real average is outside that range. You cannot be 100% certain unless you measure every man in the population. The statistician can provide an estimate that is 99% certain, but to do so he or she must widen the confidence interval. For example, the statistician may be 99% certain that the actual average height is between 5'7" and 6'5".

The statistician could be more certain if the sample size was increased, but the sample would have to be increased very significantly to make much difference. Even with a sample of 1,000 men, the confidence interval in this example would only narrow by 1 or 2 inches.

For most practical purposes, increasing the degree of inaccuracy does not alter the implications. Consider, for instance, the statement that "52% plus or minus 3% of the practice's patients will report that they are very satisfied with the service and care that they received." Because of the margin of error (or confidence interval) involved, it is just as likely that 49% of patients feel this way as that 55% do. It might be nice to know that the real number is over 50% — that more people feel well served than do not. That more precise information would not, however, change the practical implication of the finding — that close to half of the practice's patients are not satisfied with the service received. Whether the real percentage of satisfied patients is 55%, 52%, or 49% makes no real difference. The practice has to do something to increase patient satisfaction.

In this example, patients were only given two choices: They were either satisfied or dissatisfied. Many surveys give more options, such as a four-point scale: very satisfied, somewhat satisfied, somewhat dissatisfied, or very dissatisfied. One expects that the response will mirror the normal distribution, with about one-third of the respondents in each of the two middle categories (each side of the average), and one-sixth in each of the extreme categories.

Table 7-2 summarizes the results of one such study, based upon a sample of 450 patients. This tables shows that the percentage of very satisfied patients is much higher than statistically expected, even allowing for the margin of error in the sampling. The percentage rating the practice in either of the top two categories (68%) is still somewhat higher than the expected 50%, after allowing for possible sampling error. Because these percentages are higher than statistical theory expects them to be, it is reasonable to conclude that satisfaction with the practice is reasonably high.

Table 7-2 Results of a Hospital Consumer Satisfaction Survey

	% Response	
Satisfaction with Practice	Expected	Actual
Very satisfied	17	38
Somewhat satisfied	33	30
Somewhat dissatisfied	33	12
Very dissatisfied	17	20

Percentages are accurate to within approximately ± 5 at 95% confidence.

The percentage of patients who are very dissatisfied, however, is also larger than expected. This distribution is not normal, as we expected, but *bimodal*, with peaks at the two ends. Although the majority of patients are satisfied, a significant minority are very dissatisfied. That is the danger of only looking at averages: they may conceal such unusual distributions on each side of the means. It was noted in Chapter 5 that very dissatisfied patients share their negative feelings with friends much more than do very satisfied patients. This practice, therefore, has a satisfaction problem even though a significant majority of its patients are pleased with its service.

The above discussion seems to have omitted reference to one other factor. Does not the *response rate* to a survey also have a major impact on its accuracy? It is not uncommon to hear questions about surveys that focus on the implications of only getting a 20% or a 30% response.

In fact, response rate is much less important to the accuracy of survey findings than sample size, as long as the sample is broadly representative of the population. Consider, for instance, a researcher who calls 5,000 households to check which television shows members have watched in the last week, but only gets through to 1,000 of those households. The response rate is thus only 20%. Nevertheless, as long as those 1,000 households are broadly representative of the population at large, very accurate conclusions can be drawn. This is, incidentally, very close to the way that the Nielsen ratings of TV audience size are actually calculated. Various independent parallel surveys have confirmed that the Nielsen results are very accurate.

If the respondents do not seem broadly representative of the population being studied, it may be worthwhile to gather more responses from the underrepresented segment. If, for instance, it seems important to have men and women proportionately represented, and only 40% of respondents are men, it may be appropriate to seek more male respondents. Merely trying to increase the sample size may not eliminate that bias. If only 40% of the additional respondents are men, the bias will remain. In practice, the more sophisticated types of statistical software now available can weight the sample to compensate for such obvious underrepresentation.

There is a continuing debate among market research experts about so-called *respondent bias*. While it is possible to adjust a sample to correct for an underrepresented demographic segment (e.g., men, people over 65, people living in Middletown etc.), there is always a possibility that those who responded have different opinions from those who did not. Again, increasing the response rate helps to reduce this risk, but a far better approach is to run a second, smaller survey among nonrespondents to the first survey and to compare the two samples.

In any event, the risk of respondent bias leading to false conclusions may not be great in practice. As already noted, it is only wise to act upon findings that are very significant, not upon apparent fine distinctions. Several of the studies quoted in Chapter 4, for instance, found that more than 90% of respondents, when asked to rank the top two of three attributes most important in a physician, mentioned "explains things well." No other factor was mentioned by more than 70%, and quite a few factors were only chosen by handfuls of respondents (including "where he trained," and "medical school affiliation"). These percentages are far from the statistically expected levels: If people are asked to prioritize 3 of 10 attributes, the "expected" random result is that each will be mentioned by 30%. An attribute selected by 90% in several independent studies, when the expected selection rate was only 30%, is clearly an important and significant finding whatever respondent bias may have occurred. If, by contrast, all the 10 attributes offered had been selected by at most 40% at least 20%, compared to an expected 30% selection for each, it would be unwise to draw any practical conclusion other than that all these attributes are of roughly equal importance.

Often it is desirable to break down the results obtained from a sample survey. It may be useful, for instance, to compare the views of men and women, or of different age groups, or of patients coming at different times of the day. Statisticians again have techniques for performing such analyses. The basic principles are the same as those already described for looking at samples as a whole.

Statisticians call such pieces of samples *cells*. As described above, when they are asked to draw conclusions about populations from samples, they look at sample size to assess the accuracy of their conclusions, and they quote them as a range or confidence interval. They do the same when asked to compare a cell with an entire sample. Because cells are only pieces of samples, cell size is smaller than sample size. As might be expected, therefore, their confidence intervals around conclusions about individual cells are larger than those around conclusions about samples.

Indeed, if the cell sizes become too small, they become "unstable," and it may not be possible to draw conclusions about them with an real accuracy.

For example, a hospital conducted a satisfaction survey among patients discharged through the previous 3 months and received some 300 replies. The questions all used a 5-point scale, and the answers were converted to a weighted average. One of the lowest scores was given to "noise." The results were then broken out between men and women. Women gave the hospital worse ratings for noise than did men. The results were also broken out by nursing unit of which there were over 20 in all. For simplicity, Table 7-3 just shows the best- and worst-rated nursing units on the noise parameter.

As a result of these findings, the hospital reached three conclusions: (a) Noise was a problem; (b) female patients were most sensitive to it; (c) it was worst on one unit. The nursing director selected that unit for a pilot effort at noise control. It happened to be a general medical-surgical unit. What should she have done instead?

First, even though many surveys report results in terms of 4- or 5-point scales, this does not make for easy reading. Since statisticians most often express confidence intervals as percentages, or points out of 100, such an approach also makes it easier to understand their qualifying comments about such tables. The difference between the best and the worst unit looks larger than expressed as 3.4 versus 3.0 than when converted to 68 versus 60.

Table 7-3 Consumer Dissatisfaction with Hospital Noise Levels

Category	No. of Replies	Rating for Satisfaction With Noise Levels[a]
All respondents	300	3.25
Men	120	3.65
Women	180	2.95
Best of 25 nursing units	30	3.40
Worst of 25 nursing units	20	3.00

[a]Average of responses on a 5-point scale.

Second, the nursing director neither understood confidence intervals nor asked a statistician for help in reading this table. In fact, given the total sample size, the average rating of 3.25, or 65 out of 100, is accurate to within some 5%. In other words, it is better stated as 65 ± 5. Because the cell size of the number of men, or women, is smaller than the total sample size, the confidence interval widens to about 7%. Men thus rate satisfaction with noise at 73 ± 7, and women rate it at 59 ± 7. The cell sizes for the individual nursing units are so small that it is almost impossible to compare them accurately with each other or with the overall average. It is, indeed, very possible that the worst rated unit is actually the best, and vice versa.

What the director of nursing probably should have done, given that she wanted to run a pilot program on one unit first, was to select an all-female unit, not the one that appeared worst but probably was not. The data do suggest that female patients are less satisfied with noise control. The cell sizes are too small to suggest which unit is really the worst.

Psychographic changes in people's attitudes, likes, and dislikes can create new market opportunities and new market threats. The fitness craze has made it acceptable to wear warm-up suits and sneakers for routine casual wear in place of slacks and loafers, thus expanding the market for sports clothing. Concern with looking thin and young has increased the demand for light beer and hair colorants for men. The growing emancipation of women in the workplace and in social pursuits has made it profitable to market beer as a woman's drink and to offer smaller food portions in restaurants catering for business lunches.

In health care, reduced loyalty to primary physicians has expanded the demand for hospital referral services. People are less willing to accept chronic pain, and this has increased the use of chiropractors. A reduced willingness among working women to sacrifice career goals to take care of elderly parents has increased the demand for senior day centers.

Changing fashions in hair styles has posed a threat to the makers of hair creams, and opened an opportunity for makers of dry hair dressings. The psychographic reaction of many drivers to the 1970s' oil crisis was to switch to smaller cars, posing a threat that took the U.S. auto industry more than a decade to manage. The continued preference of many baby boomers for rock music has depressed the audiences of easy listening radio stations, which previously picked up listeners as people reached their 40s.

In health care, significantly lower tolerance for delays in obtaining service has stimulated the growth of faster and more convenient urgicenters and surgicenters. The trickling down of these values to the poor, together with their greater sense of entitlement, has made the classic slow and disorganized university hospital clinic struggle for patients and forced new thinking on how to give residents ambulatory care experience in other settings. Rising standards of judgment among women on what constitutes good decor, a comfortable waiting area, and privacy in changing rooms, has lowered their tolerance of many hospital outpatient facilities.

As well as reviewing and interpreting psychographic surveys critically, and seeing if the data support the conclusions, even a basic understanding of the principles of sampling and statistical analysis will help you to identify opportunities and threats more accurately.

Life-Style

As mentioned earlier, life-style is essentially a product of demographics and psychographics. With rising affluence and increased individualism, however, a variety of differing life-styles have proliferated. Any generalization about "the typical customer" is now becoming suspect. Many large enterprises have decided that general products and services for a general market are now less likely to succeed than a wide variety of special products and services tailored to *niche markets* of people with particular life-styles.

As one illustration, recent demographic changes have increased the percentage of women working outside the home. Psychographic changes have extended the period over which many couples are now spreading their childbearing years. In combination, these trends have produced a much more segmented pattern of households with distinctive life-styles. One analysis, for instance, of the 30 million or so two-income households in the United States divides them (in order of prevalence) into "full-nesters" (working spouses with children aged 6 to 17), "crowded-nesters" (working spouses with children aged 18 to 24), "new parents" (working spouses with children under 6), "honeymooners" (young working spouses with no children), "empty-nesters" (older working spouses whose children have left home), "young families" (working spouses with children of varying ages), and "just a couple" (older working spouses who have never had children) (Townsend and Riche 1987).

Add to that segmentation the fact that couples may now start a family at any time between their late teens and about age 40, and you produce a patchwork quilt of household structures that belies the notion of an archetypical model family. As one example, it is possible for four neighbors to consist of one household of "empty-nesters" in their early 40s (if they had their children in their early 20s), next to "new parents" who are actually a year or two older than them (if the started their family in their late 30s), next to "crowded nesters" in their late 50s (if they have children in their 20s still living at home), next to "just a couple" in their early 50s.

How do you market soup to this row of homes? The soup ad of the past appealed to the nonworking woman at home, waiting for the return of her spouse from work and her children from school, with a smile on her face and a can of soup on the boil. Not one of the four households described above fits that model. They either have no children at home, have grown up children capable of fixing their own soup, or have young children but both spouses work. How do you market Avon cosmetics to them? Not one of the women is likely to have the time, energy, inclination, and financial need to go selling door-to-door, and if she did, it is uncertain whom she would find at home. Campbell Soup and Avon happen to be two of the companies that have identified the threats facing them from Americans' changing life-styles and have developed both new products and new marketing methods in response.

To take a health care example, a young orthopedist completed his residency and set up a suburban sports medicine practice near the city where he had trained. A competitive runner himself, he soon developed an active practice. His early patients were fellow runners whom he had met at local races during his residency, but they soon passed news of the practice on to friends. His own involvement in the sport gave him not only contacts but immediate credibility with his patients.

After about a year in practice, the orthopedist was featured prominently in a Sunday edition of the local newspaper, which further boosted his practice. What he had done, by accident more than design, was to position his practice to appeal to a small but active life-style segment of the population: competitive runners.

One of the readers of that newspaper report was this physician's former chief of orthopedics. He had never rated the young doctor highly when a resident. He was also skeptical that there was such a subspecialty as sports medicine. It was, in his opinion, just general orthopedics by another name. The chief of orthopedics decided to launch his own sports medicine center at the university. It would meet in his offices on Tuesday afternoons, where patients would be seen by residents under his supervision. The public relations office of the university issued a press release announcing the new service. It was carried by the same newspaper that had featured his young competitor, but on a Wednesday, and as a small story on an inside page. Nine months later, University Sports Medicine Center was quietly allowed to die, having treated fewer than 10 patients.

A few years later, another large hospital in town launched a sports medicine program. By now the young orthopedist's practice was large. It still consisted mainly of runners, but word had spread to some other sports enthusiasts. The new program decided that the time had come to segment this life-style group even further. It announced different office sessions for different types of sports: tennis, swimming, weightlifting, golfing, basketball, football, skiing, and so on. It was also staffed by doctors who were active in at least one of these sports. This program also proved reasonably successful, but not at the expense of the young orthopedist, who continues to prosper.

There are many other examples of the impact of changing life-styles on health care. The increased value that some people place on their leisure time has reduced their tolerance for long waits for service. More hospital inpatients are anxious to get out as quickly as possible and return to their chosen life-styles. Increased exercise has increased the fitness of an active minority of people, but also increased the incidence of foot problems, such as minor injuries and sprains. Growing social recognition of passive smoking has led to more peer pressure on smokers to seek help in quitting. Decisions to delay childbirth until later in adulthood have increased the need for high-risk obstetrical services. The greater number of women who expect to remain "in control" of childbirth has increased the demand for alternative birthing facilities, both inside and outside hospitals.

Although life-style changes have their roots in the interaction of demographic and psychographic changes, they are worth examining in their own right. Their consequences, both good and bad, for providers of services can be profound.

Epidemiological Trends

As mentioned earlier, health care providers should also pay particular attention to epidemiological trends, just as clothing stores need to watch trends in dress and fashion, and banks need to watch trends in spending and saving behaviors.

Epidemiological trends are themselves the result of the interplay of some of the other environmental factors already discussed: advances in medical technology, changes in economic conditions, demographic shifts, and psychographic and life-style changes. Nevertheless, it may well at times be easier to detect the first clue of a new opportunity or threat in epidemiological change itself than in one of its underlying causes.

If a new phenomenon has already begun to impact epidemiological patterns, it is somewhat less speculative than if it seems about to happen because, for instance, of some shift in demographics. U.S. hospitals ought to have seen by the mid-1970s that falling length-of-stay and rising ambulatory surgery would reduce the demand for hospital beds, but many hospitals went on adding beds until these changes resulted in reduced occupancy rates.

The other environmental factors discussed above are therefore worth monitoring, because they may give an early warning signal of a coming epidemiological change, and because spotting that signal ahead of competitors may provide a real competitive advantage. Epidemiological trends are also worth studying, however, because they may show up a change that was not apparent from looking at those other aspects of the environment.

Epidemiological changes can be of two types. They may be products of real changes in medical know-how or of other environmental factors, like the increase in the percentage of deaths attributable to trauma, or the rising teenage suicide rate, or the decline in rheumatic heart disease, or the reduced need for tonsillectomies or surgical treatment of ulcers. They may also, however, be the result of improved differential diagnosis. Reflex sympathetic dystrophy was commonly confused with other causes of chronic intractable pain until the 1980s. Compulsive gambling was only officially recognized as a distinct psychiatric disorder in the early 1980s. Bulimia was recognized earlier but was not widely known among parents and even many primary doctors to be a separate and treatable condition. Male impotence was widely assumed to be psychosomatic, until improved research in the 1960s and 1970s showed that organic causes were responsible in many cases, and mixed organic and mental causes in some others. Osteoporosis has been known about for a long time, but only recently has it been closely associated with fractures in the elderly.

Even if an epidemiological change is simply the result of improved medical definition, it can still have a major impact on the pattern of health care services. Each of the examples of improved definition quoted in the previous paragraph has provided the opportunity for the creation of new treatment centers. Each major medical improvement can also pose a threat to some part of the existing delivery system. Just as there were many tuberculosis sanitoria before about 1950, there were specialized centers for the care of children and sometimes adults with rheumatic heart conditions prior to about 1960. In that same year, tonsillectomy was among the three most common inpatient surgical procedures performed in U.S. hospitals. Two decades later it had become a much less common procedure, largely performed, if at all, on a same-day basis.

Despite the growth in the under-16 population in the 1970s and early 1980s, the number of pediatric beds in hospitals has plummeted. Rapid and far-reaching improvements in pharmaceuticals and in ambulatory care now keep many more sick children out of the hospital. Those who do need inpatient care tend to be much more sick than children admitted to hospitals two decades ago. They tend to need the skills of subspecialists in various branches of pediatrics, and they tend to need very specialized nursing care. As a result, many community hospitals have cut down considerably or even eliminated their pediatric units. At the same time, many of the major university hospitals, with large and specialized pediatric staffs, have increased their pediatric census.

To take another example, the vehicular accident rate has risen and has increased the traffic through many hospital emergency rooms. Advances in trauma care, however, have at the same time made it desirable that any victim with major multisystem injury be transferred to a trauma center with specialized multidisciplinary staff on duty at all times to provide rapid treatment. Because that highly specialized care is most likely to be effective if started within the "golden hour" after traumatic injury, such trauma centers are being created in most parts of the country. Getting patients to them within that critical first hour has also required more and better trained paramedical personnel, improved emergency life-support vehicles, and air evacuation helicopters to serve the more remote areas.

Epidemiological changes can create both new opportunities and new threats for providers of health services. Even though they are nearly always caused by other environmental changes — in technology, economics, demography, psychographics, or life-style — the practical consequences may be overlooked or may be unclear, until they show up as actual changes in epidemiology. It is important, therefore, to monitor and assess such changes carefully.

References

Applebaum, W., and S. Cohen. 1961. The dynamics of store location strategy and market equilibrium. *Annals of the Association of American Geographers.*

Booz Allen and Hamilton. 1982. *New product management for the 1980s.* New York: Booz Allen and Hamilton.

Cadbury, N. D. 1975. When, where and how to test market. *Harvard Business Review* (May-June): 96-105.

Capon, N., and R. Glazer. 1987. Marketing and technology: a strategic co-alignment. *Journal of Marketing* 51(3).

Chase, C., and K. Barasch. 1977. *Marketing problem solver.* Radnor, PA: Chilton Book Company.

Dickson, P. R., and J. Giglierano. 1986. Missing the boat and sinking the boat: A conceptual model of entrepreneurial risk. *Journal of Marketing* 50(3): 58-70.

Fisk, T. 1986. *Advertising health services: What works, what fails,* pp. 10-12. Chicago: Pluribus Press.

Galton, L. 1985. *MedTech.* New York: Harper and Row.

Hamburg, M. 1974. *Basic statistics.* New York: Harcourt, Brace and Jovanovich.

Hrebiniak, L., and W. Joyce. 1986. The strategic importance of managing myopia. *Sloan Management Review* 28(1): 5-14.

Kanter, R. M. 1984. Innovation: The only hope for time ahead. *Sloan Management Review* 25(4): 51-5.

Kiplinger, A. 1986. *The Kiplinger Washington Newsletter* 63: 52.

Levitt, T. 1960. Marketing myopia. *Harvard Business Review* (July-Aug): 45-56.

Mendenhall, W., and J. Reinmuth. 1974. *Statistics for management and economics.* Scituate, MA: Duxbury Press.

Newitt, J. 1984. Where do suburbanites come from? *American Demographics* (June): 25-27.

Nielsen Marketing Services. 1980. New product success ratios. *The Nielsen Researcher* 1.

Nelson, R., M. Peck, and E. Kalachek. 1967. *Technology-economic growth and public policy.* Washington, DC: Brookings Institution.

Peters, T., and R. Waterman. 1983. *In search of excellence.* New York: Warner Books.

Porat, M. 1976. *The information economy and the economy of information.* Stanford, CA: Stanford University.

Porter, M. 1985. *Competitive advantage:*

Creating and sustaining superior performance. New York: The Free Press.

Quinn, J. B. 1979. Technological innovation, entrepreneurship and strategy. *Sloan Management Review* (Spring).

Roberts, E. 1987. *Generating technological innovation.* New York: Oxford University Press.

Townsend, B., and M. Riche. 1987. Two paychecks and seven lifestyles. *American Demographics* (August): 24-29.

Von Hippel, E. 1978. Successful industrial products from customer ideas. *Journal of Marketing* (January): 39-49.

Von Oech, R. 1983. *A whack on the side of the head: How to unlock the mind for innovation.* New York: Warner Books.

Vichas, R. P. 1982. *Complete handbook of profitable market research techniques.* Englewood Cliffs, NJ: Prentice Hall.

Witt Associates. 1983. *The physician as entrepreneur: Executive forum.* Chicago: Witt Associates.

Zarecor, W. 1975. High technology product planning. *Harvard Business Review* (January-February): 108-115.

Review Questions

1. A very large percentage of new service ideas fail. What are some of the most common reasons?

2. "Successful services offer effective and different solutions to common problems." Where might you look to identify problems for which you might have the effective and different solution?

3. What are marketing myopia and marketing presbyopia?

4. "We often talk about health care technology as if it were one thing. It is not." Discuss.

5. How does market geography influence what a health provider can and cannot do successfully?

6. "Market research can be very misleading." Discuss.

Chapter 8

Evaluating Service Ideas

Concept Screening

The purpose of the environmental analysis discussed in the previous chapter is to identify new opportunities and threats. If performed thoroughly, and if the results are added to those new ideas that surface spontaneously from people inside the enterprise, there will be far too many potentially good ideas for the enterprise to be able to pursue all of them. There may well even be too many for all to be studied seriously.

Organizations that manage innovation effectively have procedures in place to screen all such ideas very rapidly and to select just a fraction of them to study in more depth. Some of these screening systems are formalized and quantitative, such as the Boston Consulting Group's Product Portfolio Matrix or General Electric's Business Screen. Various texts (e.g., Ansoff 1976; Porter 1980; Hax 1987; Roberts and Berry 1985) describe these and other screening methods in detail. This chapter offers a broad introduction to the processes involved, and provides one relatively simply model for concept screening in the context of health care.

The key questions to ask in screening any new product or service concept are:

1. Is it compatible with the organization's mission statement?

2. Do the people within the organization already have the experience and the expertise required to implement it?

3. How closely does the potential market for this new product or service parallel those the organization already serves? What is its service compatibility?

4. Will the new product or service use channels of distribution with which the organization already deals? What is its distribution channel compatibility?

5. To what extent does this new idea compete with existing products and services of the enterprise? What internal competition does it create?

6. What are the costs involved? What is the idea's affordability?

7. To what extent might the organization be able to offer this product or service at a lower price than competitors? What is its likely price advantage?

8. What is the total need for this product or service in the service area, and what market share will be required to cover costs?

9. At what stage of its life-cycle is this product or service?

10. How does this idea rank on these nine factors compared to other ideas that the organization might pursue?

The Mission Statement

There are many ideas that an organization *could* pursue. One of the primary purposes of a mission statement is to help select those that the organization *should* pursue. Every year, bright people leave major organizations to pursue ideas that their employer would not develop. Sometimes the organization was short-sighted. Often, however, the idea just did not fit in with the priorities defined in the company's mission statement. Even when those bright ideas go on to become successful products and services, the organization was not necessarily at fault for rejecting it. It may have chosen to pursue other, equally successful ideas.

Not every idea identified in an environmental analysis, then, "belongs" in the organization that detects it. Not every bright idea suggested by people within the enterprise is a sensible one for that organization to pursue. Screening new ideas against a mission statement helps to sort out those that are really worth detailed analysis.

Organizational Experience and Expertise

It is easy for an organization to assume that its people can do anything. The purpose of the second question in the list above is to consider whether the organization has the *experience and expertise* necessary to pursue a specific new idea. As noted in Chapter 7, successful innovation requires at least an adequate competence in three areas: product or service know-how, process know-how, and relevant management know-how. It also usually requires a level of competence greater than that of potential competitors in at least one of these three areas, to give the organization a competitive advantage over those rivals.

For many health services, it makes sense to subdivide existing expertise and experience into four dimensions:

1. Physician competence

2. Nursing (or other health professional) competence

3. Technical personnel competence

4. Managerial personnel competence

To take an example, a psychiatrist at a hospital was very interested in the treatment of chronic intractable pain syndromes. He realized that such cases often have both a psychosomatic and an organic element. He therefore talked with his colleagues until he found an internal medicine specialist willing to collaborate with him in this program. The psychiatrist also assigned a psychologist in his department to help with the initial evaluation and treatment of patients. The hospital marketing staff considered this an attractive idea and one that their expertise and experience would make easy to market. They launched a mailing campaign to local doctors and soon attracted a number of referrals.

Some months later, the head of anesthesiology at a rival hospital recruited a young colleague who had just completed a fellowship at one of the few pain centers in the United States with at least a decade of experience with such programs. The new recruit had acquired substantial expertise at using nerve blocks and various other techniques to alleviate chronic pain. There were already both an internal medicine specialist and a psychiatrist on that hospital's staff who had been treating chronic pain on an individual basis. They now joined forces with the new anesthesiologist. That hospital's marketing department also promoted its pain program to local doctors. Soon this rival program proved very successful, and the original program at the other hospital lost volume.

What was the key difference between these two centers? Although treating chronic pain syndromes requires the active involvement of both an internal medicine specialist and a psychiatric staff, the roles that they play are relatively easy to match at another hospital with such doctors on staff. It is much more difficult to find an anesthesiologist with expertise in this field. Both hospitals possessed the necessary managerial and health professional expertise, and some of the necessary physician expertise. Only one of the two, however, could add the other element of physician and technical expertise needed. Indeed, one reason for the rapid success of the second center was that some patients who had tried the first center had quickly lost faith in it and reported its apparent lack of progress in relieving their pain back to their referring doctors. Those primary doctors were ready to try an alternative center that seemed to have a broader competence.

Two common fallacies to which organizations sometimes fall victim are that missing expertise and experience can be rapidly acquired by training existing staff or by hiring new personnel. Both methods of adding expertise can work, but rarely if ever do they work as fast as expected.

The so-called *learning curve* frustrates the quick development of new expertise. The early development phase of a service, process, or management technology that is new to an organization is usually quite slow. Eventually that expertise reaches a critical level from which it then expands more rapidly. The concept of the learning curve applies just as well to professional activities as to product development (Wheatley 1983).

The hiring of new personnel into an organization to give it new expertise and predeveloped experience also usually takes longer to make an impact than is often assumed. Very seldom can the new employee immediately contribute to the organization without the help and support of many of its existing personnel. This is particularly true in relatively complex activities like health care, where most practical results depend upon a complicated pattern of team effort.

The new employee is being hired to change the enterprise by adding new expertise to it. He or she may well, therefore, also encounter resistance to change. Before the new employee can really function effectively, he or she has to "educate" those whose cooperation is vital—to move them further up their own learning curve. For instance, a number of the executives hired to start first-ever marketing programs for hospitals have found that it may take 18 months to 2 years to introduce the marketing concept, as a new management technology, within the organization before they can take any significant actions. The same pattern has been noticed in non-health care organizations introducing marketing as a new activity (Costello 1987).

Because expertise and experience are, in fact, quite difficult to develop, even by hiring new personnel, it is worthwhile to examine all new ideas to see how much of the necessary know-how already exists within the enterprise. It is much easier to develop an idea successfully if there are people on board who have already advanced quite far along the relevant learning curves.

Service Compatibility

It is also less of a challenge to pursue an idea with a high level of service compatibility. The ideal new idea directly addresses benefits sought by customers who are already using the organization. For instance, it should be much easier for a hospital to promote pediatric care to mothers who elected to come there for childbirth than to mothers who did not, as long as they were very satisfied with the care and service that they received. By contrast, it is much more difficult for hospitals to sell billing services to physician practices, because, for the most part, the hospitals' prior relationships with those practices have not been concerned with issues of practice management and organization. Even though a physician may know a hospital well, he or she does not necessarily have any reason to believe that he can trust his billing and revenue collection to it.

This concept of service compatibility has been translated into a set of rules, which are carefully followed by many innovative organizations. It is easiest for an organization to expand by either

1. Introducing existing products to new markets (*market development*), or

2. Introducing new products to existing markets (*product development*).

It is much more difficult for an organization to create new products for new markets—*diversification* (Ansoff 1976). Perhaps the easiest strategy of all is to sell more of existing products to already existing markets (*market penetration*). However, that may not be as easy as it sounds if the organization already has a high market share, or if the product is already in decline. Both of these issues will be reviewed later in this chapter.

The ideas most likely to succeed are those most closely related to other services for which customers already use and value the organization. By contrast, existing customers may not readily accept the organization as a credible supplier of services that represent a radical departure from those previously supplied.

As an example, it was mentioned in the last chapter that the increased percentage of working women in the economy has dealt a triple blow to Avon Cosmetics. It has reduced the supply of Avon ladies, fewer women are at home during the day when the representatives call, and working women have more discretionary income to buy more expensive cosmetics. Avon decided to respond by an act of market development, by selling additional products to its existing market. It bought a jewelry company, Tiffany's, and started offering inexpensive jewelry under the Tiffany label. Many customers, however, accepted neither Avon as a source of jewelry nor Tiffany as a product sold in the home.

Distribution Channel Compatibility

In the above example, the new product was not accepted as service compatible, nor did it possess *distribution channel compatibility*. Tiffany products had not previously been sold in that manner.

As another example, many hospitals have advertised their capabilities in cancer treatment. The direct public response has usually been less than for other advertised services where there is at least some tradition of self-referral to hospitals. However, ads may well have benefitted the hospitals by increasing awareness of their programs among physicians and the public. Some patients looking for a second opinion about a diagnosis of cancer may also have been stimulated to respond directly. The response has been lower than for some advertised services because self-referral to a hospital for cancer diagnosis or treatment represents an unfamiliar distribution channel to many people.

It is easier to market a new idea that will use methods of distribution with which the enterprise already deals than one that requires new trading relationships.

Internal Competition

Some new ideas may not add new volume to an organization at all. They may just substitute a new service for an old one that the enterprise is providing, thus constituting *internal competition*.

Many hospitals, for example, have successfully added VIP patient suites as a new service. Others have tried to do so and failed. One hospital administration was asked by its trustees to screen such an idea. The initial screening review was inconclusive, but the administrators were skeptical that the idea would work. Rather than invest time and money in a full-scale feasibility study, they formulated a simple and quick test. They obtained the membership list of the local country club. They argued that, if this idea was to work at all, it would have to work with this group as constituting several hundred of the wealthiest people in the area.

The hospital mailed a one-page questionnaire to this list. It received almost 100 replies and revealed two major findings. First, the only people who would use the VIP suites were people for whom the hospital was already the preferred hospital. The suites were unlikely to lead to any additional patients. Second, the respondents wanted such suites to contain a wide range of amenities, which the hospital estimated would add some $200 to the daily room rate. However, fewer than 5% of the respondents were willing to pay more than $100 for all the amenities they expected, and so the service would lose money, while doing nothing to increase admissions. All the new idea would do, therefore, was to provide internal competition to existing rooms.

There are some circumstances where it makes sense to substitute a new idea for an existing one. Both computer companies and pharmaceutical firms, for instance, frequently withdraw an old product from the market and substitute an alternative. They do so, however, because they predict that someone will come out with a superior product if they do not do so themselves. By being first with the new generation of products, they can preserve their market share rather than lose it to a competitor.

It is more profitable to concentrate on ideas that expand the organization's volume of sales or services, rather than those which merely substitute for them and, thus, constitute internal competition. There may, however, be cases where it makes sense to develop a product or service, for example, when a competitor might come out with a superior product or service unless the organization does so itself.

Affordability

The main test of the *affordability* of a new idea is usually deferred until the feasibility study. However, if the issue is ignored completely during concept screening, an organization could find itself in trouble. It may have selected too many costly ideas and rejected others that were slightly less attractive but significantly less expensive.

The three most critical financial screens are:

1. What is the approximate capital cost of the project?

2. How long will it take to break even (i.e., to cover the project's operating costs)?

3. How long will it take to reach payback (i.e., to cover its operating costs and yield enough surplus to repay its initial capital costs)?

Somebody has to finance the operating expenses of any new idea until it reaches the *breakeven point* and is bringing in enough revenue to cover its own daily costs. Somebody has to finance its initial capital costs for an even longer period, until it reaches *payback* and recoups those start-up costs. The data in Table 8-1 provide an illustration of the concepts of breakeven and payback.

A hospital developed a rehabilitation satellite in a nearby suburb. Its cash flow history followed a pattern similar to that in Table 8-1. All the numbers, however, were about four times larger. By the end of the second year, its accumulated negative cash flow stood at $220,000, and the hospital trustees began to get nervous about the

Table 8-1 Cash Flows to Break Even and Payback

Year	Cash Required	Cash Earned	Cash Flow to Date
Start-up	$40,000		($40,000)
1	$20,000	$10,000	($50,000)
2	$25,000	$20,000	($55,000)
3	$30,000	$30,000 **break even**	($55,000)
4	$35,000	$50,000	($40,000)
5	$40,000	$60,000	($20,000)
6	$45,000	$65,000	**payback**

project. Closing the satellite down was seriously discussed, but in the end it was decided to give it one more year.

By the end of that year, the satellite had broken even. The trustees were still concerned about the $220,000 accumulated negative cash flow, but at least that amount had not increased in year 3. As that amount fell through the next 3 years, they became more relaxed. The satellite, now beyond its sixth year, makes a reasonable profit of some $80,000 each year.

Did the hospital make the right decision in launching this satellite? It appears that it did: The project reached breakeven, then reached payback, then became very profitable. However, the hospital did not make the right decision if it invested funds in this project instead of in some other service concept in which it could have even more success.

Many small enterprises go out of business that might, like this example, have eventually proved very successful. They do so because the owners, or their bank, cannot or will not maintain the negative cash flow long enough to get them to payback. Others go out of business because they can offer no evidence that they will eventually get there. The project in Table 8-1 had no such evidence to offer until the third year. Up to that time, its negative cash flow just kept on growing. Even in year 3, it only succeeded in stabilizing cash flow. It was not until year 4 that its cash flow deficit started to come down.

In larger organizations with multiple products or services, existing programs as well as new concepts may have cash flow needs. Even if an existing service is making a profit, it may need further capital to replace equipment that is wearing out or to expand space or personnel. The organization may therefore have to borrow from the profits of other programs or from outside to sustain that existing service.

Some new service concepts may not be affordable, even if they seem likely to become profitable in time. The organization may not be able to afford the negative cash flow required to support the new service until it reaches breakeven and payback. The new service concept may not only be in competition with other new concepts for cash. It may also have to compete with existing services that need more money injected into them.

Price Advantage

It may not be essential for a new service concept to give the enterprise a *price advantage* over its competitors. Many products and services do not succeed by price alone. Greater perceived quality, greater customer convenience, greater reliability through time, easier maintenance, and being seen as more up-to-date are all common reasons why customers may not necessarily be attracted to the lowest price option available.

As an example, a young family physician bought a practice in a small town from an elderly and well-respected physician who had decided to retire. In fact, this doctor had been in semi-retirement for some years. Recently he had only had office hours three mornings a week and saw only three or four patients on each of those mornings. The new doctor knew that he needed almost 100 office visits weekly to cover his costs, repay the bank loan that he had taken out to buy the practice, repay the loans still outstanding from his medical training, and take home an acceptable personal income.

The older doctor had not been bothered about his low office volume. He had made a lot of money over a lifetime in practice and had few financial commitments. He had mainly kept the office open as a service to a few patients of long standing.

After 6 months, the new doctor was still only seeing between 10 and 15 patients weekly and was heading deeper into debt. He decided that he needed a second source of income. He knew that many young doctors in similar circumstances had worked shifts in local emergency rooms, where they could pick up $200 or so a night. He came up with a different "new service concept." He would make house calls at night. He assumed that he would have to price such calls competitively with the charges made by local emergency rooms for walk-in patients, and so he chose a price of $40.

To market his new service, the new doctor decided on two methods. He would advertise in local papers serving the area within about 20 miles of his home. He would also write to doctors in that area offering to make house calls on their patients at night. He thought that they would welcome this offer. If they made house calls themselves, he would relieve them of doing so each time a patient asked. If they did not make house calls, his service might be a useful enhancement to their practices. He knew that doctors would be concerned that he might poach their patients for his own practice, so he promised not to do so.

After another 6 months, the new physician found that his practice was now profitable. He was averaging about 20 house calls a week referred by other doctors. His advertising was generating another 10 house calls weekly. Even though the advertising was a new cost, a number of the patients that he had met through these house calls had become regular patients, and his office volume had risen to 40 visits weekly. He had maintained his policy of not poaching patients whom he met by physician referral.

However, each of his house calls were taking an average of 60 minutes including travel, and, at 30 night-time house calls per week, he was suffering from fatigue. He decided to seek another young physician, at a similar stage of building his practice, to share in the home visits.

However, his average of some four house calls nightly produced about $160 in revenue. All the other young doctors to whom he spoke said that they could make more than that working a night in an emergency room. Some of the local emergency rooms were in fact fairly quiet after midnight, and covering them was not a strenuous task. Those that were busy offered a much more interesting variety of cases than four or five house calls could. In any event, if he gave the entire $40 for a house call to other young doctors, he would make nothing out of them for himself. He might as well never have started the service.

The new doctor therefore discovered that, although his $40 price gave him a price advantage over local emergency rooms, it was too low to be profitable for him. He had never considered that there might be other benefits to house calls in the eyes of both patients and referring doctors that made price less important. The 20 or so weekly house calls that he was getting by physician referral were bringing in $800 weekly. His advertising was costing him $200 weekly, but bringing both 10 house calls and about 30 extra office visits at $40 each. After paying for the advertising, therefore, it was producing $1,400 weekly. The office visits that he inherited from the previous practitioner added $400 weekly. In total, therefore, he was receiving, after his advertising costs, $2,600 to cover his office and other costs and to leave him with a personal income.

What this doctor probably should have done from the start was to charge more for his night-time house calls (perhaps $60) and not offered to do them by referral at all. He would have forgone the $800 that his referred house calls produced weekly, but also saved himself 20 night-time hours of work. At $60 for a house call, and $40 for an office visit, he would have made $2,000, or $1,800 after the cost of his ads. With the office visits he inherited, his revenue would have been $2,200. In other words, he would have had $400 a week less income, but 20 fewer night-time hours of work. If he felt that he could not live on that reduced income, he too could have worked in local emergency rooms at $200 a night. Two such nights a week and his income would be back at $2,600. He would still be putting in fewer hours, and he would have more flexibility to decide which nights to work and which to sleep.

A price advantage may or may not be important to the success of a new service concept, but, at the screening stage, an idea that can create such a price advantage is more attractive than one that cannot.

Total Need

The total need for a new service concept also has a major impact upon its likelihood of success. It is fairly obvious that it should be easier to market a product or service that a lot of people need than one that only a few people need. Often in health services planning, however, little attention is paid to this factor.

For example, in the mid-1980s there was a sudden proliferation of programs specializing in the treatment of bulimia and other eating disorders. The actual incidence of eating disorders among the population has not been well researched or documented. Despite publicity about a few extreme cases, the actual incidence of the problem may be quite low.

Many of these centers were defensive measures by hospitals and psychiatrists, who saw competitors announcing such programs and were afraid of losing patients to them. However, each of the centers required a certain marketing expenditure. It is questionable whether many of them have attracted enough patients to recover that marketing investment.

The incidence of even some quite well recognized diseases is quite low. You may recall in the case of the proposed regional epilepsy center (Chapter 2), only 5,000 patients with a history of seizure disorders were estimated to exist in a population of some 6 million. It is in the nature of health care that it deals with both diseases that are very common and diseases that are quite rare. The latter are likely to require a specialized program with distinctive competitive advantages to be successful. Such a program is more likely to be based at an institution that has a history of drawing patients from a very broad service area than at one that serves a restricted geographical market.

As an illustration, consider Black University Hospital, in the center of a large city. Its marketing staff has divided its broad service area into nine sales territories. The downtown area comprises one of these. The surrounding suburbs are divided into four further sales territories: the suburban northeast, southeast, southwest, and northwest. Further out, the rural areas surrounding the city are also divided into four sales territories: rural northeast, southeast, southwest, and northwest. Figure 8-1 shows these nine sales territories.

White Community Hospital is located in the middle of the suburban northeast area. There are a number of other hospitals in the city. Black University Hospital and White Community Hospital have very different market shares in each of the nine sales territories. Table 8-2 shows their market share of all hospitalizations in each area.

Both hospitals are considering major expansions in balloon angioplasty for coronary artery disease. They both estimate the annual incidence in the population of coronary artery disease for which this is a suitable treatment at 1 in 5,000. As there are 7,100,000 people in the region as a whole, 1,420 such procedures should potentially be needed annually. Both hospitals calculate that a minimum of 400 annual angioplasties is needed for a successful program.

White Community Hospital has a major market share for general hospital admissions only in the suburban northeast. The estimated annual need for angioplasties in that sales territory alone is

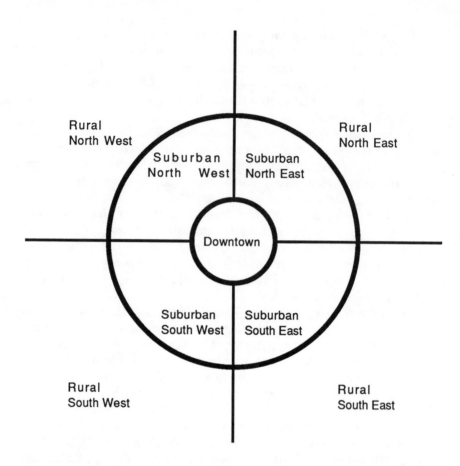

Figure 8-1 The sales territories of Black University Hospital and White Community Hospital.

only 200. Currently, White does not attract 65% of all patients admitted to hospital out of its own part of the city. It is reasonable to assume that one segment that it does not do well at attracting are those in need of specialized tertiary services such as heart surgery. It draws only very small market shares from two other territories: the suburban northwest and the rural northeast. Those two areas in combination produce another 400 potential angioplasty patients annually.

Table 8-2 Hospital Admissions and Market Share by Region

Area	Population	Total Annual Admissions to All Hospitals	Market Share (%) Black	White
Downtown	100,000	10,000	25	0
Suburban NW	1,000,000	100,000	2	1
Suburban NE	1,000,000	100,000	2	35
Suburban SE	1,000,000	100,000	5	0
Suburban SW	1,000,000	100,000	2	0
Rural NW	1,000,000	100,000	1	0
Rural NE	1,000,000	100,000	1	5
Rural SE	1,000,000	100,000	1	0

The administration at White has concluded that "the hospital needs 400 angioplasties for a successful program, and the estimated number of patients needing this procedure in the communities White serves is 600." As you will readily see, the wording of this statement is grossly misleading. White receives only a marginal number of referrals from the areas containing 400 of those 600 cases. In any event, a 66% market share is an almost impossible target.

The statement goes on to say that "this advanced program will also help to boost White's market share in other parts of the city." At the moment, White has 0% market share in other parts of the city. Even if it could attract 10% of all angioplasties from outside of its own area, that would only yield 122 cases. Even if it could also capture all the 200 annual cases in its own sales territory, it would still be well short of its target of 400 annual cases.

Black University Hospital shares one feature with White. It has quite a high market share in its own community. In this area it is a *market penetrator*. Unlike White, however, it has a broader service area, throughout which it is a *market skimmer*, drawing a small share from a large market.

Black's strong presence in the downtown area will not aid its ambitions in angioplasty very much. The expected annual number of cases in this area is only 20. To attract 400 cases, it must achieve a 28% market share of the 1,420 cases in the region. Table 8-2 above suggests at first glance that that goal may be difficult to attain.

Black's market share outside of the downtown area ranges between 1% and 5%.

However, as a university hospital, the cases Black attracts from farther away are probably nearly all for more advanced tertiary services. If such tertiary services account for only about 3% to 5% of all hospital admissions, then Black's market share among that type of admission is quite high. It may be getting between 20% (from the four rural sales territories) and 100% (from the suburban southeast) of all the tertiary care in the region.

Knowledge of how many open-heart bypasses, for which angioplasty is an alternative for some patients, are currently being performed at Black would make a more accurate conclusion possible. From the available facts, however, the total need for angioplasty and the market share needed for a viable program suggest that such a program cannot succeed at White but might be successful at Black.

In this case the calculations of market share were made in relation to the total need for angioplasty—the specific service concerned. They were not made in relation to the total need for hospital admissions. The fact that 100 per thousand in this case were admitted each year to the hospital is irrelevant when looking at angioplasty as a potential service. The market involved is not the 710,000 hospital admissions, but the 1,420 likely admissions for angioplasty.

As we have seen in earlier examples, several sponsors of fitness centers, erred in treating all those who claimed to be regular exercisers as part of their potential market. Another hospital screening a proposal for a fitness center decided to conduct a brief sample survey to test likely interest among the 400,000 people who either lived or worked within 1 mile of the proposed site. On the basis of this survey, it drew up the information in Table 8-3.

As will be seen, the total need in this example was not assumed to be 400,000 people, but only the 4,000 people who met all of the six criteria studied. The market share needed for a viable program was not calculated as a percentage of the 400,000 estimated population, but only as a percentage of those who met those six criteria. It should be. The marketing task, if this program was pursued, would not be "to persuade 0.4% of the local residential and business population to join." That challenge is exactly 100 times more difficult then it seems when stated in the first of those two ways.

Table 8-3 Results of Market Survey for a Proposed Fitness Center

Criterion	% Yes	Potential Market
Live/work within 1 mile	100	400,000
and "Regular exerciser"	80	320,000
and "Exercises enough to impact		
cardiovascular fitness"	30	120,000
and "Highly interested in idea"	10	40,000
and "Not a member of similar		
club already"	5	20,000
and "Would pay $750 per year"	1	4,000
Needed to break even		1,600
Market share to break even		40%

Conclusion: Market share probably too high to achieve.

New service concept ideas are most likely to succeed when the total need for them is high and the market share required to break even is low.

The Product Life Cycle

Life-Cycle Stages. The concept of the *product life-cycle* is perhaps one of the most important in the field of marketing science. Just like people, all products and services go through a life-cycle. It starts with birth and infancy (*service introduction*), continues with childhood and adolescence (*service growth*), turns into early adulthood (*service maturity*), and finally evolves into later adulthood (*service decline*). It ends, like life itself, in *service death* (Kotler 1972; Day 1981; Reibstein 1985). Figure 8-2 depicts this process.

The idea that products and services, like people and animals, have life-cycles seems strange at first encounter. However, it is not difficult to find real examples of products and services that are in each of those five life-cycle phases. Among the products that, as of 1988, are still in their infancy or *introduction phase* are compact disks, (CDs) and players, prescription antismoking medications, car

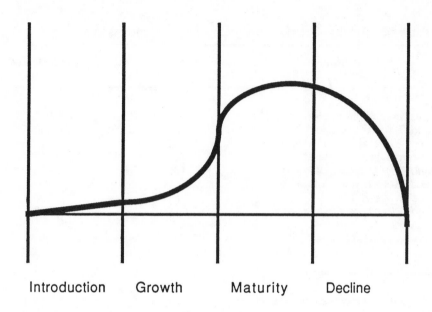

Introduction   Growth   Maturity   Decline

Figure 8-2 The service life-cycle.

telephones, holograms, Sears' Discovery credit card, telephone banking, laser weapons, and automobile computers. In health care, services in their introductory phase include PET scanning, genetic screening and engineering, extracorporeal membrane oxygenation (to sustain lung function in immature newborns), living wills, patient-administered anesthesia, preferred provider organizations, Medicare and Medicaid HMOs, plastic surgical procedures to reduce "crow's feet," same-day cardiac catheterization, home chemotherapy, intraoperative radiation, cerebral perfusion for stroke, and many more.

Among the products and services that have gone beyond their introduction phase and are into their *growth phase* are videocassette players, home movie rentals, cable TV, microwave ovens, satellite weather forecasting, supersonic commercial aircraft, time-sharing of vacation homes, automatic tellers, "all-natural" sodas, unsaturated-fat diets, and disposable paper clothing. Health care services now in their growth phase include home care, trauma centers, same-day surgery, in vitro fertilization, laser surgery, liposuction, balloon angioplasty, third-generation antibiotics, topical anesthetics, wellness programs, home dialysis, transplant surgery, the artificial tendon, and many other recent innovations.

Products and services that have reached their *maturity phase* include stainless steel tableware, telephones, portable radios, washing machines, lawnmowers, automobiles, pianos, light bulbs, paper towels, ballpoint pens, newspapers, portrait photography, and patio furniture. Health care services now in their mature phase include CT scanning, chest x-rays, aspirin, cesarean sections, and appendectomies.

Examples of products or services now in their *decline phase* include dishwashing liquids, nonpermanent press sheets, shoe repairs, canned fruit juice, hot water bottles, window air-conditioning units, flypaper, hotel valet services, live-in servants, small food stores, movie theaters, and steak knives. Health care services now in decline include ulcer surgery, inpatient pediatrics, electric shock therapy, amputation, open-heart surgery, and outpatient "clinics."

For a product or service to reach *death*, it need not disappear completely but may become very rare, or may be retained merely for its sentimental or curiosity value. Examples of products or services that have "died" include washboards, copper bathtubs, horse-drawn trolley cars, outdoor toilets, many local newspapers, vaudeville, and pawnbrokers. Health care services that have died, or virtually died, include tonsillectomies, tuberculosis hospitals, polio clinics, the iron lung, and cobalt therapy.

Starting in about 1860, phrenology, or the classification of psychiatric disorders by mapping the shape of the skull, became one of the hottest and most respectable branches of medical research and investigation. By the early 1880s, the largest attendance at any national medical meeting was at those devoted to phrenology. By around 1900, however, this medical science was in decline, and it was effectively dead by 1920. Its whole life-cycle thus lasted for about 60 years.

That is probably longer, however, than the likely life-cycles of open-heart surgery and CT scanning. The first open-heart surgery was performed in the early 1950s, and the first uses of CT scanning were in the late 1960s. Open-heart surgery will have to survive to 2015, and CT scanning to 2030, to have longer life-cycles than phrenology enjoyed. On current trends, it seems highly probable that both will have been superseded by other techniques before then.

How long do product or service life-cycles last? The answer to that question is less certain. Some products and services have very short life-cycles of just a few years, while others continue for quite a few decades. There are rare exceptions that have even shorter or longer life-cycles. Some fad products, like hula hoops, or services, like selling krugerrands as an investment, have very brief life-cycles. At the other extreme are generic products like steel and coal, which remain in use after several thousand years.

Many marketing scientists would argue, however, that neither extreme represents a true life-cycle. The hula hoop and the pet rock were "gimmick" products. Coal and steel have been around for a long time, but are two of the most abundant natural materials on earth, and their main uses have changed repetitively during that period. Steel has lived through a series of life-cycles — of handheld weapons, of early industrial machinery, of the railroads and steamships, of the age of the automobile and the steel-cased appliance. It has not, then, so much had a life-cycle of its own as it has been a generic product incorporated into others with their own shorter life-cycles.

All products and services pass through a life-cycle of introduction, growth, maturity, decline, and death. This life-cycle may last just a few years or continue for some decades, but it always occurs.

The Dynamics of the Life-Cycle

Why do product life-cycles occur? Why is their pattern so consistent? Think for a moment about human life. Although medical advances have increased the human life span, death is still inevitable. It seems to be so because the same natural forces that enable human beings to grow also, in time, lead to their degeneration. In the previous chapter, a "nonorganic" example of the same process was described. The advances in technology that created demand for the modern hospital have progressed to a stage where they have reduced the demand for hospitals. A new force did not intervene to turn the tide. The same force both generated the growth and caused the decline.

The same happens in product and service life-cycles. They start as a new concept, created by an individual or an organization. Because the concept is new, the introductory phase usually moves quite slowly. It takes time to get the new idea to work properly—to develop its product or service technology. It takes time and experimentation to discover how to produce a lot of the product, or to deliver a lot of the service economically—its process technology. It takes time, and trial and error, to work out how best to manage and market it—its management technology. While the innovator or organization is developing these areas of know-how, use of the new concept grows, but only gradually.

Sometimes a new concept never advances beyond its introductory phase. It dies in its infancy, because one or another of the technologies involved to make it successful proved too difficult, or because someone funding the project got frustrated at the slow rate of progress. As noted in Chapter 7, as many as half of all the new concepts that reach this stage fail to thrive and never go any further.

If the innovator or organization does master the new technologies involved, suddenly the product or service enters its growth phase. This transition usually occurs because a critical mass of customers has now been exposed to the innovation, like it, and pass the word along to others. The product starts growing almost under its own momentum. Now the innovator or organization faces a new challenge. In the introductory phase, the top priority was nurturing the new idea and making sure that it worked, along with the process to replicate it and the systems to manage and market it. By contrast, in the growth phase the largest challenge is to keep on feeding the project. Demand for it keeps on growing and does so quite rapidly. If the innovator or organization cannot expand output to keep pace with demand, rivals will be encouraged to enter the field. Even though these competitors may be quite a long way behind on the learning curve, if there are customers who want the product but cannot get it, some will accept a less reliable version. If the innovator or organization should fail to respond to the rising demand for the product or service, they will therefore encourage new entrants into the field. If too many such new entrants emerge, they may cut off the growth of the original innovator's market prematurely. The first pig in a litter may not grow into a big pig if he has too many brothers and sisters vying with him for the food in the trough.

Even if the innovator or organization does succeed in keeping pace with growing demand for the new idea, in time others will see its success and be motivated to act. They may see that the original innovator is making a lot of profit, as is likely to happen in the growth phase. The innovator went through most of the expensive process of learning how to produce and deliver the product or service back in its introductory phase. Now, as demand for it accelerates, the innovator only has to do what he or she has already learned to do but on a larger scale. With the high costs of developing the product or service and its market passed, the more product the innovator now makes, the lower is the average cost and the higher the profit.

Consider for a moment the handheld calculator. It can cost millions of dollars to develop and perfect a new model scientific calculator. Producing the first 100 can be very expensive. A high percentage of them may even be defective and unsellable. By the 100,000th sale, however, those early teething troubles have largely gone. Rather than 100 experimental units in a workshop, there is now an entire automated assembly line devoted to their manufacture. The same phenomenon works in health care. A center that performs 500 open-heart cases a year is likely to be less costly, more efficient, and have lower mortality rates or "product failures" than one that only performs 50.

Because innovators begin to accumulate substantial profits during the growth phase of a new product or service, and because the new market is more visible as it grows, it attracts the attention of competitors, who may take one of four actions:

1. They may conclude that the innovator is too strong to take on (a *noncompetition strategy*). In this case, the innovator will go on to control the market.

2. They may decide to enter the market with an equivalent new product (an *imitation strategy*). If they do, the original innovator may maintain the largest market share, or may lose it to one of these competitors, but will never totally control it.

3. They may decide to invest in developing a better product to steal away the market (a *substitution strategy*). The effect of this action will be commented on shortly.

4. They may decide to take over the innovator (an *acquisition strategy*). If they succeed, they will have acquired both the innovator's know-how and the innovator's established market.

Even under the most favorable of these actions for the original in-novator—a noncompetitive response—the market cannot grow forever. A time begins to draw near when most people who want the new product or service have it. The market reaches *saturation*. This happens even with products or services that are perishable, like cosmetics or batteries. The initial growth was created by people buying their first ones and then replacing them. Once everyone who is interested has bought their first one, the future market depends upon replacements only, so that total sales start to stagnate.

Even in health care, where a new group of patients might contract the disease and need the service each year, their numbers are still likely to be less than in the early growth phase of the service. When the idea was new, its patients included some who had been waiting for such a solution to their problem. Others were uncertain if they needed it but decided to try it, or at least to ask a doctor about its relevance to them. As the service matures, its annual market tends to shrink down to new cases in real need.

Once the market for the innovation reaches maturity, therefore, activity levels even off. If, as usually happens, competitors have entered the market during the growth phase, that competition now grows more intense. With sales stagnant, one organization can grow only if another declines. The various competitors also seek out particular market segments, or niches, where they see themselves as having an extra competitive advantage. In the growth phase, it was not particularly important who was buying the product or service as long as an increasing number of people were. Now that the growth has stopped, one competitor who can mount a special appeal to some segment (such as women, or older people, or empty-nesters, or the most quality conscious) may still have some room to grow by attracting this type of person away from competitors.

Once the product or service has been mature for some time, the market will actually start to decline. Two forces, separately or together, often account for this next transition in the life-cycle. If the product is durable and will last, once everyone who wants one has it, future sales will occur only as the product wears out.

Again, medicine is no exception to this rule. As the cure rates for various cancers improve, patients who previously received very regular but ineffective therapy now go into remission permanently or for long periods. As the value of prostate surgery becomes more widely recognized, patients with prolonged prostate problem necessitating periodic care are now cured of their problem for life, or at least for several decades.

Any one doctor or hospital that develops a strong reputation in a field may continue to grow by attracting a disproportionate market share of new cases with the disease. For the health care delivery system as a whole, however, the more people are cured of a disease, the lower will be the total demand for the services that made it possible.

One cause of products and services going into decline, therefore, is that they have saturated demand and their results are "durable." The other major cause was alluded to earlier: *substitution*. Any large market will attract the attention of other innovators and organizations. They will try to develop the next generation of superior products or services. In time, a few of them will succeed and create a viable new product or service starting out on its own life-cycle. When it reaches its growth stage, it will drive the old product or service out. If it does so effectively, the old product or service will die. That is what the electric blanket and central heating did to the hot water bottle, and what modern respirators did to the iron lung.

The Life-Cycle and New Concept Screening. The life-cycle stage of a particular product or service is important in the screening of new service concepts, because each stage poses special challenges to a new entrant. A conscious decision has to be made, therefore, to enter a new market at any given stage. Otherwise the enterprise is likely to encounter problems for which it is not prepared.

The *introductory stage* of a new product or service may appear to be the ideal time to become involved with it. However, there is a high failure rate among new products and services in this phase. It also requires considerable funding to develop and debug the necessary technologies and to market an unfamiliar concept to potential customers. Revenue only builds slowly as these customers begin to appreciate the benefits of the new technologies. Getting involved with a new service at this stage, therefore, takes available cash away from the expansion of existing services. The rewards for entry into a new service at its introductory stage can subsequently be very great, but so are the initial risks.

The *growth phase* of a new service also appears to be an attractive time to enter the field. The initial innovators have lived through the problems of developing the concept, and the new entrant can learn from their mistakes.

However, the real ability of a new entrant to imitate the know-how of those pioneers varies a lot. If the service requires distinct and complex technologies, it may prove impossible for a new entrant to copy them effectively. Many health care services appear much simpler to imitate than they really are. As one example, there are, as of 1988, only some six major multidisciplinary shoulder centers in the United States. The idea itself is not complex: combining the know-how of several physicians in different disciplines, but with a common interest in shoulder problems, into a collaborative team. In practice, however, the idea is unlikely to work with any five or six doctors with the relevant specialties. Unless each of them has a preestablished interest and considerable individual experience in treating such diseases and disorders, it may be many years before the new center develops any real competitive advantage over other physicians already caring for such problems. If, alternatively, the new idea does not have such major technological barriers to entry, the growth phase is an attractive time to enter a market. Hospitals that have launched special outreach programs to the elderly, for instance, often have no very distinctive competence to serve as a barrier to the entry of any number of later imitators.

The opportunity to enter a market in its growth phase may in any case not be as attractive as it seems, depending on where the market is *within* its growth phase. The very early stages of the growth phase offer a good opportunity to join in. The total market has a long way still to grow, and there are not yet an abundance of competitors. By the middle of the growth phase, however, a large number of enterprises have jumped on the bandwagon. Competition heats up, and not every new entrant is successful. Even though a new entrant may possess the needed know-how, the field has become too crowded for all to succeed.

The rise of HMOs illustrates this pattern, at least in the major metropolitan areas. The real innovators struggled for several years before their plans started to gain significant support. Their success encouraged others to join the field. Some lacked the necessary know-how to succeed. Others, however, even with the necessary know-how, found it impossible to get a viable enrollment and got out of the business by putting their small plans up for sale to larger ones. Many plans that did find buyers have come away without any profit, and some incurred sizable start-up losses before realizing that they were not going to succeed.

The very late stages of the growth phase are an even less favorable time for a new entrant. Not only is the field now crowded with competitors, but total demand for the service does not have much growth left ahead. Existing competitors in the market who sense its nearing maturity will already be intensifying their competitive tactics. Unlike the new entrant, they have usually accumulated large profits earlier in the growth phase, which they can now invest in product improvement or in defensive marketing to make entry even more risky for a new competitor.

The only circumstance in which it may be wise to enter a market even when it is nearing maturity is when the new entrant itself has developed a significant service improvement and has a program to offer that is clearly superior, or much less expensive. However, it is easy at this stage to delude oneself that one has a real service improvement to offer; often the "improvement" totally fails to impress the customers. This has proved true, for instance, of many "enhanced" features on TV sets, and of many minor revisions of surgical techniques. Market research becomes even more important at this stage of the life-cycle to establish whether such improvements are really likely to impress the customer.

The *maturity phase* of the life-cycle sounds like an unattractive time for new entrants and usually is so. It is more sensible to look for the next generation of services that may eventually replace this one and may by now be entering their growth phase. It may, however, be a good time to acquire an existing supplier to provide an established market share for a substitute technology that the buyer has in development. It is also a propitious time for innovators who do not want to face up to the risks of the introductory phase to sell an idea to an existing company in the field that realizes that the days of its present product or service are numbered.

Rarely, if ever, does it make sense to enter a field in its *decline phase*. It has usually reached that stage because some better replacement product or service is already in its growth phase.

The life-cycle occurs principally because all products and services have only finite demand and at some point reach a stage at which the market is saturated. It is also propelled by the emergence of replacement products and services. Where a product or service is in its life-cycle makes a crucial difference to the chances of success of an organization entering that market for the first time, as well as to the types of challenges for which it must be prepared.

Locating New Services on the Life-Cycle Curve. If the life-cycle stage is so important to the success of a new entrant into the market, how can you tell what stage a product or service has reached?

The first answer is a disappointing one: Often you cannot assess accurately what stage a service has reached in its life-cycle. Innovators and organizations can, however, make a more inspired estimate if they understand the dynamics of the life-cycle. If, for instance, a service is new and not yet widespread, it is probably in its introductory phase. If it is "hot" and a lot of people are talking about it, and there are quite a few people beginning to provide it, it is probably in its growth phase. If many people seem to be trying to enter the market, but a high percentage of them are unsuccessful, the product may be nearing maturity. If a product has been around for some time and seems fairly commonplace, it is probably in its maturity. If new and better concepts are beginning to come onto the market, the old concept may be entering its decline.

The second answer is more precise. It is often possible to make a more accurate assessment of the life-cycle stage that a product or service has reached if some years of data on sales, patient volumes, visits, or procedures are available.

If data are not available for a number of years, they may be for a number of past quarters. However, remember when using anything other than annual data that many services experience seasonal fluctuations in volume. Dental practices, for instance, often slump in the summer and around Christmas, making the last two quarters' volumes lower than the first two. Plastic surgery tends to boom in the early fall. Asthma programs see most patients late in the spring and early in the fall. Enrollment in health insurance plans tends to be highest in January and in June or July, because most companies ask employees to elect their benefit options in one of those two periods.

If annual data are not available for enough years, quarterly data can be quite easily adjusted for seasonal patterns. There are various ways of making such seasonal adjustments, but one simple approach can be illustrated using the data in Table 8-4.

Table 8-4 Patient Visits by Quarter, 1987-1988

Quarter	Visits
1987	
1st	50
2nd	40
3rd	60
4th	50
1988	
1st	70
2nd	50
3rd	80
4th	60

Note that visits in the latest quarter are only 20% higher than those in the first quarter in the table. This service is growing, but has it really grown by 20%?

The first step in seasonally adjusting these data is to calculate the average number of patient visits for the eight quarters. Total visits over those 2 years were 460, for a quarterly average of 460 ÷ 8, or approximately 57. Table 8-5 takes the average of the first quarters of the 2 years. It then divides 57 by that number to produce a seasonal weighing. This calculation is repeated for each of the four quarters.

Finally, Table 8-6 takes the original quarterly patient visits and multiplies them by the seasonal weights. Doing so eradicates the effect of seasonal variations.

The original, unadjusted data suggested that the service had grown by 20% between the first and last of these eight quarters. The adjusted data put that growth at almost 30%. However, the practice did not experience steady growth. It was fairly flat through the first year, on a seasonally adjusted basis, and then jumped to a higher level for the second year, during which it again stayed fairly flat.

Where might this service be in its product life-cycle? It does not seem to be in decline, or activity would be falling. It is not mature, or there would be no growth. The service could be in its growth

Table 8-5 Calculation of Seasonal Weights

Averages	Seasonal Weighting
Average of both 1st quarters = 60	57 ÷ 60 = 0.95
Average of both 2nd quarters = 45	57 ÷ 45 = 1.27
Average of both 3rd quarters = 70	57 ÷ 70 = 0.81
Average of both 4th quarters = 55	57 ÷ 55 = 1.04

Table 8-6 Seasonal Adjustment of Visits

Quarter	Unadjusted Visits	Seasonal Weighting	Adjusted Visits[a]
1987			
1st	50	0.95	48
2nd	40	1.27	51
3rd	60	0.81	49
4th	50	1.04	52
1988			
1st	70	0.95	67
2nd	50	1.27	64
3rd	80	0.81	65
4th	60	1.04	62

[a] All numbers are rounded up to nearest whole number.

phase, but the growth phase usually consists of sustained increases, not a jump from one plateau to another.

It is possible, of course, that the capacity of the service was expanded at the beginning of the second year, by adding more staff or more hours, and then quickly hit full capacity again. If that were known, it would be reasonable to conclude that the service is in its growth phase. It would also be possible to draw another conclusion:

that the practice is not expanding fast enough to keep pace with growth, because when it adds capacity it rapidly fills it up again.

If there was not such a "capacity constraint," and the practice could have handled more patients throughout this period, it is probably in its introductory phase. The increases are not sustained enough to suggest that it is in its growth phase. Sudden rises in demand like this one can happen, however, during the introductory phase. Word about a new service gets out enough to attract a surge in patients, but not widely enough to generate continual growth.

There are ways of being even more precise in estimating where a service is in its life-cycle, using data like those above, but these require some basic application of algebra.

In Figure 8-3, look first at line A. For every inch that it goes horizontally, it also goes up an inch. If you divide the vertical "rise" of a line by its horizontal "reach," you get a number known as the "slope" of the line. Like the signs on railroads and some highways, the slope tells you how fast the line is rising. Line A, therefore, has a slope of 1 divided by 1, or 1. For every inch it goes left to right, it goes up by the same amount.

Line B, on the other hand, is flat. It has no slope. For every inch that it goes left to right, it rises zero inches. Zero divided by one is zero. Therefore, the slope of line B is zero.

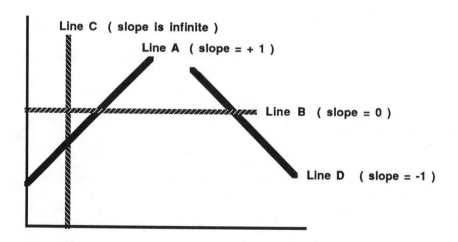

Figure 8-3 Sample lines and their slopes.

Line C is completely vertical. It does not move left to right at all, but it goes straight up forever. The slope of a vertical line is regarded as infinity (because it could go straight up forever) divided by zero (because it never travels right or left). Division by zero is an undefined mathematical operation. The slope of Line C is therefore undefined but can be thought of as infinite.

Finally, line D falls 1 inch for every inch that it goes to the right. Its slope is calculated as -1 divided by 1 or -1.

Figure 8-4 reproduces the same axes, but the typical product life-cycle curve has been added. Whereas lines A through D were all straight, the product life-cycle is represented by a curve. What is the slope of a curve? Think again about driving up a long hill. The first gradient sign that you see reads "1 in 10," or "10%," meaning that the hill rises 1 yard for every 10 yards of distance. Then you come to another sign, which reads "1 in 5," or "20%." The hill has become steeper. You are not driving up a straight line, but up a curve, and the slope of a curve changes.

Now look at the introductory phase of the product life-cycle. Which of the four straight lines is that part of the curve most like? It

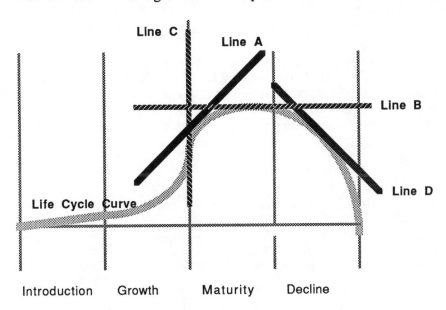

Figure 8-4 The service life-cycle showing the slope of the curve at various stages.

is somewhere close to line A. Its slope is around 1. It is certainly above zero, because it is steeper than line B. It may be slightly steeper than line A but not by much. In this introductory phase of the life-cycle, therefore, the slope of the line is greater than zero but still quite small.

The early to middle part of the growth phase of the life-cycle curve is much steeper than line A, and so its slope is much greater than 1. However, it does not go vertical like line C, and so its slope is not infinite. In this growth phase of the life-cycle, therefore, its slope is some quite large number. Note, however, that toward the end of the growth phase, the line starts to flatten. Its slope begins to drop.

In the mature phase, the curve is most like line B. It is quite flat, with a slope close to zero.

Finally, in its decline phase, the line drops. It is now most like line D, with a negative slope. The service is now "going downhill."

Different phases of the life-cycle, therefore, have different slopes. In practical terms, that means that the rate at which sales, or visits, or procedures are changing varies. Thus, if you can calculate the rate of change in sales or in number of patients, you can compare that slope with that of the product life-cycle and see where it seems to fit.

Many people would argue that home care is a growth industry — one that will continue to grow very rapidly through the next 10 to 20 years. Table 8-7 shows the actual percentage growth in home care in the United States as a whole in each of the years 1982 through 1985. Clearly, these four years represent only part of the life-cycle of home care. It existed as a service before 1982 and still does.

Table 8-7 Growth in Home Health Care, 1982-1985

Year	% Growth in Home Care	Cumulative % Growth Since 1981	Slope
1982	12	12	12
1983	17	29	17
1984	22	51	22
1985	21	72	21

However, knowing where in its total life-cycle these four years fall could be important information for home care providers.

If you were to draw this partial life-cycle, you would plot the years along the horizontal axis (1981 through 1985), and cumulative percentage growth since 1981 along the horizontal axis. You would then plot five points. The first, for 1981, would be at 0% cumulative growth, since this is the base year; the second, for 1982, would be at 12%; the third, for 1983, at 29% cumulative growth; and so on. If you then connected the five points, you would have drawn the life-cycle for home care over that five-year period.

The last column gives the slope of the life-cycle for home care in each year. How are these numbers calculated? We saw that a hill that rose 1 yard vertically for every 10 yards traveled horizontally had a slope of 1 in 10 (or 0.1). Similarly, the slope of the home care life-cycle in any year is given by how much it increases divided by how far it travels. The only difference is that the life-cycle is traveling through time, whereas a hill travels through space. That makes calculating its slope in any year easier. We merely divide the increase in home care sales in each year by one (one year).

In fact, these data come from a report by one of the largest health-related corporations in the United States (Baxter Travenol 1987). It concluded from this table that "the growth rate is expected to slow as the market enters the mature phase of its product life cycle." The corporation reached that conclusion because the changing slope of the line shown in the last column of the table looks most like that part of a life-cycle curve in the last stages of its growth phase. Arguably, four years of data are not enough to be certain that the era of rapidly increasing home care is over, but Baxter Travenol used the information that was available to decide that it could not safely assume that such fast growth would continue.

That product life-cycle dealt with an entire industry — home care in the U.S. The life-cycle can also apply, however, to individual organizations, practices, and programs. As an example of a program life-cycle, consider the example of a hospital's open-heart surgery program, now entering its 14th year (Table 8-8).

There are more numbers in this table than in the previous home care example. The data cover more years, and the actual numbers of cases are shown as well as the percentage changes. If you graph this life-cycle, you will have 14 years along the horizontal axis (including year 0 as the base year when no procedures were performed). In this example, you have a choice of units for the vertical axis of the graph.

Table 8-8 Growth and Decline in an Open-Heart Surgery Program

Year	Open Heart Cases	Increase (Decrease) From Prior Year	% Change	Rate of Change
Introductory phase				
1	100	100		
2	104	4	4	
3	110	6	5	1.25
4	118	8	7	1.40
Early growth phase				
5	135	17	14	2.00
6	173	38	28	2.00
7	280	107	62	2.20
Late growth phase				
8	540	260	93	1.50
9	1090	550	102	1.10
Mature phase				
10	1100	10	1	0.01
11	1050	(50)	(5)	
Decline phase				
12	950	(100)	(9)	(1.80)
13	700	(150)	(26)	(2.90)

You could, as in the home care example, use the cumulative percentage growth. Alternatively, you could use the actual number of operations performed (0 for year 0, 100 for year 1, 104 for year 2, and so on). In fact, this is the more common approach in graphing life-cycles, using actual units "sold" in each year. Sometimes, however, only more limited data are available.

If you were to use the actual annual number of cases in a life-cycle diagram, what would then be the slope of the line in each year? Now, the line rises or falls each year by a number of cases, not by a percentage change. Therefore, it is the second column of the table that shows the slope of the line.

Trying to determine where a service is in its life-cycle is not just an exercise in math. It can be a very important tool in decision-making. Consider, for instance, the state of this cardiac surgery program at the end of its ninth year. Through the prior two years, volumes have grown almost fourfold, from 280 cases to 1,090. In each of the previous nine years, cases have grown by a larger percentage than in the year before. The staff would apparently have every reason to believe that their program is strong. If they were thinking of spending more dollars on it (more staff, new space, etc.), their growth performance would seem to justify this action. However, the volumes for years 10 through 13 show that such optimism in year 9 about the future would have been misplaced.

Would there have been a way, in year 9, to foresee that imminent downturn in activity? There are various advanced statistical methods of forecasting the future trend of a time series of data like a life-cycle (Mendenhall and Reinmuth 1974). The last column in the table provides one relatively simple example. It is an index of the rate of change in volume. It is calculated by dividing the percentage growth in the latest year by the percentage growth in the preceding year. For example, in year 6 volume grew 28%, compared to 14% in year 5, for an index value of 2.00. A glance down the last column of the table shows that this index peaked at 2.20 in year 7. By year 9, it had fallen two years in a row. Despite the fourfold growth of cases in years 8 and 9, therefore, the program's underlying growth rate had already passed its peak. Even without going through the quite complex math of calculating the likely future trend of this index, it can be concluded that, since it has been falling for several years, the best forecast is that it will continue to do so.

This life-cycle concept seems to imply a sense of fatalism about the growth of any service, that it will inevitably, at some stage, peak and then decline. That is so, as long as the service remains the same. It will eventually be eclipsed by other providers, or by some new and better approach to meeting the same patient need. If that fate and its approximate timing are predictable, however, actions can be taken to avoid its consequences. A hospital with a major open-heart surgery program could, for instance, have been among the first to realize that balloon angioplasty would replace that procedure for many patients. It could have decided to be, itself, a pioneer of that alternative therapy.

As a final illustration of the wide applicability of the life-cycle concept, consider what has happened in recent years to patient volumes in physicians' offices. The career of an individual physician or other health care provider in private practice follows its own life-cycle.

Dr. Average, Senior, entered practice in 1950. By 1975, he was in his mid-50s and had a prosperous practice. His son, Dr. Average, Junior, followed him in becoming a physician, starting practice in 1980. He not only admired his father's dedication and professionalism, but also saw how financially rewarding medicine had been for him.

Table 8-9 shows the total annual patient visits to the average U.S. doctor's office in 1975 and 1985. The data are broken down for doctors in five different age groups (American Medical Association, 1987). The available data are more limited than in the open-heart program example, but can still yield some important practical consequences. The last two columns show the average annual growth in

Table 8-9 Annual Patient Office Visits, 1975 and 1985

Doctor's Age	Annual Office Visits		Annual Growth in Office Visits	
	1975	1985	1975	1985
Growth phase				
Early thirties[a]	6,968	6,084	1,394	1,217
Early forties	7,436	6,240	47	16
Mature phase				
Early fifties	8,206	6,344	77	10
Decline phase				
Early sixties	6,968	6,396	(124)	5
Late sixties[b]	5,096	4,992	(374)	(281)

[a]Assumed to be five years on average after entering practice.
[b]Assumed to be five years later than "early sixties."

office visits between these ages for which data are given. Since, for instance, the 1985 data show 156 more visits to a doctor in his early forties than to one in his early thirties, each of those 10 more years in practice are worth 16 more patient visits.

Figure 8-5 depicts these two professional life-cycles.

Dr. Average, Sr., entering medical practice in 1950, could look forward to a gradual but, over time, dramatic growth in his practice volume. At somewhere around 1,500 patient visits a year, he could cover his office expenses. He therefore had a substantial personal income from early on in his practice, but a portion of this went to pay off debt accumulated through his long years of training. With the high office volumes of his 40s and 50s, however, and now clear of such debt, he could become a relatively wealthy man.

In contrast, Dr. Average, Jr., entering practice in 1980, faces a very different life-cycle. His practice is mature as soon as it opens. He cannot look forward to the same rates of growth and the same high-income years in mid-career. Because of increased office and malpractice costs, it will now take him about 2,500 annual visits to break even. He therefore has less personal income from the start, often a larger debt, and the prospect of much less income growth in the future. He is by no means poor, but neither is he likely, by mid-life, to be as wealthy as his father at that stage of his career.

What has depressed the physician practice life-cycle? Just as the theory predicts, the high earnings of previous decades have led a large number of people to enter the medical profession (Graduate Medical Education National Advisory Committee 1980). With more doctors, but without substantially more patients to serve, the peak has been "sliced off" the practice life-cycle.

The doctors in this case represented the average of all physicians. The actual number of annual office visits varies by specialty. For nearly every type of doctor, however, rising competition has flattened the life-cycle as shown in Figure 8-5. Within any particular specialty, of course, 50% of doctors do better than average, but there are also 50% who do worse.

Although complete and accurate data are not always readily available, it is often possible to obtain enough information about recent trends in any service, program, or practice to draw useful and practical conclusions about its current stage in its life-cycle. In screening ideas for new services, this knowledge can be very helpful in assessing the likely success of a new service, as well as the special challenges with which it may have to contend.

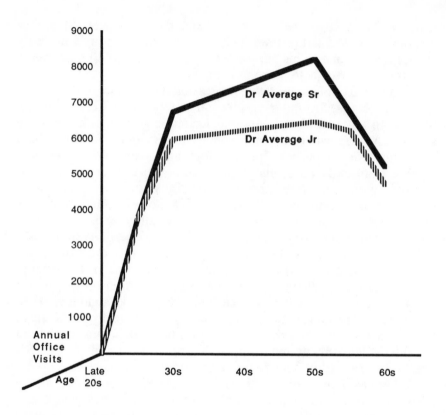

Figure 8-5 The expected professional life-cycles of doctors entering practice in 1975 and 1985.

Ranking New Service Concepts

The previous section has shown that there are several critical factors that should be considered in screening new service concepts to see if they are worthy of more detailed feasibility analysis. At the beginning of this chapter, it was noted that successfully innovative organizations tend to reject about half of all the "bright ideas" that come before them at this initial screening stage. They know that they cannot realistically afford to study every good idea in equal depth. They also know that not every good idea is "right" for them as an organization. Many just do not fit their mission or circumstances. They also know that many good ideas have inherent problems that even a brief systematic screening will show up.

How can these ideas be practically applied in health care? Table 8-10 presents one standard *service appraisal methodology*, which has been developed and employed for concept screening at Thomas Jefferson University Hospital. The 12 factors listed are identical to those discussed in this chapter. The issue of existing competence, or know-how, has been broken out into four components: managerial, physician, nursing, and technical. As a result, one-third of the 12 factors all relate to this single issue of competence. That may seem to be a lot of emphasis to place on one element out of all those discussed above, but this particular health care organization has decided that it deserves that degree of emphasis. It has concluded that the new projects that it should most readily take on are those for which it has the requisite expertise and knowledge.

If you study the five *ranking criteria* listed against each of the 12 *concept characteristics*, you will note that an attempt has been made to provide brief but fairly precise descriptions, for example, "More than 1 in 10 of the population will need such care during their lives, but not usually repetitively," or "Have no in-house nursing expertise in this field, and recruitment will be difficult."

Why create such a system? Why try to be so precise? Each new service concept that emerges in an organization will tend to have one or more "champions." These may be clinical or operational people who are convinced of the strength of their suggestion. The champion may be a planner or a market analyst who has spotted a trend during environmental analysis and feels strongly that the organization must respond. Without preestablished screening criteria, the review of a new concept can degenerate into an argument about how to evaluate it, not about its merits or drawbacks.

Table 8-10 Service Appraisal Methodology

Characteristic	Excellent (5)	Above Average (4)	Average (3)	Below Average (2)	Poor (1)
Compatibility with vision	Directly addresses a mission state-ment issue.	Is consistent with direction set in mission statement.	Has no relation to mission statement issues.	Is somewhat con-tradictory to direc-tion set in mission statement.	Is counter-productive to mission statement objective.
Intrinsic growth (stage in product life-cycle nationally)	In growth stage. Total use has grown at an increas-ing rate in recent years.	Either in develop-ment stage, or nearing maturity with total use growing, but growth rate is flat.	Mature. No significant total growth.	Early decline. Total use falling for several years.	Decline. Total use falling.
Total need	More than 1 in 10 of population sometime in life, and need repeats.	More than 1 in 10 of population but usually nonrepeti-tively.	More than 1 in 30 once-off or 1 in 20 repetitively.	Less than in 3.	Very low incidence.
Managerial competence	Have management personnel com-mitted to product with required expertise.	Have manage-ment personnel committed to project with re-lated expertise.	Have manage-ment without re-lated expertise but willing and able to learn.	Have no in-house management exper-tise but recruitment will not be difficult.	Have no in-house management ex-pertise and recruit-ment will be difficult.

Table 8-10, continued.

Characteristic	Excellent (5)	Above Average (4)	Average (3)	Below Average (2)	Poor (1)
Physician competence	Have physician personnel committed to product with required expertise.	Have physician personnel committed to project with related expertise.	Have physician personnel without related expertise but willing and able to learn.	Have no in-house physician expertise but recruitment will not be difficult.	Have no in-house physician expertise and recruitment will be difficult.
Nursing competence	Have nursing personnel committed to product with required expertise.	Have nursing personnel committed to project with related expertise.	Have nursing personnel without related expertise but willing and able to learn.	Have no in-house nursing expertise but recruitment will not be difficult.	Have no in-house nursing expertise and recruitment will be difficult.
Technical competence	Have technical personnel committed to product with required expertise.	Have technical personnel committed to project with related expertise.	Have technical personnel without related expertise but willing and able to learn.	Have no in-house technical expertise but recruitment will not be difficult.	Have no in-house technical expertise and recruitment will be difficult.
Service compatibility	Directly addresses benefits for which significant numbers already use us.	Directly addresses benefits for which some people already use us.	Addresses benefits for which doctors closely identified with us are already used.	Health care industry regarded as credible source but we have no closely allied service.	Not currently perceived as related closely to health care.

Table 8-10, continued.

Characteristic	Excellent (5)	Above Average (4)	Average (3)	Below Average (2)	Poor (1)
Internal competition	Largely draws new users with identifiable spin-off use of existing services.	Draws new users with possible spin-off use of existing services.	Draws new users but only remote spin-off.	Largely redirects existing users.	Jeopardizes viability of an existing service.
Affordability	No capital outlay. Product revenue will exceed expense during first year.	Capital outlay >$10,000. Product revenue will cover start-up costs and operating expense during first year.	Capital outlay >$10,000. Product revenue will cover start-up costs and operating expense by end of second year.	Capital outlay >$10,000. Product revenue will cover start-up costs and operating expense by end of second year.	Capital outlay >$10,000. Product revenue not expected to cover start-up costs and operating expense.
Distribution channel compatibility	Uses intermediaries already loyal.	Uses intermediaries generally loyal plus others unfamiliar with us.	Uses no intermediaries.	Uses intermediaries with no significant history of relationship.	Uses intermediaries with whom our track record is antagonistic.
Price advantage	We can definitely price at least 20% below competition.	We can price at least 10% below competition.	We can match competition and offer real nonprice advantages.	Our prices will exceed competition but within 10% and we can offer real nonprice advantages.	Our prices will exceed competition.

Organizations that regularly use this type of system usually ask the proposers to outline their case to a senior group of managers, who represent the main functions in the organization. They may also ask specialized business or planning analysts to comment. Each of these senior managers and analysts is then asked to provide a personal assessment of the idea, using this type of scoring matrix. This step ensures that the ideas has been screened from each important perspective: clinical, financial, operational, marketing, and so on. This process is sometimes called a *concurrence process,* because the person responsible for each major aspect of the organization must concur that an idea is worth studying in more depth.

Often, these separate appraisals of a new service concept are in close agreement, and a *consensus proposal,* for or against further study, can go before the head of the enterprise. If there is a lack of consensus, the head of the enterprise may meet with this senior group and hear the cases for and against.

There is no simple rule for using these criteria to identify acceptable projects. Certainly any project that is approved for detailed feasibility analysis should score high on such a system. Recall from the beginning of this chapter that only a small percentage even of those new concepts that advance to feasibility analysis are going to be successful in the end. There is no reason, therefore, to let any but the really strong ideas proceed any further.

With experience in using such systems, organizations develop a sense of what it takes at the screening stage to succeed at the later steps. They develop informal, or even formal *decision rules.* One such rule, based on the methodology shown above, might be, for instance, only to invest further effort in concepts that "score better than 45, and for which no characteristic is rated as low as 1."

Usually even systems such as these depend in the final analysis on judgment. That judgment is likely to be much better, however, if the senior decision-makers have a common and structured set of criteria and scores in front of them. The approach works even better when several new service concepts can be "batched" and presented together. Even if they have no close relationship, comparing their scores on different characteristics can aid decision-making. Projects cease to be considered in piecemeal fashion. For example, Table 8-11 shows how three projects ranked on the above system. Assuming that finances and time allow only one of these ideas to go forward for more detailed review, which one should it be? On total scores, each does quite well, but none clearly surpasses the rest.

Table 8-11 Service Appraisal Rankings of Three Proposed Projects

Characteristic	Concept A	Concept B	Concept C
Compatibility with mission	4	3	2
Intrinsic growth	3	4	5
Total need	4	5	3
Managerial competence	5	4	2
Physician competence	3	4	4
Nursing competence	5	5	5
Technical competence	4	4	3
Service compatibility	2	2	3
Internal competition	3	3	4
Affordability	4	4	5
Distribution channel compatibility	3	4	3
Price advantage	1	1	2
Total Score	41	43	41

Project C should almost certainly be rejected. Although it scores more 5s than either of the other projects, on one of those three characteristics where it scores a 5, both other projects do also, and in the other two cases it is not substantially ahead. Its major problems are that it scores low on "compatible with mission" and on "managerial competence." It sounds like a reasonable good concept but not for this organization.

Projects A and B have identical scores on 8 of the 12 characteristics. Project A is slightly more relevant to the organization's mission. Project B, at a more advantageous stage of its life-cycle, has better intrinsic growth prospects, and the organization has slightly more existing physician competence and slightly more experience in working with the distribution channels involved. Which one wins? Project B wins if the organization is willing to stray somewhat from its mission. Project A wins if the organization wants to stick by its mission more rigidly. This is exactly the type of decision that may have to be made by the head of the organization, or even by the trustees.

Employing some formal system of screening and ranking projects against these critical success variables clarifies and structures what would otherwise be extremely complex

decisions. It also approximately doubles the likelihood that those concepts that are taken seriously enough to study in depth will prove successful. It must be remembered, however, that only a minority of the ideas that do pass such initial screening go on to prove successful. Screening concepts systematically is worthwhile, therefore, but it is only the first step in successful service innovation.

Feasibility Analysis

The concept screening process described above is primarily intended to answer the question, "Is this idea worth serious study?" That serious study starts with the next step in the service development process. The purpose of *feasibility analysis* is to resolve three critical questions:

1. What resources will it really take to develop, launch, and sustain the service?
2. Can the enterprise successfully market the service?
3. Can the enterprise really afford to do it?

Any feasibility study of a new service concept seems at first glance to be heavily oriented toward answering the third question. Often the most-read part of such a study is its tables of income and expenditure forecasts and of cash flow projections: How much revenue will the service generate and by when? What will it cost to develop and launch? What will its ongoing operating costs be? How much cash will it require until it reaches breakeven and then payback?

However, those financial tables and projections are only a convenient summary of a much more complex set of issues that have to be investigated during a feasibility study. In order to calculate reasonably accurate *revenue projections*, someone has to answer two more basic questions:

1. How much of the service can we sell (e.g., how many patients can we attract)?
2. What can we charge and get paid for the service?

By definition, *revenue* means units of service times the price received. To project $100,000 of revenue in year 1 is the result, for instance, of 100 patients at $1,000 each, or 1,000 patients at $100 each, or some other combination. Consequently, the revenue forecast in a feasibility study is only as good as the projections of volume and of price.

Similarly, the *cost projections* in a feasibility study are only as reliable as the answers to two other questions:

1. What are *all* the resources that the new program will need?

2. How much will we have to pay for them?

Erroneous assumptions about these four issues — sales, prices, resources, and their cost — can easily be overlooked when they get merged into several pages of financial forecasts. Overly optimistic projections are commonplace in many feasibility studies. They may, for instance, assume a buildup of patients in a health care service that the normal working of the life-cycle shows to be highly improbable (Shanklin 1986).

As an example, a hospital's feasibility analysis for a women's care center was built on the assumption that patient visits in each of the first four quarters would be 500, 1,000, 1,500, and 2,000. One reason for those projections was that breakeven for the center was estimated at 2,500 quarterly visits. The champions of the scheme wanted to show a reasonable chance of reaching that breakeven volume by the second year. It would have been more realistic to forecast breakeven by the fourth or fifth year, but they were worried that such a forecast would kill the project's chances of approval.

Contrast these forecasts with the earlier discussion of the product life-cycle. They implied that the center would grow by 200% in its second quarter, 50% in its third quarter, and 33% in its fourth quarter. Not only are those highly improbable growth projections for any introductory service, but they also imply a decelerating rate of growth from the start.

Forecasting Sales

How does one make a realistic *sales forecast* for a new service? Three considerations are most important:

1. Assume a conservatively slow rate of buildup in the first year or so.

2. Thereafter, the rate of buildup will partly depend on the life-cycle stage of the service. If the project involves a new type of service, not many examples of which exist, the idea is still in its introductory phase and may face several years of sluggish growth. If other suppliers are already offering the service, and it seems to be in its growth phase, the new entrant may share in the rapid growth after its initial establishment in the market. If the idea is at any later stage in its life-cycle, the new entrant may never achieve significant annual growth rates unless it has some really superior competitive advantage.

3. Assume a low market share as the ceiling for the forecast.

A good illustration of the second point above is provided by the development of the market for magnetic resonance imaging (MRI) technology. The six major sellers of MRI units in the United States in 1983-1985 were Technicare, Diasonics, Picker, Siemens, General Electric, and Philips. Among them, they estimated that they would achieve sales over those 2 years of between 204 and 257 units. They actually sold 150, or only 75% of the low end of their forecast. Siemens and General Electric actually beat their upper forecast. The other four only achieved half of their lowest forecast sales. What was different about Siemens and GE that made their forecasts more accurate? "A Siemens spokesperson said it recognized the difficulty of introducing a new medical technology into a changing marketplace. A General Electric spokesperson said that the company did not want to be overly-optimistic" (Rajan, Kangun, and Rodrigues 1987).

As stated in the list above, a low market share should be set as a ceiling for the sales forecast. There actually was a corporation in the early 1970s, Equity Funding, which published a forecast for growth in the number of lives covered by its life insurance policies which would have meant that within 5 years every man, woman, and child in the United States would be insured four times over with this one company.

The earlier example about a fitness center that was not built illustrated how 400,000 adults within walking range of the proposed location were shown by market research to translate into only 4,000 real potential customers. As the center needed 40% of them to break even, the project was abandoned.

As a further example of the same principle, a realtor with experience in selling homes in retirement communities in Florida works on the conservative assumptions that only people over 70 years old will be interested; that they must already be living within 20 miles of the site, since most elderly people do not in fact move long distances; and that he can only expect to attract 1 in 20 of them. (Kunnerth 1987). In other words, he defines his maximum achievable sales as a 5% market share of people over 70 living within a service area of 20 miles.

Contrast that realtor's approach with the following example case of an urgent care center. Built in a community of 60,000, this center needed 20,000 annual visits to break even. Each person visits a doctor on average between 3 and 4 times a year. The total physician encounters in this population were thus about 200,000. Some 60% of the population had a regular doctor with whom they were satisfied, and most of these doctors were associated with the local hospital and recommended their patients to its emergency room. The new urgent care center thus needed to attract a 10% market share of all physician encounters in the community, or 25% of all visits by people without a regular doctor. It was put up for sale 2 years later, having achieved only 10,000 annual visits — a 5% market share of all physician encounters, or a 12% share of visits by those without regular doctors.

Realistic forecasting of expected volume is vital to sound feasibility analysis. It is wise to assume a slow buildup and a maximum eventual volume that represents only a small market share. It is also worthwhile to consider at what stage of the product life-cycle the new service will enter, because growth prospects vary dramatically with the life-cycle. The earlier screening process included a look at both total need and life-cycle stage among its criteria. Even for projects that seem to have promise at that screening stage, it is necessary to consider their volume potential more carefully during a subsequent feasibility analysis.

Pricing Assumptions

The *pricing* of a service assumed in a feasibility study is the other critical variable that affects the revenue projections for the proposed program.

No organization has total freedom of pricing. It may operate under one or more of three restraints:

1. Official pricing regulation and control

2. Dependence on major volume buyers (e.g., insurance companies or other major corporate buyers) with their own views about reasonable prices for services, and purchasing power with which to try to impose those views

3. What the individual customer is willing to pay.

A great many services, in health care and other sectors, are subject to regulatory pricing controls. Banks, insurance companies, hospitals, telephone companies, HMOs, and, in some states, a wide range of other businesses face price controls. If such official oversight applies to the pricing of a service undergoing a feasibility study, it must be taken into account.

The power of *oligopsonists* (a few dominant buyers) can often be overlooked during a feasibility study. Large admitters to a hospital, large referrers to a health service, corporate buyers, and others can have distinct views about the price of new services. It is often worthwhile, therefore, at least to talk to a few of them about the proposed idea, or to use an independent third party, such as a market researcher, to poll some of them without revealing the name of the sponsoring organization.

An illustration is provided by the sponsors of a proposed upscale lunchtime fitness program for executives, who paid a market research company to conduct telephone interviews with some selected target companies, which they were hopeful would sign up some of their top managers for the new service. The sponsors were concerned about how those companies might react to the price needed to break even. The researcher reported back that price was not a major issue for these companies. Much more important was the fact that some, as a matter of principle, offered no special executive perks, while some others were owned by corporations located elsewhere and did not have the freedom to confer a benefit upon their local executives that differed from what other executives in the firm received.

Perhaps the most important audience for a pricing decision is the individual customer. Marketing scientists distinguish a *buyers' market* from a *sellers' market*. In a sellers' market, demand for a product or service exceeds supply. Customers will often put up with inconvenience and pay marked-up prices to obtain the scarce commodity. That has been true for products as diverse as Trivial Pursuit, gasoline during the oil crisis, Coors beer, and hospital beds in the 1950s and 1960s. In a buyers' market, supply of the product exceeds demand for it. The product or service is in surplus. Competition now exists, because not every provider can sell all that it wants to, and power moves to the customer. The buyer now has choice, and one possible basis of choice is price.

Many health services do not seem very price sensitive. They are used mainly on the basis of their perceived quality. There are an increasing number of people who now "shop around" for at least some health services, with price as a major concern. Again, therefore, it pays to survey a sample of them to test what price the market will bear. The technical term for such pricing is *customary pricing*, or charging what customers expect to have to pay.

When an organization seems to have some freedom of choice about service pricing, there are some general findings from marketing research to be considered.

Many organizations use various types of *discounts* to attract buyers. These may be discounts for quantity purchases, or they may be special introductory offers. They may be discounts for those who pay in cash or they may be seasonal discounts to boost volume at a time when it usually slumps.

For at least some customers, price actually serves as a proxy for quality. A more expensive version of a product or service may be assumed to be better. This type of *prestige pricing* may well be a factor for at least some customers of health services.

The stage of the product life-cycle can also have an impact on pricing strategy. If a new service is genuinely innovative, a deliberate choice has to be made between two initial pricing strategies. Because the costs of developing and launching an innovation are often high, there is an understandable desire to get those costs covered as quickly as possible by pricing the service high. There may well be some buyers for it at that high price. Once sales to them seem to have stagnated, the price can be cut for those not quite willing to pay as much as the first, and so on. This tactic of *price skimming* is commonly used, for instance, by computer and electronics companies launching a new computer, stereo system, or cooker.

The alternative strategy in the introductory phase is to price the product or service low to capture as big a market as possible as quickly as possible. This approach is known as *penetration pricing*.

If the innovation is not really original, and the organization is just trying to catch up with competitors who got into a new field first, the pricing decision can be even more difficult. If the product has already entered the growth phase, competitors may well be dropping their prices, now that their high start-up costs are behind them. On the other hand, the new entrant trying to catch up may not face all the start-up costs of his or her competitors, because the new entrant can learn from their earlier mistakes, but costs are still going to be higher for some time until the new entrant gains market share.

Just as the growth phase tends to see lower prices, as providers achieve economies of scale, so prices tend to drop even further at the mature stage as providers compete with each other even more intensely.

The price to be charged for a new product or service is also crucial to the revenue projections made during its feasibility analysis. Organizations do not often have total freedom of choice on pricing. The feasibility study should not, therefore, just use price as a "fudge factor" to make the concept look profitable. The pricing assumptions used have to be rational and justifiable in terms of market conditions.

Estimating Costs

The full identification of the *resources* that a new concept will require and their proper *costing* is the other half of the challenge of feasibility analysis. It is easy to overlook important resources that will be required to develop the project effectively, to launch it, or to sustain it. It is also easy to understate their true cost.

One common mistake, for instance, is to estimate the start-up costs of a program on the assumption that certain aspects of it will be done by existing personnel. For example, a hospital started offering nurses as speakers to local voluntary organizations. It was not looking for any direct revenue out of this service, but saw it as a way to market the hospital. It planned to provide this service with existing personnel. In the first few months, requests averaged only about one a week, so that it was not difficult to find a nurse to volunteer. Then the hospital decided to advertise the service in the local press. About half of its budget advertising dollars for the next month went to promoting that offer.

The ads were very successful. Requests for nurse speakers now rose to more than 20 a month. The director of nursing went to see the head of marketing. She explained that her few volunteers were now overstretched and experiencing burnout. She felt that the only way to sustain this program was to hire two people on it full-time, at a cost, with fringes and travel, of about $60,000 a year. The head of marketing replied that he had a problem, too. He could not go on devoting half his monthly advertising budget to promoting this one program, when there were many others in need of promotion. He would need about $60,000 a year also to sustain this public education program. Thus, a new service that was going to be supplied "free" by existing resources had, in just one month, become a $120,000 decision.

One of the most frequently overlooked and underestimated of all project costs is marketing expense itself. It can be used as an example of how critical forgotten costs can be to project feasibility. The same mistakes can easily, however, arise with any other resource needs, as the case of the nurse speakers shows.

Table 8-12 shows a summary of a project feasibility study. This project looks to do somewhat better than break even. Omitted, however, are any marketing costs needed to attract the 300 to 400 expected patients. Table 8-13 recasts the data to reflect marketing considerations. The project which appeared to be probably worth pursuing in the first summary, now appears of very questionable profitability and requires a large market share. As the article in

Table 8-12 Results of Project Feasibility Study

	Year 1	Year 2	Year 3
Projected patients	300	400	400
Projected revenues	$150,000	$200,000	$200,000
Projected costs	$160,000	$180,000	$180,000
Projected surplus	($10,000)	$ 20,000	$ 20,000

Table 8-13 Revised Results of Project Feasibility Study

	Year 1	Year 2	Year 3
Projected operating costs	$160,000	$180,000	$180,000
Projected price	$500	$500	$500
Patients necessary to break even	320	360	360
Projected marketing costs	$50,000	$30,000	$30,000
Revised patients necessary to break even	420	420	420
Estimated market @ $500	2,000	2,100	2,100
Market share necessary to break even	20%	20%	20%

which that table first appeared commented, "anticipating marketing costs becomes even more important as health providers diversify. For home care agencies, for instance, marketing budgets average 5% of total costs, for billing systems vendors they average 10% and for fitness programs up to 30%. Whatever marketing advantages a provider may think that its new ventures possess, they are unlikely to be a match for this type of marketing muscle." (Bradley, Fisk, and Owens 1987).

The assumptions made about volumes and pricing are critical to a sound feasibility study. So are the assumptions made about the real resources required and their true costs. Marketing is just one of those costs of doing business that frequently get ignored or underestimated. In reviewing feasibility study reports, it is crucial to go behind the financial summaries to be sure that they rest upon sound assumptions about the service, its costs, and its markets.

References

Ansoff, I., ed. 1976. *From strategic planning to strategic management.* New York: Wiley.

Baxter Travenol. 1987. *The home DME marketplace*, pp. 1-4. Deerfield, IL: Baxter Travenol.

Bradley, M., T. Fisk, and H. Owens. 1987. The finance marketing interface in hospitals. *Health Care Strategic Management* 5 (1): 11-22.

Costello, M. 1987. Hospital marketing revisited. *Health Care Strategic Management* 5 (5): 9-12.

Day, G. S. 1981. The product life cycle: Analysis and applications. *Journal of Marketing* 45: 60-66.

Graduate Medical Education National Advisory Committee. 1980. *Report of the graduate medical education national advisory committee, Volume H.* Washington, DC: Department of Health and Human Services.

Hax, A. C. ed. 1987. *Planning strategies that work.* New York: Oxford University Press.

Kotler, P. 1972. *Marketing management*, pp. 429-438. Englewood Cliffs, NJ: Prentice Hall.

Kunerth, A. 1987. Real advice. *Modern Demographics* (August): 15.

Mendenhall, W., and J. Reinmuth. 1974. *Statistics for management and economics*, pp. 401-470. Belmont, CA: Duxbury Press.

Porter, M. 1980. *Competitive strategy*. New York: The Free Press.

Rajan, T., N. Kangun, and A. Rodrigues. 1987. A prescription for overcoming the marketing failures of MRI sellers. *Journal of Health Care Marketing* 7(2): 70-76.

Reibstein, D. 1985. *Marketing: Concepts, strategies and decisions*, pp. 313-319. Englewood Cliffs, NJ: Prentice Hall.

Roberts, E., and C. Berry. 1985. Entering new businesses: Selecting strategies for success. *Sloan Management Review* 26(3): 3-17.

Shanklin, W. 1986. Six timeless marketing blunders. *Journal of Consumer Marketing* 3(4): 31-34.

Wheatley, D. 1983. *Marketing professional services*, p. 50. Englewood Cliffs, NJ: Prentice Hall.

Review Questions

1. What are the 10 key questions to ask in screening any new service idea? Explain briefly why each is important.

2. Explain the key differences among the following four growth strategies: market development, product or service development, diversification, and market penetration.

3. What is the difference between breakeven and payback?

4. What is the difference between market skimming and market penetration?

5. How would you briefly describe the key features of the service life-cycle to someone unfamiliar with the concept? How would you explain why it is important to consider the life-cycle in a decision about a new service idea?

6. "One of the most common errors in feasibility forecasts for new health service ideas is an overly optimistic forecast of patient volumes." Discuss.

Chapter 9

Implementing New or Changed Services

The last two chapters reviewed the first three steps in the service innovation process: concept generation, concept screening, and feasibility assessment. It was noted that experience in innovative companies shows that it takes 64 innovative concepts to yield 32 ideas that pass initial screening. Those ideas then advance to a more detailed feasibility study, from which only a minority emerge that appear to be worth pursuing (Booz Allen and Hamilton 1982).

This process of attrition applies both to entirely original ideas for new services and to suggestions for upgrading present services. Organizations that are less rigorous in screening ideas and reviewing their feasibility tend to have high rates of *service failure*. In a large and complex health care organization, such as a major hospital, many services actually fail to attain their goals but are nevertheless maintained. This happens because the many not-for-profit hospitals are not so concerned with maximizing their bottom line as they are with providing as broad a range of health services as they can while ensuring their overall survival. They may, as an example, perpetuate a loss-making obstetrical program or transplant surgery service, as long as their total *product mix* of services generates enough of a surplus to keep the hospital in business.

As competition intensifies among hospitals, however, it is unlikely that they will be able to run as many loss-making programs as in the past. They will have to apply more stringent standards to the new services that they consider starting, to the enhancement of existing programs, and, in some cases, to reviewing whether certain of their programs will have to be abandoned. Dropping a program is always more difficult than avoiding its inception. The more rigorous the appraisal of ideas for service innovation, therefore, the fewer new ventures may be started, but likewise, the fewer are the ventures that will fail.

Many health care providers are much less complex organizations than these large medical centers. A small provider may only have a few, and perhaps only one, innovative concept upon which the whole enterprise seems to succeed or fail—home care, smoking cessation, or selling a preferred provider health insurance plan. The risks of failure are just as high, but the ability to cross-subsidize a loser from a winner is not there in the small enterprise. That is why more than half of all the small enterprises started up each year do not survive beyond their first or second year.

Some small and failing organizations do strike it lucky. Even though they are losing money, some other enterprise decides to buy them in the belief that it can put them onto a profitable footing. For example, one group of hospitals formed a preferred provider organization (PPO). Two years later, most of those who had joined the plan were employees of the hospitals themselves, and it was losing money. Two critical miscalculations had been made. First, the hospitals had overestimated the pace at which the idea of PPOs would catch on among employers and their workforces. Second, the hospitals had underestimated the effort, expense, and time that it would take them to develop real know-how in selling and managing health insurance. The hospitals were faced with a dilemma: Keeping the plan going would take yet more cash, but closing it would be a confession of failure to the various hospital boards and to their enrolled employees.

Fortunately, a major insurance company was in the process of developing its own PPO to sell in the area. It regarded this group of hospitals as important to its ability to offer employers a plan with broad geographical coverage. The company therefore bought the failing plan. The hospitals did not recoup all their losses, but they stopped them from growing any further.

Despite the outcome in this case, it is obviously not a wise tactic to start up a small program in the belief that, if it fails, someone will reprieve it. The high failure rate of small enterprises shows that they really need to screen and test service innovation concepts even more thoroughly than larger organizations.

Both large and small enterprises should screen and test ideas for new services, or revisions to existing services, rigorously, because the risks of failure and financial loss are high. Indeed, the smaller the organization, the less ability it has to subsidize loss-making programs from profitable ones.

Where concepts are properly screened and subjected to feasibility analysis, fewer than one in four survive to the remaining steps in the service development process: service development, service testing, and service launch.

Service Development

Despite the rigors of the screening and feasibility assessment steps discussed in the previous chapter, all that has been proved about any idea that survives them is that it fits a basic set of criteria and that it appears to be financially viable. The next questions that arise are:

1. Can the concept actually be put together so that it works?

2. What additional things have to be done to maximize its market potential?

3. Is it still financially viable after that more detailed definition?

In the late 1940s, General Electric screened and assessed the feasibility of developing an electric knife. The concept passed the company's screens as being a potentially popular electrical consumer product. Feasibility assessment showed that it could be produced at a reasonable cost and sold at an attractive price. GE product developers started to create a prototype. At the same time the market research staff investigated the likely market appeal of the product. They reported back that it was not well perceived. Only a small percentage of interviewees reported that they were likely to buy one. As a result, the marketing staff advised that the costs of promoting the product would be much higher than assumed in the feasibility study. Once these extra costs were added, the product was unlikely to prove profitable. Development work on it was halted, but as we shall see later, only for a time.

The same phenomenon can easily occur in the health care arena once an apparently feasible project becomes the subject of an actual developmental effort. In Chapter 2, for example, a proposed center for the treatment of seizure disorders was described, which appeared feasible until developmental work on it was already quite advanced, even to the point of a specialist physician having been recruited to head it. In both that case and the one concerning the electric knife, it was the real costs of promotion that sunk the project. It is just as likely, however, that operational difficulties will be encountered. The logistics of making an idea actually work may be seen, once development work commences, to be much more difficult than earlier assumed.

As an example, a hospital administrator was approached by the operator of a local executive limousine service. His limos were heavily used at night but often stood idle during the daytime hours. For a discounted fee, he was prepared to take home patients being discharged from the hospital. The administrator saw this as a good service to offer to obstetrical patients. Competition among the local hospitals for such patients was intensifying, and this "offer" would give his hospital something different to use in its promotion. He was even willing for the hospital to pick up the cost, so that it could be advertised as a free service.

The administrator asked the nursing and discharge planning staff to work out the details with the limo operator. The closer they looked into the idea, however, the less practical it appeared. The company did normally have idle limos during the day, but occasionally it received calls for daytime journeys, which would have to take priority. At times, its entire fleet of four vehicles was either in use or undergoing repairs. Also, nearly always an obstetrical patient's spouse came to take her and the new baby home.

The limo operator was uncertain whether he could extend the service to picking up the husband, bringing him to the hospital, waiting for discharge to be completed, and then driving them home. Often this whole process would take some 3 hours. The limo operator could therefore only manage some two or three such journeys a day, but the hospital discharged an average of seven OB patients daily. At times, the husband would drive to his place of work, and then leave to pick up his wife at the hospital. Even if the limo driver could afford to pick up the spouse at work, the spouse's car would then be stranded there. Sometimes a husband would bring older siblings to collect the mother and baby, and the hospital could not assure the limo operator how clean his autos would be after a few hours' occupancy by a young and excited family. Finally, the hospital's own liability for the safety of mother and baby might extend to the journey home if it was providing the transport.

As these cases illustrate, some concepts do not survive their development phase, even though they appeared both desirable and feasible beforehand. Even those concepts that are successfully developed often undergo major changes of format, scope, and cost during their detailed development.

One frequent reason for such changes is that more detailed review shows a necessity of revising one of three service dimensions (Kotler 1972). Any service is an amalgam of:

1. The *generic service*, or the benefit it delivers to the user (e.g., relief from pain, a longer life, improved appearance, or improved functionality in daily living skills)

2. The *tangible service*, which is the process that delivers the benefit (e.g., neurological testing and treatment, plastic surgery, or occupational therapy)

3. The *extended service*, or the functional features that are added on to meet incidental benefits sought by customers and to give the service stronger appeal (e.g., social work support, patient education, evening hours, changing rooms that afford greater privacy).

For instance, the costs of efficient data or word processing (the generic product) by IBM computers and terminals (the tangible product) are increased by that company's deliberate commitment to high reliability, extensive customer training, rapid servicing availability, and the broadest possible availability of compatible software (the extended product). Similarly, the costs of quick relief from pain caused by minor trauma and other medical problems (the generic service) in urgicenters (the tangible service) are expanded by having highly visible, and therefore somewhat more expensive, locations, adjacent parking, and longer hours than doctors' offices (the extended service).

The Generic Service

Perhaps the two most common generic service issues that arise in the development of health programs concern:

1. The novelty of the benefit
2. The degree of quality to be incorporated into the service.

Novelty. The greater the novelty of the benefit of a health service, the higher will be the costs of its initial marketing. It is true of all truly original products and services that their benefits are not instantly apparent to the customer. The benefit of an automobile is readily accessible and reasonably rapid personal mobility. Now that automobiles are familiar products, a company launching a new model does not have to convince customers of this benefit. Its marketing concentrates more upon explaining unique features of the extended product that a particular model incorporates. The early auto makers, however, faced a 20-year process of convincing a critical number of customers that the benefit of the generic product was worth obtaining.

The typical health customer now has an equivalent understanding of the value of such established medical services as open-heart surgery, emergency rooms, intensive care units, cosmetic surgery, childbirth in a hospital, or care by a licensed nurse. However, a century ago the benefits of hospitals and nurses were almost as obscure to the majority of the public as those of automobiles. Hospitals mainly catered to the poor and the terminally ill. Fewer than 2% of doctors had hospital privileges, because most care was delivered in the home. Hospital nursing was "a menial occupation, taken up by women of the lower classes, some of whom were conscripted from the penitentiary or the almshouse" (Starr 1982). Earlier in the nineteenth century, physicians had faced a similar challenge in convincing the public of their superiority over "traveling bonemen," surgeon barbers, and herbalists.

The generic service of a very innovative product or service is not self-evident. It will take added cost and time to communicate it to people. This is one reason why innovations tend to face a slow and risky introductory phase in their life-cycle.

A multidisciplinary team of physicians interested in dementia and its accurate differential diagnosis and treatment founded a center for patients with Alzheimer's disease. This center built up a small monthly volume of cases through its first 6 years. They came by referral from other doctors and from health agencies with which these doctors had made personal contact. The founders were, however, disappointed at this low volume of cases.

As public knowledge of Alzheimer's disease grew through increased media attention in the mid-1980s, the physicians were hopeful of receiving more referrals. Unfortunately, that publicity also led many people to believe that all memory loss is attributable to Alzheimer's, rather than to treatable conditions, and that nothing can be done to aid Alzheimer's patients and their caregivers. It took an advertising campaign by the center, primarily aimed at correcting these false impressions, to increase its activity levels.

The more innovative a health service really is, the greater will be the initial effort required to convince customers, in the medical community or the general public, of the value of the generic service. The benefit will not usually be obvious to them without a major communications and promotion effort. This task inflates the cost of real innovation and may at times make an otherwise strong concept financially unviable.

Levels of Quality. The level of *quality assurance* to be built into a service is also critical to its development. Marketing scientists distinguish four broad approaches to quality in fields other than health care (Lele 1986). An innovator may elect one of the following methods of translating the concept into an actual product:

1. A *disposable product* that is not to be promoted as of continuing reliability (e.g., many small appliances)

2. A *repairable product*, which customers will expect to work most of the time, but also to require periodic maintenance and repair (e.g., automobiles, washers)

3. A *rapid-response repairable product*, similar to the preceding category but which is supported by quickly available servicing (e.g., photocopiers, farm tractors)

4. A *"never-fails" product*, which is designed only to fail in the most extreme of circumstances (e.g., airplanes, seat belts, telephone systems, paging systems, medical monitors).

Customer expectations of most medical programs are that they will be "never-fails" services. Meeting these expectations, whether in health care or another field, tends to require built-in redundancy (e.g., backup resources if the primary circuitry in electronic equipment fails, or some other predefined protocol or referral arrangement, if a medical service does not work). It may also require more frequent maintenance and greater inspection and monitoring. Because of these needs, "never-fails" products and services all tend to have both higher fixed costs and higher variable costs. They tend to be both capital intensive and labor intensive.

The extent to which an innovative health service concept requires such features to ensure its quality often does not become apparent until the detailed development stage. For example, the earliest surgicenters and the earliest alternative birthing centers in many states found, at quite a late stage of development, that regulatory agencies required documentary proof of preagreed transfer protocols to a nearby hospital for the very small projected percentage of patients who would face complications that were unmanageable at a free-standing center. The earliest HMOs discovered that they needed "re-insurance" — a policy with a major insurance company to cover them if they had an unexpected number of patients requiring the most expensive types of hospital care before they were large enough to spread these costs over many thousands of enrollees.

The level of quality to be incorporated into a new health service, or into an extension or revision of an existing service, is thus a critical issue in its development. It is not a question that the enterprise can answer for itself in a vacuum, without regard to the expectations of the potential customers.

For instance, how might a hospital approach the development of a smoking cessation program? The failure or recidivism rate for such programs is over 50%. Will enrollees have higher expectations of such a program when sponsored by a hospital, particularly one that enjoys an image of high quality? If so, will those who fail in this program lower their image of the quality of other hospital programs? What can the hospital's program do to lower the recidivism rate? Can backup resources be made available for those who fail, which try a different approach? Have those backup techniques been tested and demonstrated, or are they just a theoretical but untried application of existing behavior modification techniques? Do the extra costs of a program with a projected lower recidivism rate destroy its marketability?

The level of quality to be built into a new health service, or a revision of an existing service, and how to ensure that level of quality, are important issues in their detailed development. The internal quality philosophy of the enterprise is not the only issue at stake. The quality expectations of potential customers should also be considered, and they may well have to be researched and tested. It should not be assumed that the public expects all health services to operate at the "never-fails" level, but, without investigation, it may also be risky to assume that they do not expect that level of assurance. The financial viability of the program may have to be reassessed once actual quality assurance requirements have been identified.

The Tangible Service

This issue of quality may, of course, also impact the development of the tangible service, which may have to take a different form from that originally conceptualized. Several alternative birthing centers developed by nurse midwives, for instance, discovered that, to satisfy both their own quality standards and, in some cases, those demanded by regulatory agencies, they had to appoint a physician medical director, contrary to their initial plans. Their challenge then became to find a doctor who would play this role but leave them with the maximum professional latitude.

Identifying a Leader. This example illustrates another issue in service development. The actual format of many services depends crucially on the personalities, interests, and temperaments of their key personnel. That tends to be just as true outside of health care as within it. Many enterprises are, in large measure, a reflection of their key leader or leaders. IBM is still heavily influenced by the legacy of Tom Watson, ITT by the past role of Harold Geneen, and McDonald's by that of Ray Kroc.

Often health services grow out of the goals of a particular physician or other health professional. Their private visions often have to be somewhat remolded to fall in with practical operational or marketing considerations, but the tangible service is largely of their own making. Many innovative concepts, in health care and elsewhere, come from someone or some group of people who "want" to do something.

The reverse situation also often applies: An innovative idea arises from an organization's formal review of its opportunities and threats. The idea seems desirable and feasible, but it lacks an obvious leadership. In such circumstances, a major task in the development phase should be the identification and early involvement of a potential individual or group leader. The concept often cannot be finally developed without allowing for modification of its tangible service to accommodate the style and ideas of those who will provide it. That is one drawback that frequently inhibits the success of "imitation" services, designed to match an apparently successful initiative by a major competitor. If that initiative was largely born out of the personal aspirations of someone at the rival organization, it may not be possible to replicate its effectiveness.

One hospital that conducted a public survey identified a potential market for a specialized center treating a particular neurological disorder. A nearby rival hospital had a well-known specialist in that field, but had not chosen to promote that capability in its public marketing because that physician already had a very busy referral practice.

The first hospital saw this situation as an opportunity. It logically assessed that demand for treatment of that disorder was increasing as the public heard more about it in the media. It also rightly concluded that treatment of the disease was in its growth phase, creating room for new entrants. It even correctly saw that the specialist at the rival hospital was committing one common mistake of medical innovators: He had seen some new methods of treating this disease through their difficult introductory phase. Now that they were in their growth phase, however, rather than expand his own practice by taking on a partner and sharing his know-how, he had created an opening for another practice to enter on his coattails.

The hospital sounded out its own neurologists. None was initially enthusiastic about heading up a new center with this narrow focus. After some 6 months of discussion, however, one neurologist was persuaded to head it up in return for a guaranteed income. The program was launched and advertised, and it attracted some initial patients. The hospital expected that after such support with its launch, the center would have patients and families who would then spread news of it. After a critical mass of such patients had been treated, the marketing support could be reduced as word-of-mouth "marketing" by patients themselves took over.

Twelve months later, that stage had still not been reached. Although quite a few patients had been seen, nearly all the new ones were still being generated by advertising. When the hospital administration examined why, they realized that this had never been the "volunteer" physician's real field of interest. He had been talked into running the program. As a result, he had less interest in the center's patients than in those coming to his private practice with a broader range of neurological problems. He had given the patients at the center the lowest priority in scheduling and follow-up, creating low patient and family satisfaction as a result.

Even in quite large enterprises, successful products and services are, more than is often realized, driven by the enthusiasm of particular people. The final development of a tangible health service innovation should reflect the input and ideas of those who will give it professional leadership as far as financial, operational, and marketing realities can allow.

Location and Access. In the development of any service where the consumer must travel to the site to receive the service, location is another vital aspect of the tangible service. Where it is may be at least as important as what it is.

Some formalized methods of reviewing service location options were discussed in the previous chapter. They were based on mapping the residential pattern of the intended target audience and using a gravity model to determine the location or locations most accessible to the largest number of them. These concepts are equally applicable to locating health services (Eaton, Church, and Revelle 1977).

The best location for a hospital-associated ambulatory service may not be at the hospital itself if the residential pattern of the target audience differs from that of hospital patients as a whole. Even if their residential pattern is similar to that of the hospital's inpatients, they may well have different attitudes toward regular travel for ambulatory service than they have toward a very infrequent hospital admission. Often there seem to be overwhelming reasons for locating a new ambulatory program within the hospital: Space may be available; it may be more convenient for the professional staff; it may seem to be a useful way of introducing more patients to the hospital facilities. It should not be taken for granted, though, that these considerations are more important than a location that minimizes travel for the maximum number of people.

The nursing staff at one hospital were disappointed at the quite small percentage of women delivering at the hospital who enrolled in its childbirth education classes. The nurses were even more disappointed that some women who came to their hospital for childbirth attended other hospitals' childbirth education courses. When they investigated why this was happening, they saw that a large number of their obstetrical patients were admitted by two physician groups whose offices were close together but some 15 miles from the hospital. They interviewed some of the recent mothers, who explained that a hospital 15 miles from home was acceptable for a 2- or 3-day inpatient stay, but not for repetitive attendance through their pregnancy at childbirth education classes. The nurses therefore started some classes closer to these patients' homes. Not only did enrollment increase, but their classes now attracted some women from that community who were planning to deliver at rival hospitals.

One primary issue in location, therefore, is proximity to the target audience for the service. Often of equal importance is the degree of competition present in different locations. One consultant on physician marketing, for instance, has calculated population requirements for a successful new practice location. A family medicine specialist should look for a pocket of 3,000 people without a nearer competitor; an allergist needs to be nearer than any competitor to 26,000 people; a pediatrician needs to be more accessible than any competitors to 12,000 people, and so on (Korneluk 1985).

The third most important locational factor for a service, especially one that depends upon a large volume of self-referred patients, is visibility. Some of the more successful developers of urgicenters, for instance, follow a strict rule: Their centers must be located on major highways with a certain minimum daily traffic volume past the door. If they cannot find a location in a target community that satisfies that criterion, they do not develop in that area. Some of these for-profit developers have learned that lesson by experience.

One, for instance, started a number of highly successful centers in the South and Midwest. He then tried to develop some in the Northeast. None of the first six he opened in the Northeast proved profitable. The developer had taken care to distance himself from hospitals with emergency rooms and to seek out communities with the lowest numbers of primary physicians. To locate near a reasonably high density of population, however, meant going into established suburbs where the best major highway locations were all occupied. His least successful location was literally visible from four major highways where they intersected, but accessible from any of them only by a convoluted and badly signed route.

The enthusiasm that develops for a new service can easily lead its advocates, when they find that no ideal location exists, to compromise on a second-best location. It may be off major highways, or it may be distant from the center of gravity of the target population. If a service seems to depend on self-referral and patient convenience, a suboptimal location may be enough to destroy its viability.

For many ambulatory services, vehicular access and parking may also be critical to successful design and development. If this appears to be less than optimal at any location, it may be worthwhile moving, or at least building in some compensating service feature. For example, an optometrist in downtown Los Angeles suspected that lack of immediately adjacent free parking was inhibiting his practice. He spoke to the building owner, who agreed to park his patients free in the basement garage in exchange for $200 monthly from the doctor. Rather than commit to this decision without further consideration, the doctor mailed a self-designed, one-page survey to past patients. Forty-four percent identified parking as a major complaint about his practice. Fewer than 5% mentioned any other complaint at all. The survey itself cost him $175 in total. Based on the results, he instituted the free parking deal, and his practice grew (Review of Optometry 1982).

In services for which customers must travel to the site of delivery, location is a vital ingredient in the tangible service design. It is even more important if the service depends, wholly or partly, on self-referral. The four most important aspects of location for health services are typically:

1. *Proximity to the target audience*

2. *Degree of competition in a location*

3. *Visibility from well-traveled routes*

4. *Vehicular access and parking.*

The Extended Service

The third aspect of service development concerns the extended service. The generic and tangible components of any service usually need to be supplemented by added "functional features," for three principal reasons (Stewart 1959).

First, as discussed in Chapter 3, customers rarely utilize a service for one benefit only. They seek to satisfy a bundle of benefits simultaneously. The generic and tangible aspects of a service address the primary benefit sought (e.g., relief from pain, improved appearance, a longer life). It is the added functional features built into the service that address their other, ancillary needs (e.g., for information, reassurance, convenience). Since most customers have multiple benefits in mind in selecting health services, programs that lack added functional features constitute an "incomplete" market offering.

In reality, a failure to consider these extra customer needs in service design can result in something worse than an incomplete offering. It can result in a service that actually contains dysfunctional features, or real barriers to customer usage. In the previous chapter, for instance, it was shown how a university hospital's department of orthopedics created a sports medicine program unthinkingly modeled on traditional outpatient clinic lines, with limited hours and initial workup by residents. This application of an inappropriate clinical model to a new service doomed it by building in features that made it dysfunctional in attracting injured athletes in a very competitive market.

The second reason for planning extended service features is that they serve to position the new program in the market. They help the new service to seem different from its competitors. Most innovators of new services strive to make their program superior in clinical quality to its rivals, but communicating actual proof of greater quality to the potential customer is not easy. By contrast, special functional features of the new service can make it stand out in the minds of customers as having one or more distinctive attributes.

A hospital found that it was losing patients to two urgent care centers that had opened in its community. These centers were advertising that they offered quality urgent care (the tangible service) with shorter waits (the extended service). The hospital reorganized its emergency room in response. It strengthened the initial triage staff and created a separate urgent care area. Previously, patients with minor emergencies faced the longest waits when the emergency room was busy, because true emergent cases received priority. Now, with the distinct urgent service, they were also seen reasonably quickly. The hospital now advertised its quality emergency care (the tangible service) as "always quick, never closed." It now matched the urgent care centers in their extended service claim of quick treatment, and surpassed them with the added benefit of being "never closed." The urgent care centers considered whether they could move from 16-hour to 24-hour daily operations, but concluded that they could not do so.

The third possible advantage to be gained by added functional features is in securing free publicity in the media. It may well be the unusual but relatively inexpensive added functional feature that makes a program newsworthy.

Many such functional features are also much easier to add to or delete from a service than its more central components. Marketers in other fields often build functional features into a new product or service to strengthen its market launch, knowing that they can drop them subsequently if they are not needed on a continuing basis. In health care, some diagnostic services have similarly offered "free screening" to some audiences during their start-up period to help build traffic. It is usually important, however, to publicize such start-up extended services as *limited-time offers.* Public response is greater for offers that are seen to have an expiration date, and setting such time limits can also protect against some customers claiming the free service after a long delay when the new program cannot so readily accommodate them.

> *The comprehensive development and design of a new or revised health service should include deliberate decisions about the extended service features it will incorporate. Such added functional features enable a service to better address the benefit bundles customers seek. They can also help to position the service as different from its competitors and may, on occasion, aid in securing free publicity.*

Four critical extended service features of health care programs that often seem to receive inadequate attention during this developmental process are service scope, service name, patient information, and hours of operation.

Scope. The declared *scope* of a service can be crucial to its marketing success. The earliest entrants into a new service field can usually afford to target a broader audience of customers than can later entrants. Once a service has entered the growth phase in a particular geographical market, a new entrant may be unwise to try to compete with established suppliers across the board. They are often tempted to do so because of a belief in the superiority of their own new service. It is usually safer, however, to position the late-entering service to appeal to a specific segment.

For instance, there are currently only a limited number of well-organized centers diagnosing and treating sleep disorders in the United States, yet the incidence of such problems in the population is estimated to be quite high. Because of the small number of existing programs, each is able to promote itself as concerned with the full spectrum of such disorders. Epidemiologically, however, there are a number of such disorders, of which only sleep apnea has so far achieved any widespread public attention. It is very likely, as this field of clinical care grows, that subspecialist centers will emerge. If there is already a strong center of this sort in a local market, a new entrant may be more successful in attempting to take a slice of this market as its own. It might target a particular type of sleep disorder, or all sleep disorders but concentrating on one gender or age group. Insomnia in the elderly patient, for instance, may constitute a viable segment upon which to build the scope of such a new service.

There is often pressure in new health services design to resist this concept of a segmented service scope. The resources involved in diagnosing or treating one disease, or in treating one gender or age group, may well be clinically suitable for diagnosing and treating others. As a result, it seems to make sense to target a new service as broadly as possible. However, because customers in competitive markets look for centers with a specialized scope relevant to their perceived special needs, the reverse is often true. Getting a new service accepted in the market is often easier if its focus is narrow (MacStravic 1977).

Consider the decision of Atlantic Richfield to withdraw its gasoline credit card. Careful market research suggested that about 60% of auto owners use their gasoline credit cards regularly and are not particularly sensitive to the price of gasoline. The other 40% do not use credit cards often or at all, and shop around for low-priced gas. Atlantic Richfield decided that it would turn its back on the 60% card-using segment, and position itself as the gasoline company of choice for the other 40%. That seems like a dangerous strategy, but it is not if the enterprise ends up with a strong competitive advantage in that particular market segment.

Another example is that of a hospital that saw that several of its competitors had opened satellites around the area, each with a different service scope. One competitor had two sports medicine satellites, another had three family medicine satellites, and a third had started an industrial medicine satellite. The first hospital decided that it should do likewise. It reasoned, however, that, if it could build patient traffic to a satellite, it was preferable for it to have a multiplicity of services rather than a narrow service scope. It therefore put several different types of physician practices in its own satellite, complete with a free-standing radiology unit.

Despite a significant public marketing effort, the satellite's performance in its first year was very poor, partly because the public was confused about the purpose and service scope of the center. It developed an image of being just another medical office building with an assortment of doctors, no better or worse than those who could be found elsewhere.

A final example is that of a Catholic hospital that operates in a very competitive market, with some 10 other hospitals within 15 miles. It is, however, the only Catholic hospital among them. The hospital has a 5% market share of all hospital admissions in the area. Before 1980 it was operating at a reasonable annual surplus with this 5% share. In line with the rest of the United States, however, total area admissions to hospitals in this area were declining. In 1980, still with 5% of all local admissions, the hospital incurred its first-ever bottom line loss. It rightly concluded that, if total admissions to hospitals were falling, it had to increase its market share to keep its volume steady.

A survey showed the hospital that 30% of the local population was Catholic and that about half of them, or 15% of the whole population, felt strongly that they should use a Catholic hospital. The hospital calculated that it needed to increase its market share from 5% to 7% to remain viable. Since only 15% of the population actually preferred a Catholic hospital, it decided to deemphasize its religious ties in order to broaden its appeal. It launched an advertising campaign that concentrated on its clinical services and played down its religious connection.

Over the next year, despite this advertising, the hospital's market share stayed constant. The hospital therefore reassessed its strategy. It noted that only half of its admitted patients were in fact Catholic. Thus, among the 85% of the population who did not prefer a Catholic hospital it had a 3% market share. A further survey among this population showed that they continued to prefer the hospital, but for reasons other than its religious ties. Principally, it happened to be the nearest hospital for this non-Catholic population. None of them objected to its religious nature. Among the 15% of the population who were Catholic and preferred a Catholic hospital, it had a 16% market share. In other words, 84% of those who preferred a Catholic hospital were going elsewhere.

To achieve its goal of increasing its overall market share from 5% to 7%, the hospital could either try to increase its share among those who did not prefer a Catholic hospital from 3% to 6%, or try to increase its share among those who did prefer a Catholic hospital from 16% to 28%. The first task sounded simpler, but they had been trying it with no success. The administrators now realized why: Among that population they were no different than nine other hospitals. Indeed, for most of that population they were not only no different but also further from home. For the segment that preferred a Catholic hospital, even though they were further from many of their homes, they alone could satisfy that extended service.

Consequently, the hospital changed its strategy and started emphasizing its religious ties. Its market share started to rise. Interestingly, it rose not only among Catholics who preferred a Catholic hospital, but also among Catholics who claimed that they were indifferent to this attribute. Its market share even increased slightly among non-Catholics. Why? It was now projecting an image that made it different from its competitors, not just an imitation of them. It therefore achieved higher recognition among all segments of the population.

The declared scope of a health service can have a major impact on customer recognition of its purpose and value to them. It can also position the service to appeal more effectively than competitors to segments of the population with distinct benefit bundles that they seek from health care providers.

Naming the Service. The above cases also help to illustrate the importance of *name* in service design and development. The all-purpose satellite in the example above failed to achieve the market recognition of competitors with clearly descriptive names such as a "sports medicine center" or an "industrial medicine center." The Catholic hospital's name happened to make it clear that it was a religious institution, and its initial advertising, which sought to play this element in its image down, just did not work.

In other industries, corporate innovators go to considerable lengths to decide on and, if necessary, test product or service names during the development stage. They do so for two principal purposes: to define a name that will help to position the product or service as different, and to look for a name that will be easy to promote (Levitt 1980).

There are four commonly employed approaches to *service branding*:

1. Emphasizing the overall corporate name (e.g., Heinz, General Electric, or Sony)

2. Combining the corporate name with a specific product name (e.g., Kellogg's Special K or CitiDining, a Citibank restaurant discount program)

3. Creating a separate brand for a class of corporate products or services (e.g., Sears' Kenmore brand or Thrift Drugs' Treasury brand)

4. Using distinct names for major products without the parent company's name (e.g., Tide, Bold, and Dash, all made by Procter & Gamble; or Comtrex, Bufferin, Excedrin, and Sal Hepactica, all products of Bristol-Myers).

Why are so many different approaches employed in product or service branding? In some cases, the parent enterprise has such strong name recognition and such a reputation for quality that it makes sense to emphasize it in all service or product names. That approach is only wise, however, if the parent's reputation is really strong and is also relevant to the new program. In the case of the all-purpose satellite discussed above, the new satellite was called "The [hospital name] Medical Center." Not only was the meaning of medical center unclear, but also this hospital had little name recognition in the suburb where it opened the satellite. Indeed, part of its logic in developing the center was to boost local recognition of the hospital. In attempting to do so, however, it handicapped the project with a poor choice of name.

In other situations, both the parent's quality image and the specific features of a particular product need to be combined. This approach is commonly used in health care (e.g., Travenol Home Health Services, HCA International Hospital, Temple University Sports Medicine Center). This branding concept again, however, presupposes name recognition and a quality image on the part of the parent organization. More subtly, it also assumes that the customer sees that parent as a credible supplier of the new service. Images of competence in one field are not necessarily carried over by customers into other services that seem only peripherally related to those in which an organization built its reputation. How attracted, for instance, would you be personally to dining in an Exxon restaurant, or flying with Bank of America Airlines, or opening a savings account with the Walt Disney Bank?

One hospital designing a fitness center learned, through some focus group sessions with representative executives, that they saw it as in "the sickness business," and not particularly credible as a sponsor of a health spa. The hospital then teamed up with a local hotel, which had a strong recreational image and underutilized gym and pool facilities. The new program bore the hotel's name. Only once potential customers called for details did they learn that the hospital was also involved.

One fairly common technique for bridging this credibility gap between an organization with a strong image in one field and its desire to move into another is to create a new brand name for these new ventures. Thus, Thrift Drugs invented the Treasury label for products it wanted to sell in its stores but that were not directly drug related. In doing so, it also countered the implication of "thrift" as implying "inexpensive" with another concept of "treasure," connoting "more expensive but of great value." There are similar circumstances in health care where it may be appropriate to create a new brand name for services that seem tangential to a provider's previous scope of services. One hospital, as an example, gives its associated urgent care centers the brand name Urgi-Care, and only makes minor mention of their connection with the hospital in promoting them.

Finally, there are circumstances where specific products or services from one organization must compete with strong rivals in a number of largely unassociated markets. It often then makes sense to promote individual product names alone. The goal in doing so is to build customer loyalty to a specific product vis-a-vis its competitors, rather than a broad loyalty to the parent supplier. In pharmaceuticals, for instance, Parke-Davis competes in the market for antitussives with its product Benylin, in the market for antacids with its Gelusil, in the market for laxatives with its Agoral, in the market for hemorrhoid medication with its Anusol, in the market for acne medication with its Therapads, in the market for insect bite medication with its Benadryl, and so on. Only two of these names, Benylin and Benadryl have any similarity.

There are at least early signs in health care of the use of this concept of branding. Several companies now offer programs nationwide under which a hospital or other supplier can become the local franchise holder for a service, which is then advertised throughout the country. One example is "You're Becoming," a cosmetic surgery program.

Experience with products and services outside health care shows a quite wide range of approaches to naming, or branding, services. Which approach is best depends on the level of name recognition and credibility of the parent enterprise and the nature of the competition for each product or service.

The other major purpose of branding is to select a name that aids in establishing recognition of the service among its potential customers. The best name for a service, therefore, is one that:

1. Says, in clearly understood words, what the service does and proclaims one distinguishing feature of it (e.g., Guaranteed Overnight Delivery or Smith Same-Day Surgicenter)

2. Can be pronounced (when answering the phone, or recommending it to a friend) exactly the same way that it always appears in print (e.g., McDonald's or Chicago Home Care)

3. Is never longer than three words, and preferably fewer. Otherwise, it will get abbreviated both by its own staff and by customers. They will not necessarily abbreviate it

in the same way. If this happens, someone reading about the service may not mentally connect it with the name that they may have heard from friends.

4. Avoids obscure medical jargon, relying instead on common words (e.g., "heart" instead of "cardiac," "children's" instead of "pediatric")

5. Never employs initials. Even though IBM and AT&T are household names, it took several decades and multimillion dollar promotion campaigns to achieve that awareness. In one service area in the United States, rival hospitals refer to themselves *internally* as CHUMC, OLOL, ZMH, MHBC, and UMH. Fortunately, each has realized the wisdom of not using such initials in their *external* promotion.

The names, or brands, used for health services should be short and descriptive and use common words. This approach not only aids in creating name recognition, but also conveys to potential customers that the service understands the basics of effective communication.

Consider, as a contrasting example, "The Eye Institute of the Pennsylvania College of Optometry in Association with the Feinbloom Center." That is the name under which one health service tries to promote itself, including in radio ads where the listener is not even aided by seeing the name in print. One of its major competitors goes under the simple name of EyeLab. It is not difficult to project which will win the battle for name recognition.

Patient Information. Since effective communication (explaining things, listening to and answering questions) seems to be part of the benefit bundle sought by a very large majority of health care customers, planning it into the service should ideally be considered during, rather than after, the development stage. Satisfying this need may well change the way in which the service is to be delivered, and therefore alter its operating costs.

National data show that the average physician office visit in primary care lasts some 15 minutes, with a significant percentage lasting under 10 minutes (Doyle and Ware 1977). Lack of effective explanation is also the major cause of patient dissatisfaction with physicians. Recognizing this situation, several new centers devoted specifically to women's health have set up schedules that permit patients significantly longer visits.

There is some evidence that many health customers, although wanting greater explanation of what is being done for them and why, do not necessarily need this information through more time with a doctor, nurse, or other health professional. Other instructional media, such as brochures, films, and tapes, are often acceptable, as long as a health professional "prescribes" them as relevant to the patient (Brown 1980). Once again, however, provision of such an extended service has to be designed into the program rather than added as an afterthought. It may, for instance, impact space needs and configuration, operational staffing, and budget. It is not uncommon in fields outside health care for such customer service and education features to comprise a major component of service design (Shycon and Sprague 1975).

Methods of meeting health customers' needs for service information and explanation may well have to be planned into a service while it is still in development. It is common in other industries for customer service and education techniques to be an integral feature of product or service design, rather than a later afterthought.

Hours of Operation. The *hours of operation* of a health program can also be an important component of the extended service it offers potential customers. Financial logic often suggests that a new service, or an expansion of an existing service, should start out with the minimum possible fixed costs, and expand on them as demand builds. Marketing logic, however, can suggest the opposite: that the service needs to be as available as possible to meet the needs of its customers. Thus, the financial argument is to start with limited hours and expand them as needed, while the marketing argument is to start with longer hours and cut them back if they prove unneeded.

At the heart of this difference of philosophy lies the *inventory paradox*. It is a complex concept, but a significant one in service development.

Consider first the case of two jewelry stores in a large town about 100 miles from the nearest major city. At one time, there was only one jewelry store in town. The storeowner thus enjoyed a monopoly. If local residents wanted to buy jewelry, they either bought from him or undertook the 200-mile round trip to the city.

In this privileged position, the jeweler could limit his opening hours. Most people who found his store closed would try again rather than set off for the city. He could also carry a quite small inventory. A customer who wanted an engagement ring could either select one from among the 20 or so that the jeweler carried, or again face a long journey for a wider choice of rings.

In time, another jeweler learned of this town where competition was nonexistent and decided to move there himself. He opened his new store right across the street from the old jeweler, with longer hours and a larger inventory. Now the first jeweler began to see his sales slide. Even people who had always shopped at his store started trying his competitor, particularly when the first jeweler's store was closed or they could not find a choice that appealed to them there.

The first jeweler talked to the accountant who helped him keep his books. The accountant had a very logical answer to his problems. Sales were down by 10%, so the jeweler had to cut costs by 10% if he wanted to maintain his previous level of profits. There were two obvious ways to cut costs. The storekeeper had money tied up in his inventory of jewelry. He bought this inventory from traveling salespersons, but items often sat in the store for months before someone bought them. If the jeweler could reduce his inventory, he would free up some cash. He would cut his *inventory carrying costs*. The other way he could cut costs would be by reducing his hours of operation. In a sense, those opening hours are an inventory also. It takes money to heat and light the store and to pay salespeople. If the jeweler shortened his hours, he could cut back on these costs.

The storekeeper next discussed his problem with the owner of a local business who had spent his career contending with competition and was experienced at marketing. He pointed out that the accountant's suggestions would only make the problem worse. The reason why sales were slipping, now that there was a competitor in town, was that some customers found the first jeweler's store closed when they wanted to buy some jewelry, but his competitor's store open. Other customers found his store open, but could not find a piece of jewelry that they liked. They therefore looked in his competitor's store. If a customer cannot find what he or she wants in the inventory of a business, marketing scientists call that a *stockout*. The jeweler's limited hours and limited inventory were creating two types of stockout: one of convenient shopping times and the other of appropriate jewelry. If the jeweler reduced his inventory of opening hours and reduced his inventory of jewelry, he would only succeed in producing more stockouts. He would lose even more customers.

In all probability, the businessman advised, the jeweler could not restore the former high profits of his business. Before the competitive store opened, the jeweler had enjoyed exceptional monopoly profits. It was unlikely he could do so again. His one hope was to outperform the new jeweler. That, however, would involve longer hours and a larger inventory.

Thus, the inventory paradox states that:

1. As competition increases, sales are likely to fall.

2. As sales fall, it seems logical to cut costs, including inventory costs.

3. Cutting inventories, however, leads to more customers who cannot get what they want, when they want it (stockouts).

4. More stockouts force sales down even further.

5. Therefore, the apparently logical step of cutting inventories as competition intensifies is in fact not logical, but makes matters worse. As competition intensifies, a business may have to increase costs and accept lower profits just to serve the same number of customers.

A number of textbooks explore these inventory management problems in more detail (e.g., Bierman, Bonini, and Hausman, 1973; Buffa and Taubert 1972). They show, for instance, some advanced methods of determining hours of operation and inventory levels that minimize the risks of stockouts, or determine the point at which the cost of higher inventory exceeds the extra revenue to be gained by staying open. The basic lesson, however, is that hours of operation are crucial to the success of service activities, and it may be very unwise to minimize them.

In many health services, the customer is purchasing a unit of professional time. The service may therefore only have one important inventory: its hours of operation. Table 9-1 shows, for the years 1975 through 1985, the average office hours of primary care physicians in the United States, their average weekly visits, and their

Table 9-1 Physician Weekly Office Hours, Visits, and Fees, 1975-1985

Year	Weekly Office Hours	Weekly Visits	First Visit Fee	Repeat Visit Fee
1975	30	101	$20	$12
1976	30	98	$23	$14
1977		Not available		
1978	31	99	$25	$15
1979	28	91	$28	$18
1980	28	87	$31	$18
1981		Not available		
1982	27	82	$42	$23
1983	27	80	$47	$25
1984	25	75	$47	$26
1985	25	75	$50	$28

average office visit fees for a new patient and for an established patient (American Medical Association 1987).

The first two columns of Table 9-1 show the inventory paradox in operation. As average weekly visits per primary care doctor have fallen, physicians have cut back office hours. The last two columns seem to suggest that they have also responded to reduced volumes by increasing fees to maintain their incomes. That conclusion, however, would be misleading. Because of inflation, the real value of those fees has remained almost level. Doctors' office incomes have, in fact, fallen in real terms. The higher fees have protected them from inflation, but not from falling office visits. In cutting back office hours by some 17%, the average doctor has almost certainly incurred more stockouts, or patients that could not get a timely appointment and went elsewhere. The costs that they have saved by an average of 5 fewer office hours weekly may well be less than the extra revenue that they could have earned by being available to see patients for those extra hours.

The hours of operation of a health service can be critical to its success and should be consciously planned as part of the overall service design.

The developmental phase of the service innovation process is the time to reach detailed decisions about the generic service (the benefit that it will deliver), the tangible service (how it will deliver it), and the extended service (what extra benefits it will also offer customers).

Service Testing

About half of all the new service innovations that are screened and then pass a feasibility study are abandoned at some point during their developmental phase. Some critical factor, not previously considered in depth, is seen to make the idea unviable. Of those new service concepts that do survive such development, only about half survive subsequent *test marketing*.

It does not necessarily make sense to test all new services prior to their actual launch. Those innovations that are low in cost, apparently low in risk, and easy to abandon if they fail can probably be put directly into operation. Conversely, service innovations should be subjected to formal testing:

1. If they are of relatively high cost,

2. If they are of relatively high risk,

3. If subsequent withdrawal will be particulary embarrassing or difficult.

The principal purpose of testing is, of course, to see if the concepts hold up in practice. One study of 17 products that failed in testing found that the most common cause of failure, accounting for more than half of the cases, was faulty development and design (Cadbury 1975).

An example is that of a company that introduced a brand of instant potato croquettes. The company concerned had, several years earlier, launched a very successful "instant" mashed potato. The company was eager to follow up this success by extending the concept to an instant form of some other potato dish, and decided on croquettes. The idea proved feasible and went into development. From that development stage emerged a viable prototype. Heated for a minute or two immersed in vegetable oil, it turned into a good-looking and tasty croquette. The product was then tested out in one market area. Sales were very poor. When the failure was investigated, it was found that the product worked best when heated in a pan of a particular size and shape. This had been realized during the development phase, and appropriate instructions were printed on the package. What was not realized until the test failure was investigated, however, was that very few households possessed a pan of those dimensions, and even fewer were willing to buy one just for this product.

While the major purpose of product testing is to discover such unforeseen complications, the process can also serve other useful purposes. It can help to refine the sales forecast to make it more accurate. It can enable variations of the product or service to be tested. It can also allow marketing variations to be tested.

Probably not enough health services are formally tested prior to a final decision to launch them. There usually is some viable way of testing such services, such as trying an innovation in inpatient care on one nursing unit first, or offering a new service to a sample of patients or of referral sources, before offering it on a wider basis.

To cite one example, a physician with a very unusual field of special interest approached the marketing staff at the hospital where he principally worked. The hospital had previously mailed information about this doctor's program to potential referral sources in its service area. The doctor believed that his program could have wider geographical appeal, and might draw referrals from a much broader area than the hospital did for other services. He suggested mailing information throughout the United States to physicians in two specialties most likely to refer. As a test, it was agreed to mail details to a sample of 200 such physicians and to measure the response. If the revenues that resulted exceed the costs of treating these patients plus the costs of the mailing, it would be extended to a broader mailing list.

In those rare cases where an actual test cannot be designed, it is usually possible to substitute a further formal market research study. The study can focus narrowly on describing the planned service and measuring likely interest. This approach has been used, for instance, to test a proposed industrial medicine program (Emery and Stuart 1987).

One caution that should be stated about such *acceptance surveys*, however, is that they usually overstate actual usage intentions. Enterprises that make regular use of this method therefore usually heavily discount the results they obtain.

One hospital, for example, asked physicians how likely they were to refer patients to a proposed rehabilitation satellite. Their responses are presented in Table 9-2. The report concluded that "30% of physicians in the service area report that they are likely to refer to this new center, and it only needs an estimated 10% to refer to break even." In fact, enterprises familiar with this type of survey would be more likely to look only at the percentage "very likely" to refer, and they would want that percentage to be at least two to three times as large as needed for break even. Far from suggesting the success of this proposed project, therefore, these data almost certainly predict its failure.

All service innovations should be tested in some manner, unless they are very low in cost, low in risk, and easy to abandon. There are many different ways to structure such tests. If a real-world test seems completely impossible, an acceptance survey among a sample of the proposed audience can substitute, but its results need to be interpreted conservatively.

Table 9-2 Physicians' Responses to a Rehabilitation Satellite Acceptance Survey

Response	%
Very likely to refer	15
Somewhat likely to refer	15
Unsure	20
Somewhat unlikely to refer	30
Unlikely to refer	20

Market Launch

The approaches discussed above to the methodical screening of new service innovation concepts, their careful feasibility analysis, their detailed development, and their systematic testing still do not guarantee a successful market launch. About half of all new products and services launched do not survive their first year or so of actual marketing. That risk of failure does, however, drop considerably when these four prelaunch steps are taken. Conversely, the failure rate of new products and services that have not received such thorough prelaunch assessment is even higher than 50%.

Those innovations that have been carefully studied, planned, and prepared, but nevertheless fail in the marketplace, do so largely because the marketing tactics used to support their launch were either misdirected or inadequate. The three most frequent types of market launch error are:

1. Misinterpreting the main benefits of the product or service to potential customers, and therefore miscommunicating with them

2. Incorrectly defining the relevant target audience(s) for the product or service, and therefore communicating with the wrong people

3. Underestimating the reach and frequency of communication needed to achieve a viable market share, and therefore underbudgeting the market launch.

Since the money available to communicate knowledge about a new service to relevant customers is limited, it is vital that it be spent purposefully. Misinterpreting the major benefits that a service offers its customers can easily lead to communicating information that they regard as irrelevant, and to which they consequently pay no attention.

Du Pont almost withdrew Teflon pans from the market because of poor initial sales. Just in time, the company discovered that the main benefit of the product in the opinion of its potential buyers was not, as had been assumed, that it was an aid to healthy cooking, but that the no-stick surface was easy to clean.

Another example is that of a hospital that received designation as a regional trauma center. It knew that the real success of the program would lie in the willingness of emergency room doctors at other hospitals, and of ambulance and emergency medical squads, to bring seriously injured patients to its hospital who would previously have been treated elsewhere. It did launch a communications program directed specifically at these groups, but it also invested in an expensive 2-minute TV ad. It calculated that this extra visibility would enhance the hospital's overall image as well as reinforce its message to those health professionals who should initiate referral to the center.

The ad dramatically depicted a Med-Evac helicopter journey to the new center, and the reception and immediate treatment of the patient. Inevitably that treatment included some fast-paced and visually upsetting surgical activities. This message completely failed to communicate the real benefit of trauma care, which is not rapid and skilled treatment but surviving and recovering from serious accidents. It showed only the tangible service, not the generic service. For viewers among the general public, it failed to demonstrate the value of trauma care, and even for health professionals it failed to explain why they should refer (because a higher percentage of their multisystem trauma patients would live).

The second main cause of ineffective market launches is targeting the wrong audience. You will recall from Chapter 7 that General Electric decided, in the late 1940s, not to launch an electric knife onto the market because an acceptance survey suggested that very few households would buy one. Several years later, a new senior executive at the company heard of this incident and pointed out that the research had asked the wrong question. He commented on an important aspect of changing demographics in the 1950s. More young people were relocating to schools or to first jobs distant from their family homes. Rising affluence was assisting this trend by making it possible for more families to finance a son or daughter through college away from home. The growth of employment in the Sun Belt was also contributing to this trend by attracting first-time job seekers from the northeast. One challenge that people who live some distance from their parents face is in selecting a gift for their birthdays or the holiday season. A new product was attractive because it was unlikely that parents owned one yet. A kitchen utensil was an attractive gift because few mothers in that generation had jobs outside the home. As a result of the executive's comments, the market research was repeated but now asked if people would buy an electric knife as a gift for a relative. The new survey showed very high public acceptance. The electric knife was launched, heavily promoted as a gift purchase, and proved very successful. Had General Electric targeted the product to people as "buyers of kitchen gadgets," it would, as the earlier research indicated, have almost certainly failed. Its subsequent launch to people as "buyers of gifts for their relatives" proved very successful.

A contrasting example is that of a health care organization that launched a package of programs targeted at the elderly. The package included senior day care, geriatric evaluation, a wellness newsletter for seniors, and preregistration at the local hospital's emergency room. It promoted the program by mailing to senior citizens. Response was very poor. The sponsors then realized that the initiator of usage of such services may not be the elderly themselves but their adult children caregivers. It was not possible to get a good mailing list of people with elderly parents, and so the enterprise switched from direct mail to local newspaper advertising. It was still uncertain of the wisdom of this change, and so it hedged its bets by addressing both seniors and caregivers in the same ad. It achieved a good response, and more than 80% of the inquiries came from caregivers.

The third most frequent cause of an ineffective market launch of a new service innovation is underestimating, and therefore underbudgeting, the communications program that will be needed to inform and motivate potential customers. A detailed discussion of the techniques of successful marketing communication is found in the next chapter, since they apply to both the launch of new services and the maintenance of demand for existing programs.

However, there are some important differences between *missionary marketing*, or introducing new services, and *maintenance marketing*, or supporting existing programs (de Kluyver and Pessemier 1986). Missionary marketing almost always requires a larger budget. In launching new food products, for instance, it is common for marketing and sales costs to constitute 60% of the entire first-year budget for the product, or four times the level (15% of total budget) that will be required later in the life of the product to maintain its market position.

Most health services do not require a marketing budget equal to 15% of total budget once they reach their maintenance phase. A range of between 1% and 5% of total budget is a typical current realistic maintenance marketing allocation. The principle still applies, however, that start-up marketing costs may have to be between two and four times that level.

There are several reasons why market launch costs tend to be much higher than subsequent maintenance costs:

1. If the new service is genuinely innovative, the benefits that it offers customers will take more explanation than those of an established service. If the new service is to compete with other providers who have previously entered that field, it will take additional effort for the new supplier to match their visibility and credibility. If the new entrant has built in a distinctive feature that should differentiate the new service as superior to existing ones, it may take extra effort to convince customers of this added value.

2. Effective communications depend on *reach*. They have to get to a large enough percentage of the target audience to create a viable level of response. The response rate to all forms of marketing communication is usually quite low. For instance, large enterprises that rely heavily on direct mail for sales typically regard a 2% or greater response as successful. They plan and budget accordingly. For example, if they need to sell 1,000 units to break even, they build in the costs of mailing to between 50,000 households (assuming a 2% response) and 100,000 households (assuming a 1% response). Many new services that fail do so because their marketing fails to achieve such a critical reach.

3. Effective communication depends upon *frequency*. To motivate an average customer, via marketing communications to respond requires getting the message to him or her at least four times. Many successful marketing campaigns in fact aim for a much higher frequency. Effective market launches often achieve a frequency of between 10 and 20 exposures to the audience reached.

4. The members of the intended target audience vary in their *venturesomeness*, or willingness to try a new service. For the average new service, about 2.5% of the audience are expected to be "innovators," who will try out the new

concept early. Another 13.5% are expected to be "early adopters," who try out the new product once an innovator whom they know recommends it. Another 34% constitute the "early majority," who use it once several people whom they know have tried it. A further 34% constitute the "late majority," who adopt the idea once it is in widespread use. The final 16% constitute "laggards," who try the service very late, or may never adopt it (Rogers 1962). Individuals may be in different segments for different types of service. Thus, a person who tends to set trends in clothes may be a laggard in trying new restaurants. A physician who is an early referrer to a specialized center for osteoporosis may be a late adopter of referrals to a specialized hip replacement program. For a really attractive idea, the distribution of these segments may be more favorable, with larger percentages of innovators and early adopters. Conversely, other innovations may have a much more adverse distribution among these groups. However, even a favorable distribution has two practical consequences: It takes time for any new concept to be adopted by a critical mass of customers. It is also likely that marketing tactics will have to be altered to appeal to these different groups. For instance, it is quite common for new electronics products to be initially promoted to innovators by emphasizing their newness, and then to early adopters by showing that people who set trends in this market have already adopted the concept.

In the aggregate, these special challenges that confront new services inflate the costs of their market launch. For example, a radiology group based at a hospital had been spending about 2% of its budget on marketing communications to potential referral sources. It decided to develop a free-standing imaging satellite some 10 miles away. Unfortunately, it assumed during the feasibility study and service development phase of this project that the new center could also be successfully marketed for 2% of budget. The new center was under construction and just 2 months away from opening before the group called in a marketing consultant to advise on its market launch. She advised that a successful launch would take between 4% and 8% of the first-year budget, which was close to $1 million. The main reason for this extra initial cost was that the new satellite needed the support of physicians with no history of referral to the group's other location.

An additional 6% for first-year marketing would inflate the budget for that initial 12 months by $60,000. The 10 physicians who comprised the group had each put up $50,000 for the project, and each of them had personally guaranteed another $50,000 in bank loans. The head of the group now had the embarrassing task of explaining to his colleagues that he might require a further investment of $6,000 from each of them to cover these unforeseen start-up marketing costs, without which they may have to wait much longer to see any return on their investment in the new center.

In this case, the radiologists were only planning to do what they had always done, but in a new location. Many new service innovations by health care providers take them into fields different from those in which they have traditionally operated. In such cases, even multiplying their established marketing expenditures as percentage of sales by two or four may not provide an adequate market launch budget.

New entrants into a field should not calculate their necessary initial marketing costs as a multiple of their maintenance marketing allocation from existing programs. To succeed in a new field, they must compete with established providers in that activity. The field they have chosen to enter may well have intrinsically higher marketing costs. They should, therefore, try to discover the competition's marketing allocations. Because they are new entrants and have yet to establish awareness and credibility among customers in that new field, they will still probably have to multiply that competitive marketing budget by between two and four for the start-up period.

A group of hospitals got together to form their own preferred provider organization. In doing so they were branching out of the health care business into the health insurance business. Each was used to spending about 1% of its total budget on marketing. They knew that established health insurers spend between 10% and 20% of their total budget on marketing and sales. They planned the launch of the new health insurance plan in two phases. For the first year they would concentrate on selling the new plan to their own employees. Since they had direct contact with this group, they concluded that their typical 1% of sales allocation for marketing would suffice.

After that first year, they would start selling the program to local companies, but they thought that since their hospitals already had high visibility and credibility in their communities, they could get by with matching the lower end of that 10% to 20% range. Early in that first year, the hospitals recognized that they were encountering sales resistance among their employees, and so they immediately increased the marketing allocation from 1% to 5% of projected first-year sales. Their fundamental miscalculation was in assuming that employees would prefer to buy from their employer. Even with this increased allocation, the first year proved very disappointing, with only 3% of employees joining.

The hospitals decided nevertheless to embark on the planned second launch phase of offering the plan to local companies. As originally decided, the allocated 10% of the second-year budget to this marketing effort. The results were again disappointing. They had miscalculated the extent to which their established credibility as hospitals would create instant credibility for them as health insurers. They also misinterpreted the information that "health insurers typically allocate between 10% and 20% of budget to marketing." That figure was an average of spending levels among both long-established insurers and new entrants. It was also an allocation that had been growing for several years because of intensifying competition in health insurance. By the end of the second year, the consortium realized that it should probably have allocated well in excess of 20% of that year's projected sales to marketing.

While new service innovations tend to require temporarily high marketing budgets, there is also a danger of overselling a new service, and creating more demand than can be handled. Often the internal champions of a new innovation are happy to see this situation develop. It helps to justify a case for expanding resources in a program if it can demonstrate more demand than it can handle. There is, however, a very serious risk in overselling. It can create dissatisfaction among potential customers, which is then very difficult to reverse.

An optometry practice decided to open a new location. Because of construction delays, the new center opened 2 months later than planned. The doctors decided to compensate by spending on advertising in 2 months the amount originally intended to be spread over 4 months. They were pleased with the response to the ads, which in each of the first 8 weeks generated some 200 calls for appointments. However, one in every four callers could not be scheduled for an appointment within an acceptable time period. Of those who were scheduled, a later survey showed that 20% were very dissatisfied with the amount of time they had to wait at the center before seeing the optometrist. The other 80% were very satisfied with their visits.

Thus, of every 100 patients calling the center, 25 were dissatisfied because they could not be scheduled within an acceptable time frame, 15 were dissatisfied with the waiting time at the center, and 60 were satisfied with their visits. Some studies suggest that a satisfied customer praises a service to an average of three friends, while a dissatisfied customer criticizes a service to an average of some 20 friends (TARP 1986). Thus, for every 100 patients calling the center in response to its ads, 800 people (40 dissatisfied callers times 20 friends) were hearing negative comments about it, while only 180 people (60 satisfied callers times 3 friends) were hearing positive comments about it. Very rapidly, the response rate to the ads began to diminish because of these negative reports circulating in the community.

The most practical means of avoiding this danger is to design the market launch in steps, starting off with one level of marketing, which can be supplemented if insufficient demand is generated. The argument that "more demand for a service than it can handle is healthy" is false. Enterprises experienced in new product launches try to match generated demand as closely as possible to available capacity. They do not try to prove the case for further expansion by creating unmet demand. They prove it instead by documenting what one level of marketing has accomplished and projecting what further efforts might achieve.

Even when service innovations are carefully screened, assessed, developed, and tested, there is still a risk that they will fail once launched. The most common reasons for failure are design faults and ineffective marketing. The marketing of innovations poses challenges not present in the marketing of established services. The benefits of the innovation have to be communicated to a large enough audience and frequently enough to match the competition provided by established alternatives. This effort temporarily requires a higher budget than that of competitors and one higher than the subsequent maintenance of market share will necessitate. Care must also be taken, however, not to generate demand that cannot be satisfied.

References

American Medical Association. 1987. *The socioeconomic characteristics of medical practice*. Chicago: American Medical Association.

Bierman, H., C. Bonini, and W. Hausman. 1973. *Quantitative analysis for business decisions*. Homewood, Ill.: Richard Irwin.

Booz Allen and Hamilton. 1982. *New product management for the 1980s*. New York: Booz Allen and Hamilton.

Brown, S. 1980. Comparing attitudes and opinions of Arizona physicians and consumers. *Arizona Medicine* 17(3):174-178.

Buffa, E. S., and W. Taubot. 1972. *Production-inventory systems: Planning and control*. Homewood, Ill.: Richard Irwin.

Cadbury, N. D. 1975. Where when and how to test market. *Harvard Business Review* (May-June): 96-105

DeKluyver, C., and E. Pessemier. 1986. Benefits of a marketing budgeting model: Two case studies. *Sloan Management Review* 28(1):27-38.

Doyle, B., and J. Ware. 1977. Physician conduct and other factors that influence consumer satisfaction with health care. *Journal of Medical Education* 52(10):743-801.

Eaton, D., R. Church, and C. Revelle. 1977. *Locational analysis: A new tool for health planning. Methodological working document #53*. Washington, D.C.: Agency for International Development.

Emery, J., and B. Stuart. 1987. Using market research to test acceptability and awareness of proposed free-standing hospital programs. *Journal of Hospital Marketing* 1(3/4):61-70.

Korneluk, G. N. 1985. *Practice enhancement*, pp. 42-50. New York: Macmillan.

Kotler, P. 1972. *Marketing management*, pp. 243-245. Englewood Cliffs, N.J.: Prentice Hall.

Lele, M. 1986. How service needs influence product strategy. *Sloan Management Review* (Fall).

Levitt, T. 1980. Marketing success through differentiation—of anything. *Harvard Business Review* 58(1):83-90.

MacStravic, R. E. 1977. *Marketing health care*. Germantown, Md.: Aspen Systems.

Review of Optometry. 1982. The savvy marketer. *Review of Optometry* (June 15).

Rogers, E. M. 1962. *Diffusion of innovations*. New York: Free Press.

Shycon, H., and C. Sprague. 1975. Put a price tag on your customer service levels. *Harvard Business Review* 53(4):71-78.

Starr, P. 1982. *The social transformation of American medicine*. New York: Basic Books.

Stewart, J. B. 1959. Functional features in product strategy. *Harvard Business Review* 37(2):65-78.

TARP (Technical Assistance Research Programs Institute). 1986. *Consumer complaint handling in America: An update study*. Consumer Affairs Council of the U.S. Office of Consumer Affairs. Washington, D.C.: Department of Health and Human Services.

Review Questions

1. What is the difference between service development and service testing?

2. Select any health service with which you are familiar and describe briefly its generic service, its tangible service, and its extended service features.

3. What are the four approaches to incorporating quality assurance into the design of a health service?

4. What are the most important considerations in naming a health service?

5. What is the inventory paradox?

6. What are the three most common errors in the launch of new service ideas?

Part IV

Communicating with Customers

Chapter 10

Marketing Communications: The Challenge

As was discussed in Chapter 3, customers select services through a five-step process of need recognition, followed by information search, followed by decision, actual usage, and subsequent evaluation. The supplier of a health service can seek to influence any or all of these steps in the process by communication with the customer. Indeed, even if no conscious effort is made to initiate and structure such communications, they will occur anyway through the contact of nurses and other health professionals involved in the service with its patients and their families, and through random, secondhand accounts of the service passed on by word-of-mouth by past customers. As one marketing authority, Theodore Levitt, has noted, "The purpose of a business is to create and keep a customer. No enterprise can do this by instinct or accident" (Levitt 1983).

Any organization that seeks to be effective must therefore have a conscious and planned marketing communications strategy.

What Are Marketing Communications?

Marketing communication can take many forms. Advertising tends to come to mind first, because it is both widespread and visible in modern society. It is, however, only one of many possible options in marketing communication. Marketing scientists often divide these options into four main types: advertising, publicity, personal selling, and sales promotion (Reibstein 1985).

Advertising does not just consist of space bought in the media to deliver a message, but includes "any paid form of non-personal

presentation and promotion of ideas, goods, or services by an identified sponsor" (American Marketing Association 1960). Advertising thus extends to sending letters to individual customers, direct
mailing to large numbers of potential customers, handing out
brochures, and any other activity that is nonpersonal and paid for.

Publicity consists in trying to obtain favorable coverage of a service in the media. Effective publicity often, like advertising, entails a
cost. Occasionally, a service may obtain media coverage that is
genuinely free. For example, a local newspaper journalist happened
to be among the first to enroll in a new fitness center. Through the
subsequent year, he reported on his progress regularly in his
column. This publicity generated a large number of other members.
That case is, however, exceptional. Usually, it takes the expense of
at least issuing a press release, or calling on media personnel, to
create even one significant item of publicity for a health service.

Even then, such a proactive effort may be unsuccessful. For example, one hospital found that the opening of a new service, which it
had invited the local media to cover, coincided with a visit by President Reagan to town. As with many major media stories, the visit
was only announced at the last minute, but it wiped out any
coverage of the hospital's story. Organizations that regularly obtain
significant media publicity often have large media relations staffs.
Publicity for these organizations thus does not come free.

Personal selling consists of personal and oral presentations to
customers, as individuals or in groups. It can therefore include
telephone calls, sales visits, counseling sessions, and even health
education lectures. Unlike either advertising or publicity, it permits
two-way communication with potential customers. It also allows the
emphasis of the marketing communication to be tailored to individual needs and interests.

Sales promotion consists of all other forms of marketing communication that do not fit into one of the three preceding
categories. For a health service, it may include free screenings, participation in health fairs, open houses, receptions for referral sources, supporting events of other local organizations, and so on.

The activities of Blue Cross and Blue Shield exemplify all four
types of marketing communication. Throughout the United States,
Blue Cross and Blue Shield are major users of media advertising.
They also attempt to secure media publicity for their annual results,
new plans, plan changes, and other events. They engage heavily in
personal selling through visits to corporate clients and participation

in their employee enrollment sessions. They also sponsor local sports, sometimes even organizing their own athletic events, as methods of sales promotion.

The promotion mix of an enterprise is the way in which it chooses to combine advertising, publicity, personal selling, and sales promotion, or specific components of them, to support its products or services.

It is by no means uncommon for organizations with similar services to select very different promotion mixes (Wright, Winter, and Zeyler 1982). They may define different messages to deliver, to different market segments, and in different combinations. As an example, the sponsors of a new HMO in an area where Blue Cross and Blue Shield is the current market leader might look at its rival's promotion mix and conclude that it cannot match the Blues in publicity, and does not want to match them in sales promotion because such visible spending may not fit well with its lower cost image, but will try to match them in advertising and outperform them in personal selling.

Why Marketing Communication is Difficult

All communications follow a common model. Their *source* must *encode* the intended message in some symbols. These may be pictures, written words, spoken words, mathematical notations, a scientific formula, or other symbols. The encoded message must then be *transmitted* through some medium, for example print, an audio recording, a video recording, or a personal conversation. That message must then be *decoded* by the *receiver* if it is to be effective (de Vito 1971). Figure 10-1 depicts this *basic communications model.*

Marketing communications are a special form of communications. To accomplish their goal effectively, marketing communications must contend with a number of specific barriers.

Communicating to Different Receivers

First, the nature of the receiver can vary widely. As noted in Chapters 3 through 5, a variety of people may be influential in the service selection process, ranging from the potential patient to a referring physician, a payer, a family influencer, a surrogate

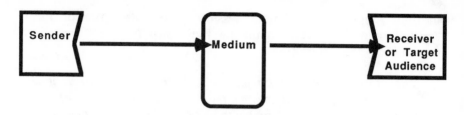

Figure 10-1 The basic communications model.

decision-maker, or a gatekeeper. In other fields of marketing, it is quite common to divide communications into two types, depending upon the nature of the targeted receiver. *Consumer marketing communications* attempt to persuade individual consumers, households, or families. *Business-to-business marketing communications* attempt to persuade companies that make purchases, or act as intermediaries, surrogates, or influencers, for consumers. For instance, a hospital that tries to attract potential patients directly engages in consumer marketing communication, while one that focuses on promoting itself to doctors is emphasizing business-to-business marketing communications.

The same communications concepts apply to both types of marketing (Fern and Brown 1984). The rest of the marketing communications model described below is therefore equally applicable to both types of receivers. The specific skills needed to modify those concepts to suit the intended receiver, however, may well vary. A particular technique that has proven effective in consumer marketing communications may not work well in business-to-business communications, and vice versa. As one illustration of this dichotomy, it is becoming increasingly common for advertising agencies to specialize in one or the other of these two fields, or for the largest agencies to have distinct groups specializing in each of these areas.

The revision of the basic communication model shown in Figure 10-2 incorporates this first barrier to effective marketing communication, the distinct type of receiver involved.

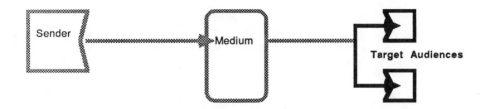

Figure 10-2 The basic communications model showing multiple target audiences.

Persuading the Receiver: The Hierarchy of Effects

Marketing communications have an objective that is lacking in some other types of communication, namely, persuasion. Their purpose is to persuade the receiver to do something. That is not true, for instance, of education, where the objective is the transference of knowledge, or of entertainment, where the objective is the pleasure of the receiver, or of communicating with relatives, where the objective is often "keeping in touch."

Other forms of communication share persuasion as their principal goal, for instance, political campaigning, explaining misbehavior to children, seeking to motivate employees, and some psychiatric therapies. The uniqueness of marketing communications, however, is that they attempt to persuade the audience to use the products or services of the sponsor (Schramm 1965; Stanley 1982). The revision of the communication model in Figure 10-3 therefore builds in a feedback loop to demonstrate that marketing communications only work when such a response is obtained. To generate such a response, marketing communications must take the receiver through the so-called *hierarchy of effects* (Panda 1966).

First, the message must *capture the attention* of the receiver. The typical person discards many letters without paying much attention to them, skips over many ads in newspapers and magazines, ignores many billboards and radio and TV ads, bypasses many booths at health fairs, is not attracted to many pamphlets they see displayed, and does not return some telephone calls that seem unimportant.

Second, the message must *create awareness* of the organization or service and of the benefits that it offers.

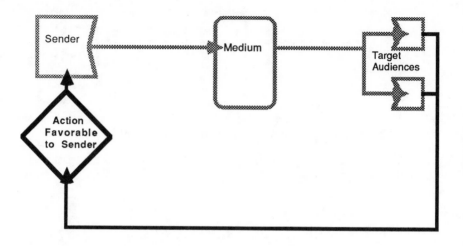

Figure 10-3 The communications model showing feedback.

Third, the message must *create preference* for the organization or service. Otherwise, capturing the receiver's attention and engendering awareness of the benefits available may lead him or her to contact a competitor rather than the sender of the message (Fisk 1986).

Finally, the message must *motivate action*. Without such action by the receiver, the desired feedback does not occur.

Not every marketing communication, however, has to accomplish all four of these tasks. Each communication must certainly succeed at *capturing attention*, without which its message is literally lost. As a practical matter, however, individual marketing communications may vary in which, or which combination, of the other three steps they are intended to achieve. The goal of specific marketing communications may therefore differ (Ray 1982).

Some marketing communications are primarily intended to *create awareness*. Particularly in the launch of new services, the major initial task confronting the provider may be to get potential customers to realize that the benefit offered is now obtainable. For example, until a few years ago, a relatively safe, quick, and effective means of surgically removing undesirable body fat did not exist. With the advent of modern liposuction, many plastic surgeons found that their largest challenge was to communicate the availability of this service. They did not particularly need to explain why they themselves were preferable suppliers of this treatment or how they could be reached. There were, at least initially, enough people looking for such a benefit that, if they saw a message about liposuction, they did not seek reasons to prefer its sponsor over other cosmetic surgeons, and they were prepared to look up the sponsor's number in the phone directory. Only as the procedure became more commonplace did it become crucial for an individual doctor to explain what differentiated him from others and to make responding as easy as possible.

Some marketing communications, by contrast, are primarily focused on *creating preference*. There may be widespread awareness that a type of service exists, but insufficient information in the minds of potential customers to make an informed selection of provider. In many geographical areas, the first one or two HMOs focused their advertising and personal selling on creating awareness of the product that they offered. There were enough people interested in the concept for them to achieve significant initial sales through this strategy. As other HMOs entered the local market, however, they often imitated this tactic with large-scale awareness campaigns, including advertising that focused primarily on name recognition. Many of these later HMOs found it much more difficult to gain market share with this strategy. The earlier HMOs were now well known, and potential customers were more interested in reasons to prefer the new plans that in knowing of their existence.

There are two variations to marketing communications that focus upon creating preference. Some communications may be *product line* specific, while others attempt to boost the general *image* of the sponsor in the belief that a strong image will spill over onto specific services. As an example, the first two hospitals to start kidney stone lithotripsy in a particular region were a large and well-renowned university hospital and a medium-sized community hospital. The latter was not well known outside of its immediate area but needed to draw from further afield to make its lithotripter pay for itself. The university hospital concentrated on reinforcing its overall image and mentioning the addition of this new service, while the community hospital undertook a major promotion campaign addressing lithotripsy specifically, without much reference to the hospital itself.

Some marketing communications focus on *motivating action*. Their sponsors perceive that potential customers are aware of the benefit of the service and have a preestablished preference for them, but need more assistance in accessing the service, ordering the product, or arranging an appointment. Many of the better known and best regarded department stores and specialty stores, for example, invest heavily in direct mail of catalogs to households both within and beyond their immediate service areas. They do so because they perceive that more people would like to buy from an L.L. Bean, a Neiman-Marcus, or a Macy's than can conveniently get to one of their retail locations. Similarly, many hospitals now offer printed medical staff lists and telephone referral services, in the belief that some people would prefer a doctor associated with the hospital but cannot easily obtain such information.

Many marketing communications try to take the receiver through the entire hierarchy of effects. It is entirely possible to do so, for instance, in a letter, a direct mail package, or a print ad, if it is properly designed. There are three potential reasons for such *combined-purpose* marketing communications. First, they protect against the danger of the sponsor overestimating the degree of established awareness or preference among their receivers. Marketing messages focusing, for instance, on motivating action may be ineffective for a sponsor who does not really enjoy a commanding preference in the market. Second, no enterprise enjoys a 100% preference among potential customers, and a composite message may both motivate those who already prefer the sender and contribute to converting some others. Third, a receiver who accepts the partial message of a limited marketing communication may not be sufficiently motivated to reference other material for the missing information he or she needs to act. Someone, for instance, impressed by a publicity story in a local newspaper may not bother to consult the phone book to discover how to contact the service. He or she may instead mention the story to a friend, who may recommend another supplier.

In recent years, marketing scientists have identified a possible value in yet a further type of marketing communication, which addresses a fifth step in the hierarchy of needs: building loyalty among existing users of a service (Puto and Wells 1984). As was noted earlier, satisfied service customers do not necessarily become loyal repeat users. Among hospital inpatients, for instance, only some 50% on average would prefer to reuse the hospital to which they were last admitted (Fisk and Brown 1987).

It should be both easier and less costly to attract previous satisfied patients either to reuse a service or to use a new service than to attract patients who have no prior experience of the provider (Mac-Stravic 1987). One value of building customer loyalty is therefore the potential for personal reuse. The other value of loyalty is that word-of-mouth testimonial remains supreme in shaping the views of new customers, even for services that are heavily promoted by other means (Berelson and Steiner 1964).

The term now becoming widely used for promotion aimed at building the loyalty of existing customers is *transformational marketing communication* (Westbrook 1987). Thus, transformation can be regarded as a further step in the hierarchy of effects.

Yet another type of marketing communication has received attention recently among some marketing scientists. So-called *preneed marketing communications* attempt to reach people who are unlikely to have an imminent need for service, but perceive that they may at a later date (Jayacharandran and Kyi 1987). It is important to note that preneed marketing communications are not aimed at just anyone; the receiver is expected to have a reasonable awareness that he or she is "at risk" in the future. The term is thus applied to people who buy life insurance, or call for a free health pamphlet, or participate in screening programs.

There are very few documented cases of people who received a marketing message but took action based upon it after a long delay. One leading authority on advertising, for instance, reports cases of people buying Steinway pianos in the 1970s who stated that they were influenced to do so by ads seen in their childhood some 30 years earlier (Ogilvy 1985). As a practical matter, it is unwise to assume such delayed response to marketing communications. Nearly all response occurs within a few months at the latest, and most even more rapidly. The advocates of preneed marketing communications do not, therefore, argue in favor of targeting people who may be at risk some time in the future. They focus on those who already see themselves as at future risk and who are disposed to do something now to limit that risk or its consequences. One example of such a preneed market is that for home diagnostic kits for various health risks. Sales of such kits were projected to quadruple in the United States between 1983 and 1988 (*Medical World News* 1985).

Specific preneed marketing communications, like those designed to address current needs, may focus on one, several, or all of the steps in the hierarchy of effects. They may concentrate on spreading awareness that a method of satisfying a preneed exists, such as the value of base-line mammography. They may focus on creating preference for one particular supplier of preneed services, such as one hospital's health awareness programs. They may focus on motivating action to satisfy a specific preneed, such as participating in a free screening program. They may focus on transformation of those who have participated in a preneed program into loyal users of the sponsor's services, such as a follow-up letter to those who called previously for a free home diagnostic kit.

The further revision of the marketing communications model shown in Figure 10-4 incorporates these several concepts about the hierarchy of effects. It shows capturing attention as a prerequisite for the receiver absorbing and retaining any message. Then it recognizes that any specific marketing communication might address either of two types of need: preneed or current need. Under each of those two headings, it allows for the possibility that the message may be focused on creating awareness, or creating preference, on motivating action, or on transforming past users into loyal users.

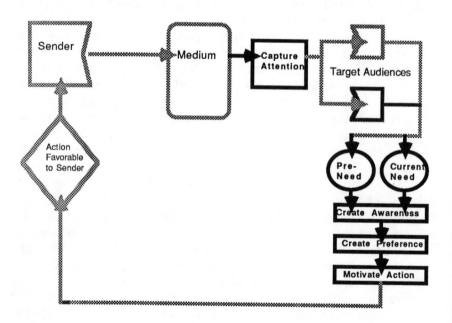

Figure 10-4 The communications model showing the hierarchy of effects.

Transmitting the Message

The next set of challenges confronted by all marketing communications lies in the transmission process. The four principal problems in transmitting any message are symbolism, media limitations, image conflict, and noise (Fisk 1986).

Symbolism can contaminate the effective communication of a message. Both verbal and visual images are imprecise and can therefore be ambiguous. The receiver may not decode a message with the meaning the sender had in mind when encoding it. For example, both Campbell Soup and Gerber products lost large sums trying to promote their products to Brazilian mothers, among whom the image of feeding children from a can or jar rather than with food prepared from scratch was interpreted as a sign of a lazy and uncaring parent. Another example is that of a pediatric surgicenter whose nurses decided to put together a very simple third-graders' introduction to the center, to put them at ease about upcoming visits for surgery. Only at a late stage in drafting this booklet was it pointed out that "You take a nap" was a better way to describe anesthesia for this young audience than "You are put to sleep" (*Healthcare Marketing Report* 1987). A common problem in marketing communications for health services is that many words that nurses and other health professionals regard as neutral descriptions of procedures are inherently frightening to the potential patient—for example, "surgery," "intravenous therapy," "blood tests," "enemas," and "life support systems."

Media limitations are inherent in any method chosen for a particular marketing communication. There is no such thing as a perfect method of communicating. It is sometimes argued that face-to-face conversation is the best means of communicating, and that any other medium is therefore always a second-best alternative when talking personally to each potential customer is not practical. That argument is questionable, because face-to-face conversation also has its limitations. The receiver hears and sees a complex combination of words, voice tone, gesture, and body language. He or she also sees the sender, and the receipt of the message may well be contaminated by how the receiver responds to the sender as a person. At times it is also argued that personal letters are a good medium for marketing communication, but they lack one ability that can be vital to some marketing messages: demonstration of the service. Mailing a videotape could in some cases compensate for this deficiency if demonstrating the service is important. However, videotapes are expensive compared to letters, are less likely to be watched, and seem to leave the viewer with less awareness of the sender's name than does a letter (Caples, 1983). Table 10-1 presents a partial list of common marketing communication options and their principal media limitations. This list is not intended to be comprehensive, but to illustrate the concept that every medium has limitations with which a marketing message must contend if it is to be effective.

Image conflict occurs when the content of a marketing communication clashes with the receiver's established perception of the sender. Certain messages coming from certain senders may lack convincing source credibility. Many enterprises and organizations have well-established images among potential customers that are hard to change. For instance, faced with declining sales, Woolworth's attempted to portray its Woolco stores as having wide variety and superior merchandise. This desired image conflicted with the image that Woolworth's had successfully built through previous decades as a lower-choice, lower-quality, but lower-priced store. The new campaign failed.

Consider also the case of the Ford Mustang. The original design sold well and was highly rated in successive consumer surveys for its modern styling, high performance, and modest price. Ford then lost sight of the Mustang's market image. Over the next 6 years the car was modified until it was 8 inches longer, 6 inches wider, and 600 pounds heavier. As these modifications became more extreme, Ford's marketing communications about the new models lacked credibility, and sales of the Mustang steadily declined, because "it was no longer a Mustang." Eventually, Ford saw its error and redesigned the Mustang closer to its original characteristics (Heller 1987).

Hospitals may often have equally well developed images, and the images of different hospitals in a particular service area may vary considerably (Fisk 1987). If such perceptions are strongly established among potential customers, the sender may have to limit its messages to those that work within its existing image, rather than attempt to modify it radically (MacMillan 1981). Even small or new suppliers of services, without any strongly established image, may face problems of source credibility if they make claims in marketing communications that clash with potential customers' current knowledge.

Table 10-1 Some Commonly Used Marketing Media and Their Limitations

Medium	Limitation(s)
Person-to-person dialogue	Little control of impression created
Telephone call	Audio only, so unable to demonstrate service, and recall of message can be low
Business lunch	Time-consuming, little control of impression created
Letter	Strong competition for attention, inability to demonstrate service
Media publicity	Uncertain use and audience reach, very little control of content
TV ads	High cost, may not get the attention of target receivers
Cable TV ads	Usually very low reach
Radio ads	Audio only, receiver is often engaged in other activities
Newspaper ads	Strong competition for attention, "short life"
Magazine ads	Strong competition for attention, competition for reader attention is often from high-quality ads by national advertisers
Billboards	Limited ability to handle complex message
Direct mail	Strong competition for attention
Displays	Receiver often in the process of satisfying other needs, and may be in a hurry
Brochure displays	Very dependent upon initial impression created, and on the environment

One hospital enjoyed a strong reputation in its community as a good and lower-priced supplier for more routine health care needs. It then, however, started a radio ad campaign, which declared that it was "nationally renowned as a leading center in treating breast cancer." None of its potential or even its past customers had previously heard such a claim made on behalf of "their" local hospital by any of its doctors or by any friends whom they knew to have used it. They largely dismissed this exaggerated claim of national renown. It also made them more wary of other, more supportable, marketing communications from the hospital. A subsequent survey showed that, among people who could recall the hospital's ads, almost one in four now doubted their veracity and value.

Noise in any form of communication consists of any extraneous messages that compete with or distort reception of the intended signal. The term is used in radio electronics to describe any interference that the listener picks up because of inability to tune into the precise waveband, or because other messages are being transmitted on that waveband. In marketing communication, noise is the collection of competing messages, often from other marketing sources, that compete with and confuse the message the sponsor seeks to deliver. Although precise estimates vary, several marketing authorities report that only a small percentage of marketing communications actually succeed in capturing the attention of the intended receivers, because of all the competing messages being directed at them by other marketers. An even smaller percentage of marketing communications succeed at the total hierarchy of effects, by actually motivating a response — perhaps as few as three or four of the many hundreds of marketing messages to which each person is exposed each day (Ogilvy 1985).

Symbolism, media limitations, image conflict, and noise all create barriers to the effective transmission of marketing communications from their sender to their intended receiver.

The revision of the marketing communications model in Figure 10-5 therefore incorporates these barriers to effective transmission.

Barriers to Response

Similar barriers can impair the feedback from potential customers who are convinced by the marketing communication and now wish to use the described service. There are four such common barriers to customer response.

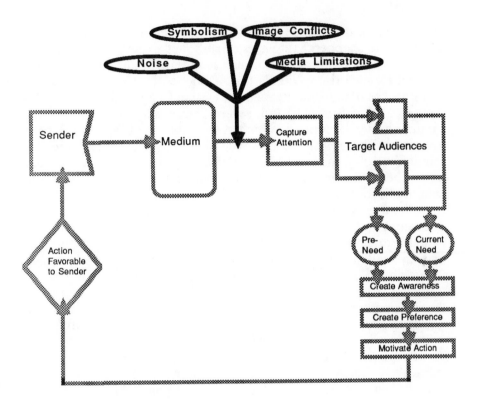

Figure 10-5 The communications model showing barriers to effective transmission.

Access deficiencies occur when a potential customer wants to follow up on a marketing communication, but cannot access the supplier or the service conveniently. The access of potential customers may be restricted by geography. It is not uncommon for mass media to have *spill-out*; that is, they reach people beyond their intended market area (Urdang 1983). Some of those people may desire the service, but discover that it is not readily available to them. For example, although the *New York Times* achieves most of its circulation within about a 50-mile radius of New York City, it attracts quite a few subscribers from Maine to Virginia. An advertiser like Macy's, with locations both inside and beyond the New York metropolitan area, has to exercise caution, therefore, in using the *Times* to promote a product that is not available at all of its stores throughout this wider circulation area. An advertiser like Tiffany's may have to ensure that it can respond to telephone orders for advertised items as well as to shoppers visiting its stores.

An example from health care is that of a new HMO, which elected to advertise in media that happened to reach into a neighboring state. Its largest competitors — Blue Cross and Blue Shield, a long-established HMO, and several large commercial insurance companies — all operated in both states. The new HMO faced a real dilemma. The reach of its advertising into the other state was probably aiding the rival HMO, but opting out of these media and into others with smaller reach in its own market area would lower its communications effectiveness.

Handling deficiencies arise when potential customers can access the service but inquiries are mismanaged and customers lost as a result. For example, a toll-free 800 telephone line for customer contact appears to be a valuable convenience to offer. It is usually beneficial to the supplier of a health service, but there is a subtle problem. Customers seem, logically, to expect 800 numbers to be busy less frequently than other lines. One study (*Direct Marketing* 1987) showed that, among callers who find an 800 line busy, 48% will try again and 24% will try to find some other method to reach the supplier. However, 16% decide to call another supplier of an equivalent service, and 12% give up completely and do not pursue either the supplier or an alternative. Thus, if an 800 line is regularly overloaded, the supplier may lose as many as 28% of the potential customers who have been convinced to call by the supplier's marketing communications.

Supply deficiencies occur when the provider cannot keep pace with the demand generated by marketing communications. This situation is quite common: Rolls-Royce automobiles, the Trivial Pursuits game, Bartles and Jaymes wine coolers, Wilkinson Sword razor blades, Cabbage Patch dolls, and Atari video games are among the documented examples of products that at one time or another became scarce goods, because supply failed to keep up with demand. The danger here is that potential customers will try, and become loyal to, rival services if they cannot be served quickly enough. They may even develop an image of the promoted service as permanently unobtainable.

Many suppliers have expanded capacity once they detected such unmet demand, only to discover, when ready to handle more demand, that they had lost the market to others. One hospital developed an advanced program for the care of newborns with certain extreme problems at birth. It took only a modest effort at marketing communication for the hospital's neonatalogists to find themselves overloaded with requests to accept transfers from colleagues at other intensive care nurseries. Soon they were rejecting more requests than they accepted. They decided to expand capacity, but it took more than a year to amass the necessary additional staff and equipment. It then took a quite extensive communications effort to convince other neonatalogists that it was now worthwhile calling the center if they had such a neonate in their care.

Noise can also occur in the response process, just as it can, as noted earlier, in the transmission process (Schultz 1981). A potential customer may be convinced by a marketing communication, but may discuss his or her intent with a friend, who offers an alternative recommendation. Similarly, a potential customer may forget the details of a marketing communication, and in attempting to retrieve them encounter a competitor's message.

The attempt of a potential customer, convinced by marketing communication, to respond may be impeded by deficiencies in access to the service, in the handling of inquiries, or in the available supply of the service. Efforts to respond may also be distracted by the noise of competitive marketing communications and recommendations. The revision of the marketing communications model in Figure 10-6 builds in these possible barriers to effective response.

Controlling the Message

The final source of difficulty in marketing communications lies in the sender's lack of control over the complete message that will reach the receiver. A Yale psychologist, John Luft developed a model of the sender of any message (Luft, 1961). He termed it "the Johari window." According to this model, the typical communication source is like a window with four panes. An MIT organizational psychologist, Ed Schein later pointed out that this model also applies when the communication source is an organization, or the supplier of a service (Schein, 1969).

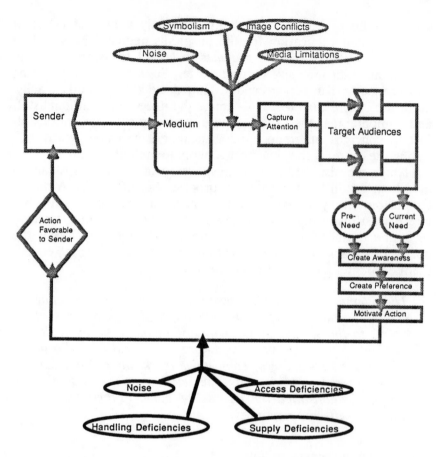

Figure 10-6 The communications model showing barriers to effective response.

As Figure 10-7 illustrates, a communications source consists of:

1. An "open" component, consisting of those aspects of its organization or services that it wants to communicate (such as, "We give good care in Community General's emergency room.")

2. A "concealed" component, consisting of those aspects that the communications source is aware of, but prefers

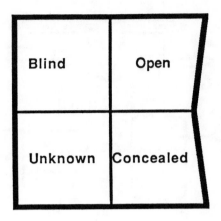

Figure 10-7 The communicator as a "Johari window".

to omit from the message because they qualify its value (such as, "Because of the nursing shortage, Community General's emergency room its not fully staffed for peak hours.")

3. A "blind" component, consisting of those aspects of which the communication source is unaware (such as, "It is impossible to get to Community General's emergency room from Centerville in less than 30 minutes on summer weekends because of traffic congestion on the turnpike.")

The communications source wishes to send the open message. However, that message may be contaminated by "leaks" from the concealed or the blind aspects of the service. The communications source, therefore, lacks total control over the message that it transmits. In the example above, the best case result is that only the planned message gets through. The worst-case result occurs if both qualifiers to this claim also reach the intended receivers.

Suppliers of services lack total control over the messages that they communicate to potential customers. Their intended messages may be qualified by the leakage of other information that

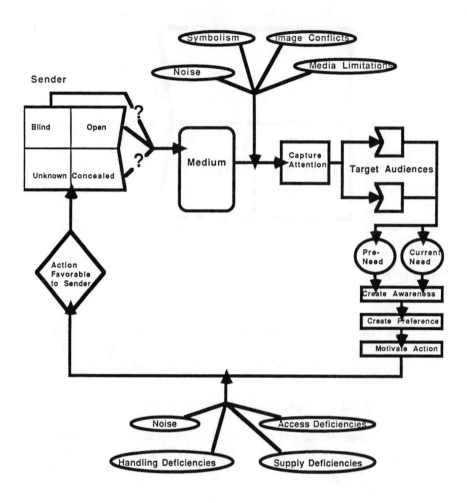

Figure 10-8 The complete persuasive communications model.

they prefer to omit, or of which they may be unaware. The final version of the marketing communications model, presented in Figure 10-8, incorporates this further potential limitation to communications effectiveness.

Despite all of the barriers standing in the way of effective marketing communications, many enterprises have learned how to minimize their impact. They do communicate effectively, at least most of the time, with their potential customers. Other suppliers, which ignore these barriers or fail to respond to them properly, have wasted large sums on ineffective communication with their markets. Chapter 11 will explore the question of what distinguishes effective from ineffective marketing communication.

References

American Marketing Association. 1960. *Marketing definitions: A glossary of marketing terms.* New York: American Management Association.

Berelson, B., and G. Steiner. 1964. *Human behavior: An inventory of scientific findings.* New York: Harcourt Brace and World.

Caples, J. 1983. *How to make your advertising make money.* Englewood Cliffs, N.J.: Prentice Hall.

DeVito, J. 1971. *Communication: Concept and processes.* Englewood Cliffs, N.J.: Prentice Hall.

Direct Marketing. 1987. Behavior and attitudes of telephone shoppers. *Direct Marketing* (September).

Fern, E., and J. Brown. 1984. The industrial/consumer marketing dichotomy: A case of insufficient justification. *Journal of Marketing* 48:68-77.

Fisk, T. 1986. *Advertising health services: What works, what fails.* Chicago: Pluribus Press.

Fisk, T. 1987. *Perceptual mapping: Hospitals' competitive images.* Paper presented at the College of Health Care Marketing Annual Symposium, February 16-18, Orlando, Fla.

Fisk, T., and C. Brown. 1987. *Practice marketing: An introduction for radiologists.* Reston, Va.: American College of Radiology.

Healthcare Marketing Report. 1987. Day surgery campaign part of marketing services for not so sick children. *Healthcare Marketing Report* 5(9).

Heller, R. 1987. *The supermarketers.* New York: Macmillan.

Jayacharandran, C., and M. Kyi, 1987. Preneed purchasing behavior: An overlooked dimension in consumer marketing. *Journal of Consumer Marketing*

4(3):59-66.

Levitt, T. 1983. *The marketing imagination.* New York: Free Press.

Luft, J. 1961. The Johari window. *Human Relations Training News* 5:6-7.

MacMillan, N. 1981. *Marketing your hospital: A strategy for survival.* Chicago: American Hospital Association.

MacStravic, R. 1987. Loyalty of hospital patients: A vital marketing objective. *Health Care Management Review* 12(2).

Medical World News. 1985. The home test movements shift into high gear. *Medical World News* (February 11).

Ogilvy, D. 1985. *Ogilvy on advertising.* New York: Random House.

Panda, K. 1966. The hypothesis of a hierarchy of effects. *Journal of Market Research* (February):13-24.

Puto, C., and W. Wells. 1984. Informational and transformational advertising: The differing effects of time. In *Advances in consumer research, Vol. 11.* ed. T. Kinnear, Ann Arbor, Mich.: Association for Consumer Research.

Ray, M. 1982. *Advertising and communications management,* p. 176. Englewood Cliffs, N.J.: Prentice Hall.

Reibstein, D. 1985. *Marketing: Concepts, strategies and decisions,* pp. 401-440. Englewood Cliffs, N.J.: Prentice Hall.

Schein, E. 1969. *Process consultation,* pp. 21-26. Reading, Mass.: Addison-Wesley.

Schramm, W. 1965. *The process and effect of mass communication.* Urbana, Ill.: University of Illinois Press.

Schultz, D. 1981. *Essentials of advertising strategy.* Lincolnwood, Ill.: Crain Books.

Stanley, R. 1982. *Promotion.* 2d ed., p. 136. Englewood Cliffs, N.J.: Prentice Hall.

Urdang, L. 1983. *Dictionary of advertising terms.* 3d ed. Chicago: Crain Books.

Westbrook, R. 1987. Product/consumption-based effective responses and postpurchase processes. *Journal of Market Research* 14:258-270.

Wright, J., W. Winter, and S. Zeyler. 1982. *Advertising.* New York: McGraw-Hill.

Review Questions

1. "Advertising is just one type of marketing communication." Comment.

2. Describe the hierarchy-of-effects model.

3. What is transformational marketing communication?

4. Make a list of all the barriers to effective marketing communication that you can recall from the chapter.

5. Select any written health marketing communication that you can find (e.g., an ad, a mailing, a brochure) and comment on how well you think it overcomes each of the barriers to effective communication.

6. "Some health marketing messages just don't fit with the image of the provider that originates them." Discuss.

Chapter 11

Basics of Effective Marketing Communications

Suppliers of services who have established a good track record of effective marketing communications tend to have followed 10 basic steps:

1. They advertise.

2. They plan their advertising communications.

3. They budget for their advertising communications realistically.

4. They implement their advertising well.

5. They nearly always get expert help with their advertising.

6. They monitor and measure the results of their advertising communications.

7. They often seek to reinforce their advertising communications by publicity, but they do not regard such publicity as a substitute for advertising.

8. They often reinforce their advertising by sales promotion, but again they do not treat sales promotion as a substitute.

9. They nearly always support their marketing communications by personal selling.

10. They nearly always support their marketing communications with a major focus on customer service.

The first statement in this list may seem confusing. As noted in Chapter 10, however, advertising consists of any marketing communication that is paid for and is not presented in person. Many effective marketing communicators do advertise in the mass media, but there are others who adopt a low profile in such media while relying on alternative advertising methods such as mail or telephone sales. In fact, by 1982, combined spending nationally on direct mail ($11 billion) and telemarketing ($13 billion) approached half the amount ($55 billion) spent on mass media advertising (Reibstein 1985; Stone 1987).

Some form of advertising, through the mass media or by other means, is almost always essential to any marketing communications strategy. The market share that any product or service can aspire to achieve is usually fairly small. Indeed, as noted in Chapter 8, it is very risky to pursue a venture that depends on an abnormally high market share to be financially viable. Most successful products and services thrive with relatively low market shares. Also, even when the target audience for a particular service can be fairly precisely defined, it is usually impossible to predict which individual members of that audience are the best prospects as potential customers. Very often, therefore, it becomes necessary to communicate with quite a large number of people in order to find the fairly small number most interested in the service.

A hospital with a major open-heart surgery and cardiac catheterization program had experienced diminishing referrals for several years. It launched a marketing communications effort targeted at primary care physicians in its service area, of whom there were some 3,000. It soon realized that calling in person on each of these physicians would prove impossibly time consuming. One person assigned full-time to this task, and averaging three visits daily, would take some 4 years to visit them all. The hospital therefore started a mailing program, a form of advertising, inviting those interested to call. The smaller number of doctors who prequalified themselves as more likely customers, by making the effort of responding, represented a more manageable schedule for a personal visit.

Planning for Marketing Communications

The three most critical questions to be addressed in a marketing communications plan are:

1. What should be promoted?
2. To whom?
3. How?

Defining the Message

Enterprises differ widely as to where they place the emphasis in their marketing communications. Some concentrate on boosting their overall image, while others focus on promoting specific services. Still others combine an element of both organization image building and specific product line promotion in their marketing.

A *product line* is a specific service that the organization offers. To take an example: Faced with increasing local competition among providers of rehabilitation services, a hospital found that its general image marketing was not proving very effective. It therefore analyzed its services and decided that they fell into 15 product lines. (*Hospital Product Line Report* 1987): pediatric rehab, brain injury rehab, stroke rehab, arthritis rehab, amputee rehab, burn rehab, back rehab, sexuality rehab, work capacity assessment, work reentry program, handicapped driver assessment, biofeedback, augmentative communication, dysphagia, and pain rehab. At a financial level, such product line systems can help to distinguish activities that are successful from those that are not. In terms of marketing, a product line system can form a basis for a more detailed strategy than an approach that treats the enterprise as if each part of it faces the same marketing challenges.

The choice between an organizational image building strategy and a product-specific strategy is usually based on four considerations:

1. What seems to be the enterprise's major marketing challenge? Preneed marketing or current need marketing? Inadequate awareness by potential customers, inadequate preference, or lack of familarity with how to access its services? Does the enterprise have enough one-time customers but a problem in transforming them into loyal repeat users?

2. The extent of competition facing the enterprise. The more extreme the competition, the easier it may be to

build demand for specific services that competitors are not emphasizing, rather than for the enterprise as a whole.

3. The relative levels of unused capacity of the enterprise's different services. If the enterprise has spare capacity in all product lines, it may not matter which gain most new customers. If, however, some services are fully utilized while others are underutilized, it often makes more sense to concentrate on the latter in marketing communications, even if the product lines that are operating at full capacity are the most prestigious. Attracting more patients to such a service who cannot be accommodated or served quickly may, in fact, harm the image of those programs rather than boost it further.

4. The relative profitability of the enterprise's different services. Many not-for-profit health providers lose money on treating some patients, but must offset these losses by earning a surplus from treating others. A general marketing communications strategy may endanger this often precarious payer mix by attracting a disproportionately large number of underinsured patients, while a more selective strategy can maintain or improve use by adequately insured patients.

An example of the use of image-building marketing communications is that of a renowned university hospital that acquired two smaller hospitals with much weaker reputations. Both acquisitions also had unused capacity. The university hospital therefore launched a general image campaign to publicize the fact that these two other hospitals were now part of its system.

An example of good product line-oriented marketing communications strategy is that of a Kansas hospital that found via a survey that it had a good image but low "product identification" — the public was unsure where it excelled. The hospital selected three services — obstetrics, adolescent psychiatry, and seizure disorders — where it had unused capacity and which were profitable, and launched campaigns for these three specific product lines. It succeeded in raising volumes in adolescent psychiatry and seizure disorders to full capacity and increased obstetrical admissions by 25%.

Effective marketing communications must be planned, and that planning begins by deciding where those communications should be focused. What is their central objective? Identifying the organization's main challenge, assessing its competitive threats, and deciding where it has the capacity to handle growth, and where growth is profitable, should all play a role in that analysis.

Identifying the Audience

The next step in planning marketing communications is to make a list of the key audiences that are important to the desired goal. Those audiences may well differ depending on the objective that has been defined. For some objectives, doctors alone may constitute the crucial target audience. For another objective, women of childbearing age as well as doctors may be crucial. For yet another objective only local school nurses may be really critical, and so on.

There may be many audiences that are of some relevance to an objective. The fewer the audiences that a marketing campaign has to reach, however, the easier and more effective it is likely to be. Usually, therefore, the key audiences for any communications effort have to be not only identified but also prioritized. This process of prioritization represents an important distinction between marketing communications and public relations activities. The objective of public relations is to foster and maintain goodwill among all of an enterprise's "constituencies." The public relations approach to a communications task is therefore usually to ensure that every constituency is somehow involved. By contrast, the objective of marketing communications is to attract users. Typically, that is best done by repetitive communication with those audiences that are most vital in the selection process for the service in question.

Consider the case of a hospital that wanted to increase use of its emergency room. Two people with public relations, not marketing, backgrounds were asked to develop a program. They identified 10 different audiences for the campaign: past patients, potential patients, hospital physicians, other local physicians, employees, hospital volunteers, neighborhood groups, ambulance services, industry, and other local health agencies (Rubright and MacDonald 1981). Again adopting a common public relations formula, they then identified between 5 and 10 affordable initiatives to reach each of those audiences.

A thorough marketing approach to that problem would have been very different. It would still have started by trying to list all the possible key audiences, but it would then have tried to narrow the list down to the few most critical audiences. In this case, for instance, hospital physicians, ambulance services, past patients, potential patients, and other community doctors would seem to be much more involved in emergency room selection than the other groups. Even among the remaining five groups, the hospital's physicians, past patients, and ambulance services may well be more likely to refer to this hospital than other community groups or people who have not previously visited the hospital. It might, therefore, be sensible to concentrate on these first three important and better-disposed target audiences initially. Perhaps that effort alone will be sufficient. Since marketing communications work through repetition, it may well also be better to reach these priority audiences 20 times each, rather than a broader audience just 5 to 10 times.

Another hospital emergency room, faced with a similar challenge, started by researching among its own doctors. It found that, on average, they recommended more than half their patients to other emergency rooms because of some quite minor but irritating organizational problems in their own hospital's emergency room. Fixing those problems, and then writing a letter monthly for a year to the 250 doctors on its own medical staff telling them about the improvements, resulted in a 15% growth of visits.

The next step in planning marketing communications is to identify and then prioritize the audiences who are crucial to the desired objective. It usually pays to communicate more frequently to a few people who are most important in service selection than to communicate with less frequency to a larger number of audiences of only marginal relevance to the objective.

Media Options

Once the priority audiences for the planned marketing communications program are identified, the next task is to itemize some possible methods of actually reaching them with the desired message. The objective should be to define a communications strategy that will achieve a good reach and frequency in the most cost-effective way.

Marketing experts use the concept of *reach* to describe the percentage of the target audience who will be exposed to a marketing communication. If, for instance, the only priority audience for a particular project is a hospital's own doctors, a letter sent to all of them will achieve a 100% reach among the target audience.

The priority audience for a pediatric asthma program was determined to be "parents of asthmatic children within 25 miles of the service." There were estimated to be 10,000 such families. A local newspaper with a circulation of 250,000 among a total of 1,000,000 households in the area is therefore only likely to achieve a 25% reach among the priority audience.

For most marketing campaigns, the actual percentage *response* among the priority audience is usually quite low. Indeed, a response rate of between 3% and 5% is normally considered excellent even for a very well planned and executed campaign (Robertson and Vortzel 1977).

Consider how this fairly low predictable response applies in this case. With an estimated 10,000 families in the service area with an asthmatic child, even a communications strategy that achieved a 100% reach among them could only be reasonably expected to yield about 400 responses (4% of 10,000). If the campaign relied entirely upon a local newspaper with a 25% reach, the predicted responses would fall to 100 (4% of 25% of 10,000).

If 100 responses are insufficient to make the planned program viable, there are only three real options available. The first is to add media in order to increase the reach beyond 25%. The second option is to expand the service area of the program in order to enlarge the size of the target population, if, in fact, it is realistic to attempt to do so. The third option is to abandon the program as nonviable.

There would appear to be a fourth option. Might it not be safe to assume more than a 4% response rate? After all, if a 10% response was attainable, the local paper, reaching 25% of the 10,000 estimated target families, would yield 250 responses (10% of 25% of 10,000). Although many campaigns do succeed in beating the 4% average response, there are just as many that fail even to secure that level of response. It is therefore risky to assume an inflated response rate for any marketing communication.

The reach needed to draw a desired response may dictate which media will have to be used (Fisk 1986). Contrast the following three situations.:

1. The sole priority audience for a program is defined as 35 gynecologists, whose names are known. The most effec-

tive communications strategy is likely to be some combination of letters and personal selling to these 35
known doctors.

2. The sole priority audience for a program is defined as
   1,000 past patients, whose names are known, and a 4%
   response is assessed as adequate. This number is too
   large for each patient to be approached in person. The
   most effective communications strategy is likely to be
   direct mail, with personal follow-up (in person or by
   phone) to those who express some interest in response
   to the mailing.

3. Four thousand responses are needed to make another
   program viable. The identity of those likely to need the
   service is not known. The only viable communications
   strategy is likely to be some form of advertising, in the
   media or by mass mailing, that reaches 100,000 eligible
   people.

Because situations such as the third one described above may exist
from time to time in any enterprise, those that establish arbitrary
policy barriers to certain types of marketing communications may
well, in effect, jeopardize the viability of some of their programs.
They deny themselves access to the only strategy that will achieve
certain program objectives, as the following case illustrates.

Because its parent university received a large amount of direct
state funding, a state university hospital decided to ban any media
advertising. It was concerned that such advertising would be called
into question by state legislators when debating future appropria-
tions to the university. They might argue that an institution that
"had dollars to spare for media ads" did not need so much state
support. The university hospital was committed to a new service that
would depend heavily on direct patient self-referral. It needed 1,000
responses from frail elderly patients with a prior history of hip replacement. Fewer than 200 hip replacements had been performed at
the hospital itself over the prior 3 years. It decided as a first step to
write to these patients, but only five responded. The hospital attributed this low response to several factors: It knew that only a 4%
response was predictable. It found that some 15% of the frail elderly
patients had died since their operation; indeed, it received several
angry letters from spouses and children of such patients accusing the

hospital of insensitivity to their grief. It also realized from this experience that the adult caregivers of frail elderly patients may be as crucial—perhaps more crucial—to the desired referrals, but its medical records on past hip replacement patients lacked information on their adult children.

The hospital then tried writing to family doctors in its service area, seeking referrals for the new program. It spent more than $20,000 on this communications effort, but it yielded only a further 30 patients.

The hospital then belatedly called in a marketing consultant. He advised that the most cost-effective strategy would be ads in the regional paper, because they could reach the 25,000 adult caregivers, whose identity was unknown, at a cost of about $3,000 each time the ad ran. The university hospital explained its policy ban on media ads. The marketing consultant then advised that the only viable option was a direct mail campaign. Even though that was also advertising, it might be less "visible" to the legislators. However, it was not possible to get a mailing list that consisted purely of adult caregivers of frail elderly parents. No such list existed. It was only possible to get a list of households where the spouses were between 45 and 55, and might therefore have a surviving frail elderly parent.

To maximize the prospects of reaching the needed 25,000 such caregivers, the mailing should probably go to at least 75,000 households in the target age range. The unit cost per household would, depending on the design of the mailing, range between one and three dollars. The total program would therefore cost between $75,000 and $225,000 each time the mailing went out, to achieve what a $3,000 media ad could probably do better.

Just as important as the reach of a planned marketing communications strategy is its *frequency*. As already noted, persuasive communication usually depends upon repetition of a message (de Vito, 1971; Wright, Winter, and Zeyler 1982). The basic minimum number of exposures of the target audience to a message to make the communication effective is usually quoted as being about four in a relatively short period of time; however, it is not uncommon for major marketing campaigns, particularly for new services, to strive for upward of 10 exposures (Surmanek 1980).

To plan an effective marketing communications strategy, it is therefore necessary to decide upon the frequency of exposure at which to aim. In the example above, the marketing consultant went on to advise that the hospital should plan for an absolute minimum of four exposures to the target audience of caregivers. This consideration would widen yet further the case for print ads. Four repeats of such an ad would total some $12,000. Even allowing for some $5,000 of ad production cost, this strategic option would only cost some $17,000. By contrast, four repeat mailings to 75,000 households would cost a minimum of $300,000, and a maximum of $900,000. Faced with this choice between a media ad strategy that violated its policy, and a direct mail program it judged to be prohibitively expensive, the hospital rejected the consultant's advice. Instead, it embarked on intensified mailing to doctors in the area and tried to obtain some free media publicity. Twelve months and $15,000 later, it had only attracted a further 10 patients to the program.

To provide a consistent basis for comparing the costs of different communication options, marketers usually adopt the convention of expressing them in terms of cost per thousand (CPM) exposures. In the above example, for instance, the minimum cost of the direct mail option was $300,000 to achieve four exposures to an estimated 25,000 eligible households. The CPM was therefore $6,000 ($300,000 divided by 25). Note that only these 25,000 households should be used in the calculation, not the full 75,000. The consultant had suggested that, because of imperfections in the available mailing lists, it would take 75,000 households reached to yield 25,000 with a frail elderly parent. The CPM for the media ad option was $580 ($17,000 divided by 25).

CPM may not be the only measure to consider. Two communication options may have different levels of reach or frequency. In the above case the hospital eventually chose a strategy (letters to doctors plus attempted free media publicity) that had a much lower CPM, but also proved to have insufficient reach or frequency to work.

The next step in planning a marketing communications strategy is to list optional methods of communicating with the target audiences. These options must each allow for an adequate reach and frequency in order to obtain the necessary level of response. The relative costs of these options can then be compared, to identify the most effective strategy or combination of strategies. By convention, it is normal to express such costs for comparative purposes in terms of cost per thousand exposures.

Comparisons of CPMs, however, must also be interpreted against the relative reach and frequency of each option.

Budgeting for Marketing Communications

The preceding section illustrated one method of budgeting for marketing communications. In the example quoted, the lowest-cost option of achieving the needed reach and frequency was calculated. In principle, an enterprise that has various key marketing communications priorities could adopt this approach to budgeting for each of them, and then add the individual amounts needed to derive its total marketing communications budget for an accounting period (e.g., a year). This *objective-and-task approach* is, in fact, just one of four commonly used methods (Dean 1951).

Perhaps the least scientific method, but one that is commonly employed, is the *affordable approach*. In its annual budgeting, an enterprise reaches an agreement on how much it can afford to spend on marketing communication. The obvious weakness of this method is that many marketing communications can and should be a direct investment in generating higher utilization. If the enterprise has the option of a communications strategy that generates more revenue than it costs, it may deprive itself of additional profits by artificially limiting the communications budget.

Another common method of budgeting attempts to address this problem. It fixes its marketing communications budget by a *percent-of-sales approach*. Thus, if last year the organization achieved $500,000 in sales with $25,000 spent on marketing communications, its percentage-of-sales allocation was 5%. If next year it plans to achieve $600,000 of sales, it will, under this approach, allocate $30,000 to marketing communications (5% of $600,000).

The weaknesses of the percentage-of-sales approach are twofold. First, circumstances may change in the market. Competitors, for instance, may decide to increase their own marketing communications budgets as a percentage of their projected sales. If so, the enterprise might find that it is now underspending relative to its competitors. Second, the enterprise may be planning to enter a new field of service where established competitors customarily spend more of their budget on marketing communications. Its own historical percentage-of-sales allocation may be inadequate to compete in a new field. As a matter of fact, the percentage of sales that organizations allocate to marketing communications does vary considerably from one type of effort to another (Vladimir and Vladimir 1984).

To address these shortcomings, some organizations budget for marketing communications using a *competitive approach*. They watch how much competitors are spending and plan to match it. They may even plan to outspend a competitor who is more established than they themselves are in a particular market (Chase and Barasch 1977).

Despite the logic that underlies the objective-and-task, percentage-of-sales, and competitive approaches, it is understandable that disagreement often surfaces between marketing staff and financial staff when enterprises prepare their annual budgets. How much spending on marketing communications will really be enough to meet planned volume targets? One other approach affords a basis of compromise between the affordability approach and these other methods. It is known as the *sales response and decay approach* (Simon 1965), or the *plowback approach* (Bradley, Fisk, and Owens 1987). It consists of agreeing on a sales target and on a marketing communications budget to support it. However, it is also agreed that progress will be reviewed periodically during the year. If sales are ahead of target, more will be allocated to marketing communications.

The logic behind this approach is that successful marketing communications strategies draw further funding as long as they remain successful. Once extra spending fails to secure extra sales, the strategy loses some of its funding. The approach is therefore, in principle, self-regulating. The following case illustrates this approach.

A home care program had target sales for the next year of $800,000 spread over four equal quarters. It was agreed, under the percentage-of-sales method, that 5% was a reasonable allocation for marketing communications. The budget for that activity was therefore set at $40,000 for the year, or $10,000 per quarter. The marketing staff argued, however, that it had developed a promising new campaign for the program, which, if properly funded, could raise sales to $900,000 for the coming year. The finance staff noted that, if sales went $100,000 over budget, operating costs would rise as well, but only by some $50,000. The extra $100,000 of sales was well worthwhile, given that level of profitability. It consequently proposed that performance be examined quarterly, and if actual sales were over budget, the 5% of sales allocation would be recalculated for the next quarter. The actual results are presented in Table 11-1.

Table 11-1 Quarterly Marketing Allocations and Actual Sales

Quarter	Allocation	Sales	Excess	Added to Next Quarter Allocation
1	$10,000	$240,000	$40,000	$2,000
2	$12,000	$260,000	$60,000	$3,000
3	$13,000	$250,000	$50,000	$2,500
4	$12,500	$250,000	$50,000	New budget year

As will be noted, this approach adds resources to marketing communications when sales exceeded budget, but also reduces this extra allocation when the campaign stopped adding further growth. At the end of the fourth quarter, a new round of annual budget discussions took place to decide what to do for the following year.

Several approaches are commonly adopted to establishing budgets for marketing communications and reconciling them with available resources in an organization. None of these methods is perfect, and each has different practical implications, which should be understood and agreed to in advance.

Executing Effective Advertising Communications

Even well-planned and adequately budgeted marketing communications will fail unless they are also well executed. This section focuses on the execution of advertising communications. Later sections look at the requirements of effective publicity, sales promotion, and personal selling.

As already explained, advertising includes any form of marketing communication that is paid for and that is not delivered in person. Many of the concepts discussed below were first discovered through research into advertising in the mass media. However, they apply equally to other forms of advertising in which nurses and other health professionals may be quite frequently engaged. These activities may include such things as writing letters to referral sources, drafting written information for patients about tests and procedures, scripting a videotape introduction to a health service, assisting in developing a service brochure, writing an announcement of a health education event, or drafting instructions for new professional staff.

The key to effective advertising communication lies in answering four questions (Fisk and Brown 1984). To *whom* shall we say *what* using *which verbal or visual images* through *which media?"*

Defining the Target Audience

The "to whom," the *target audience* for the communication, should have been defined as part of the initial planning of any communications strategy. That target audience may be immediate potential customers for a health service, such as referral sources, families, or payers. It may be future potential customers, such as medical residents, who may make referrals in their subsequent careers. It may be immediate potential consumers, such as patients with the disease in question. It may be future potential consumers, such as today's healthy teenagers who will, within a few years, control much of the demand for routine obstetrical services. It may be influencers of other people's health service selection decisions, such as health professionals or adult caregivers with elderly parents. It may be gatekeepers who are the first people to whom someone turns in a medical emergency, like a school nurse or a paramedic. It may be existing users of the service who could be repeat users, like asthmatics, or who could be users of an associated service, like new mothers considering where to seek well-baby care.

The fewer the number of target audiences identified as priorities for any service, the more focused its marketing communications can be. Similarly, the more precisely the audience can be defined, the easier it becomes to execute advertising communications effectively.

People pay most attention to messages that seem narrowly designed for people "just like them." There are three main reasons why this is so:

1. Most people do not actively read, listen to, or watch institutional messages as a source of general news. They satisfy that need largely through newspapers, magazines, and radio and TV shows. Rather, they tend to scan an institutionally sponsored message to see if it is of direct value to them. Narrowly targeted communications tend,

therefore, to be studied more by those for whom they are intended.

2. All communication, as already noted, is competitive. People are much more likely to have their attention captured by messages that seem directly intended for them.

3. People generally absorb information most readily if it appears to be meant for them individually, and not as a member of some group. The most effective advertising communications therefore read, or sound, as if they are addressing someone as "you" in the singular. The more narrowly defined the audience, the more the message can be structured for that type of person and be regarded by them as credible.

An adolescent psychiatry program sent out a mailing to households where both spouses were aged 35 to 50, and were most likely therefore to have adolescent children. The letter was headlined, "An Important Message for Parents!" It might better have been headlined, "An Important Message for Parents of Teenage Boys and Girls!" That version specifies the age of the children in question.

Advertising communications are easier to execute well when the target audience is defined as narrowly and precisely as possible.

Defining the Task

The next challenge is to define *what* the advertising communication should say, what type of task is it intended to perform. As noted in Chapter 10, a specific communication may be directed at either a preneed or a current need. It may be intended to create awareness, to create preference, motivate response, or transform existing users into loyal users. Determining which of these tasks, or which combination of them, is the principal purpose of the communication has major implications for its successful execution.

Advertising communications are easier to execute well when the principal task that they are intended to accomplish has been well defined.

A Virginia hospital ran an ad for its magnetic resonance imaging (MRI) facility with a large photo of a magnet and the headline, "If It Could Pick Up Hidden Diseases, Would It Attract Your Attention?" The body copy explained that the hospital was one of the first in the state to offer MRI. It did not specifically invite readers to do anything. It seems reasonable to assume, therefore, that the ad was intended to create preference for this hospital by distinguishing it from others. The problem with this execution lies in the fact that capturing a reader's attention is the most difficult task in any advertising. In a print ad, that task falls most to the illustration and the headline, since they are its most instantly visible elements. In fact, very few people read the detailed body copy of ads. If this hospital had really focused on the task of this ad — using its acquisition of MRI to build preference — it would have conveyed that key message in the headline and graphic, not as one of some 40 sentences in the body copy.

Contrast that case with the following one: A local Blue Cross and Blue Shield launched an HMO in an area with several established competitive plans. It also defined its central task as creating preference for its own plan. It saw the main advantage of its plan as being the very large number of doctors and hospitals with which it had contracted and the comprehensive family coverage that it offered. It therefore ran an ad that showed the face of a large friendly dog with the headline, "Under Our Health Plan, This Is the Only Member of the Family Who Doesn't Have a Choice of 400 Family Doctors, 6,500 Specialists, and All Area Hospitals" (*Health Care Advertising Review*, 1986). This ad shows a strong definition of, and focus on, the central message.

As these cases also illustrate, differences in the defined task of an advertising communication should lead to different points of emphasis in the message (Lavidge and Steiner 1961). For instance:

1. Preneed communications should normally emphasize the risks of the disease and the value of taking precautions.

2. Ads intended to create awareness among current potential patients should normally emphasize description of the service and its benefits.

3. Ads intended to create preference among current potential patients should normally emphasize arguments for selecting the service instead of competitors.

4. Ads intended to motivate action among current potential patients should normally emphasize how to access the service and contain further prompts to action ("action reminders").

5. Ads intended to transform users into loyal customers should usually emphasize confirming the wisdom of their selection, explaining how complaints will be handled, explaining follow-up customer service, or making a "special offer" available only to established customers.

Different advertising communications tasks usually call for different points of emphasis to be effective. In many unsuccessful advertising communications an original creative idea has been forced to fit an incompatible task.

Positioning

The central message of any advertising communication faces another challenge if there is a high level of competition for that service. The message must also *position* the service as different from, and preferable to, its rivals (Ries and Trout 1981). The best *position statements* convey one simple but powerful idea, such as "We're #2: We Try Harder," or "Peanut M&Ms Melt in Your Mouth Not in Your Hand," or "Coke—It's The Real Thing" (Dobrow 1984).

It was shown in an earlier chapter that the initial launch of Teflon pans nearly flopped because Du Pont misjudged their true appeal. Belatedly, it did discover "The Non-Stick Pan," and Teflon dominated the market for many years under that position statement. However, Teflon always suffered from the drawback that the surface scratches easily and wears out after about 2 years' use. By 1980, two rival and harder wearing products had entered the market, T-Plus and Greblon. Du Pont retaliated with its own superior coating, Silverstone. It decided, however, that the market for nonstick pans was now mature. Silverstone would not succeed, as Teflon had done earlier, by emphasizing its properties. Du Pont elected instead to market three lines of pan, each using Teflon's successor, but positioned differently by appearance and price. The top-of-the-line version was Le Creuset, which had wooden handles. Bourgeat pans had cast-iron handles and were less heat resistant than Le Creuset, but priced a few dollars less. Wear-Ever pans had plastic handles, which were as heat resistant as the wooden handles but looked less appealing than either Le Creuset or Bourgeat. Wear-Ever pans sold for only about a quarter of the price of Le Creuset.

Another example: It has been suggested that HMOs attract three types of enrollee. The first type is almost exclusively concerned with price, the second is concerned primarily with quality but doubts his or her own ability to make prudent selection decisions, and the third type is concerned with both price and quality (Akaah and Becherer, 1983). There is also, possibly, a fourth group who find that HMOs are easier to understand and their claims process more straightforward. Different HMOs have therefore adopted varying position statements, depending on which of these groups they most plan to attract. Some have also tried to summarize their position statement in their name. HMO Florida, for instance, primarily seeks the price-sensitive segment, and so it emphasizes the term HMO in its name. Gold Plus is an HMO name that seeks to emphasize quality. Several Blue Cross organizations have launched HMOs or PPOs that seek to combine the traditional quality and choice image of Blue Cross with the money-saving idea of an HMO. They have used names like Blue Choice and Blue Cross/Personal Choice, and slogans such as "At Last an HMO Good Enough to be Blue Cross." Other plans, seeking to emphasize their simplicity, have employed names like Independence and slogans like "Bye Bye Blues."

To take a final example: Dentists who have chosen to emphasize the cosmetic value of regular dental attention have employed position statements such as "We Put the Sunshine in Your Smile," while others choose to emphasize their sensitivity to patient dislike of dental treatment with slogans like "We Cater to Cowards" and "Even Chickens Need Check-Ups."

If an organization can incorporate its position statement in its name, it can simplify its advertising communications. A brief statement that promotes awareness of its name can then also convey a basic reason for preference. This practice is commonly followed in the naming of consumer products, such as Head and Shoulders shampoo, Intensive Care skin lotion, or Close-Up toothpaste. Several of the HMO names mentioned above incorporate basic position statements in this manner.

Particularly where a service faces strong competition, the central theme of its advertising communications should include a position statement that helps to differentiate it from rivals. Often that position statement is incorporated in one central slogan. In certain cases, it is even possible to embody that central position statement in the name of the service.

Choosing Verbal Images

The next challenge in effectively executing advertising communications is to determine which verbal or visual images to employ (Fisk and Brown 1984). The names and slogans mentioned above are examples of important *verbal images*. Indeed, the name of a service is likely to be its most widely read, seen, and heard verbal component. Well-communicated slogans can similarly become widely recognized.

Headlines, whether in a mass media ad, a letter, or a brochure, are also likely to be much more widely read than detailed body copy. As already noted, only a small percentage of ad readers actually take in even the main points of body copy, while many at least register the headline (Caples 1974). Even with a letter, not all recipients will fully read the details, but most will at least scan a headline. Indeed, it has been suggested that any medium of communication, even a telephone call, can conceptually contain a "headline," or its equivalent, if the author takes the trouble to define and include one (Caples 1983).

The two most important considerations in developing a headline are that it should relate to a benefit that is meaningful to the target audience, and that it should be worded to be as interesting as possible to them. For example, a medical practice in Phoenix ran ads with the headline, "Family practice medicine has changed over the years." That headline does not describe a benefit to potential patients, nor would it be particularly interesting to them. Similarly, a Catholic hospital ran ads headlined, "The Patients of a Saint" — a clever play on words, but scoring low on both describing a meaningful benefit and being of compelling interest.

There is a widespread belief that the ideal headline should consist of between five and eight words — long enough to make a meaningful statement, but short enough to be memorable. This notion is, however, strongly disputed by other advertising authorities (Ogilvy 1985). As a practical matter, there are many examples of headlines of very different lengths. Consider, for instance, "Co-ordinated Health Care for Seniors" (a headline from ElderMed, a national program for older adults), or "For Things That Get Bumped in the Night" (a headline for an urgent care center at Columbia Hospital, Milwaukee). Both of these examples conform to this arbitrary guideline on headline length, but just as effective is "Energize" (from a hospital fitness program in Newport News, Virginia) or "There Are Over 1,600 Doctors in the Memphis Area, But You Only Have to Make One Phone Call to Find the Right One" (from a physician referral service at Baptist Memorial Hospital in Tennessee).

Headlines can be of any length, but effective headlines are always interesting and usually summarize a key benefit that a service offers its customers.

One systematic study of headlines (Caples 1983) shows that the most effective tend to be couched in one of three styles. No fewer than 27 of the 106 headlines found to have been effective offered solutions to problems (e.g., "How To . . ."). The next most common formula (16 out of the 106) was a question (e.g., "Will you . . .?"). Other experimental studies in effective communication have also found that this approach of playing on the target audience's curiosity is a powerful means of capturing its attention and arousing interest in the message (Berlyne 1960). Again, however, the question must be interesting and concerned with an important benefit for the audience. Curiosity alone does not make an effective headline.

The third most common type of effective headline contains news (e.g., "New!" or "Announcing"). Such headlines accounted for 11 of the 106 effective examples found in the study quoted above. Once more, however, the news must be interesting and about a customer benefit. "New! St. Swithin's Opens New Lab" is, for example, a questionable application of this formula. It assumes that the benefit to patients is self-evident, which it may not be.

Three common formats for effective headlines are stating solutions to problems, posing questions, and announcing news. The content must, however, still be interesting to the target audience and mention a benefit.

Although the examples quoted above are taken from mass media ads, the concepts are just as applicable to letters, patient information bulletins, headings and subheadings in brochures, posters, public service announcements, and even signage.

For example, a hospital decided to do something about the dollars that it was losing through petty pilferage of supplies. It estimated that as much as $500,000 a year was at stake, and it strongly suspected that its own employees were the principal offenders. It decided on a poster and flyer campaign in the cafeteria, where most employees ate at least two or three times weekly. This location would also keep the campaign largely invisible to patients and visitors, who might interpret it as a poor reflection on the health professionals delivering their care. The first thought was a simple text on the posters and flyers that read, "Help Us Stop Pilferage. It's Costing Community Half-a-Million Dollars a Year." Two main objections were raised to this proposal: It lacked interest and it did not appeal to employees' self-interest. The revised version depicted a half-burnt twenty-dollar bill, with the text, "Would You Burn A Twenty-Dollar Bill? Each year at Community, we burn 25,000 of them! That's how much petty pilferage costs all of us. Without it, we'd all have more of the supplies and equipment that we need to do our jobs as we'd like to. Even more dollars in our pay packets. Let's use dollars, not burn them. Stop pilferage!"

Choosing Visual Images

Visual images in advertising communications can make as significant a statement as verbal images. Although again many of the guidelines for visuals have been most studied and tested in relation to mass media ads, they can be applied to a wide range of communications, from brochures to posters, and from illustrations in patient education materials to examples of diagnostic images used to market new services to physicians.

The most important consideration in selecting visuals is their relevance to the target audience. The visuals used in a brochure, for instance, make a direct statement to the reader of how well the enterprise understands the interests and outlook of the target audience.

Potential patients seek health care to obtain certain benefits, such as living longer, or being able to live a full life, or looking better. They can also find medical and surgical processes anxiety producing. Illustrations that demonstrate the outcome of health care are therefore more relevant to them than those that show its techniques (Fisk, 1986). If it is desirable to illustrate a medical or surgical technique so that patients are more fully informed, care may have to be taken to make any photos or graphics as free as possible of anxiety-provoking features.

Doctors are more welcoming of medical illustrations and photos that illustrate a service. However, they rarely make referrals without some thought of possible patient and family reaction to the experience. They may well, therefore, also look for visual evidence that the provider is sensitive to patients' nonclinical needs and concerns.

As a practical matter, people tend to identify most with illustrations of other people who share their interests and life-style, but are about 10 years younger (Ogilvy 1985). Thus, in an illustration intended to convey the idea that a health service can return its patients to a "normal life," it may be best to show someone slightly younger than the target audience engaged in an activity that many people share and find pleasurable, rather than one that is only a minority interest or one they perceive as a chore.

Illustrations should be relevant to the audience. They should make a statement that the provider understands the outlook, goals, and anxieties of the patient.

Advanced studies of effective illustrations show that they often achieve a *multimeaning profile* (Durgee and Stuart 1987). That is, their content relates to the desired image of the service at more than just one level. For example, a company was searching for a spokesperson for a TV ad for batteries. It concluded that the best choice was Olympic gymnast Mary Lou Retton. The company had found that customers for batteries identified the ideal product as being "small, high-energy, versatile, reliable, and a winner in its field." Mary Lou Retton shared this image. To take another example, Hush Puppies seems like a bizarre choice of name for a shoe, but a similar word association test found that customers most want their casual shoes to be "soft, warm, and friendly to their feet."

A contrasting example is that of an ad for an eye hospital, which featured a popular local comic whose own mother had been a patient there. Although the comic helped to attract viewer attention, "young, funny, and flippant" was not ideal imagery to associate with a serious health issue. On the other hand, a health care plan once featured comedian George Burns in ads for its senior citizen program. Although he was a comic, too, his public image is one of being "long-lived, respected, and sincere" — good imagery for the service.

Since illustrations can have multiple levels of meaning, they should be carefully chosen to convey several desirable features of the service. Conversely, they must avoid giving any message that is inconsistent with the intended image.

Several of the cases described above also raise another important consideration, that of selecting spokespersons for illustrations. A spokesperson may be someone from within the service who symbolizes one of its main attributes (like a woman doctor for a women's health service). It might be someone who symbolizes a successfully treated patient. It might be a celebrity whose image supports that of the service (like Mary Lou Retton). It is vital that the people portrayed in illustrations be well chosen. Celebrities, in particular, can be poor choices unless very carefully selected. They may aid in capturing the attention of the target audience, but may well impede their acceptance of the message if they lack credibility. On average, the use of celebrities has been found to increase recall of the content of ads by 22%, but to *reduce* preference for the service or product by 21% (Heller 1987). It is therefore much more important that spokespersons be credible than that they be known. A credible spokesperson can improve the response to an advertising communication by as much as 300% compared to another spokesperson with low credibility (Hovland and Mandell 1953).

One hospital ad showed its administrator comforting a waiting relative in the surgical waiting room. Most potential patients do not perceive this activity as part of a hospital administrator's normal activities. If they need comforting, they would perceive a doctor or nurse as a more assuring and credible source of support. The chosen illustration also leaves unclear why the relative needs comforting — because of the normal anxiety of awaiting the results of surgery on a loved one, or because she has just been told that this operation was unsuccessful?

The spokespersons used in marketing communications, including the people depicted in illustrations, must be credible to the target audience. Spokespersons lacking full credibility have been found to lower the results of advertising messages appreciably.

Emotion and Information

Both verbal and visual symbols inevitably convey both an emotional and a factual message, because words and pictures are usually emotionally charged. Since it is impossible to avoid conveying emotional messages, these effects of any marketing communication need to be considered as carefully as its informational content.

The emotional dimensions of marketing communication are particularly present in health care, because most of the benefits (e.g., staying alive, or being able to breath easier) it seeks to deliver are intrinsically both functional and emotional. That concept is, for instance, at the heart of the "holistic" concept of medicine. Since health care inevitably raises emotional issues, they must also be "cared for." Similarly, any communication about health care is inevitably about emotional, as much as informational, issues. Where should the balance between emotional and informational content be struck?

It should be recognized that there are three separate but related reasons to include some emotional elements in marketing communications. First, such elements directly help to convey an image of the service provider. For instance, the absence of a concern with children may be perceived as a fault in a pediatric program; the absence of a concern for the quality of life may be detrimental to the image of a program dealing with the frail elderly.

Second, the benefits provided by many health services are, as noted above, inevitably emotional (e.g., saving a child from death). Since it is impossible to sterilize discussion of health care to remove such emotional influences, they are best recognized and consciously managed in any marketing communication (Plummer and Holman 1981; Holbrook and O'Shaughnessy 1984; Mizerski and White 1986).

Third, an emotional element in a marketing communication can actually enhance message delivery, its committal to memory, and subsequent retrieval (Bettman 1979). The retention of any message seems to be a function of how deeply it is committed to memory, and messages that contain emotional as well as logical data are more likely to be retained (Cermak and Craik 1979). The retrieval of any information from memory seems to be enhanced when both emotional and logical cues can be employed to locate it (Cole and Means 1981). The use of emotional imagery to aid in both message encoding and retrieval may be particularly important in marketing communications to the elderly (Cole and Houston 1987). There is some disagreement whether memory problems in the elderly are a factor of either encoding deficiencies or retrieval deficits, but as a practical matter, the richer the message, the more likely it will be remembered.

A hospital ran a series of TV ads for its emergency room, each of which visually portrayed immediate care being rendered. The visuals thus included intravenous lines being put in, "crowd scenes" of emergency personnel making haste to carry out life-saving procedures, and patients who were clearly suffering from major trauma. These TV shots were dramatic, but they were also repulsive. Viewers tended to disengage from rather than engage in watching the spots.

As a contrasting example, the editors of *Readers' Digest* know from careful research that good health is one of the 26 most sought-after consumer benefits. Other items on that list of 26 that are also, directly or indirectly, related to certain health care services include reducing body fat, improving appearance, having a happy marriage, caring for children, improving one's knowledge, avoiding worry, avoiding embarrassment, and avoiding discomfort (Caples 1983). In this knowledge that good health is such a commonly desired benefit, the *Readers' Digest* cover story was health related in no fewer than 29 out of 120 consecutive monthly issues.

Emotional content plays several important roles in marketing communications. Because good health is among the most desired of all consumer benefits, and because most health services have an unavoidable emotional element, it is important to manage how it is visually presented.

How safe is it for the visuals in health marketing communications to imply a guarantee of outcome, by showing healthy and cured patients? This approach is less problematic in visuals than in words, yet in practice, the creators of some health marketing communications seem to pay more attention to the lesser issue of avoiding implicit guarantees in visuals than to avoiding explicit guarantees in words.

One ad for depression treatment pictured an unhappy woman with the caption, "She doesn't want to cry all the time. But she does. In two weeks, she won't" (*Modern Healthcare* 1987). It thus appears to have tried to imitate the advertising concept of providing an explicit guarantee of results. In reality, advertisers in other fields do not give guarantees as often as is sometimes assumed. Among the 106 effective headlines mentioned earlier, only 5 contained an explicit guarantee (e.g., "your money back"), and only another 10 contained even implied guarantees (Caples 1983).

If a marketing communication seems to call for some form of guarantee, it is quite uncommon to see an explicit guarantee of results. It is much more common to see a qualified guarantee statement, or a testimonial by one satisfied consumer, or a guarantee of service rather than of outcome.

Even if health care marketing communications inevitably include content that is directly or indirectly emotional, it is nevertheless important to balance it with informational content. Generally, potential consumers of health services have a very high demand for factual information in the marketing communications they see (Shapiro and Majewski 1983).

In visuals, information is best communicated in a logical order and sequence (Britton, Meyer, Hodge, and Glynn 1980). Flashbacks, for instance, tend to confuse viewer receptivity of TV messages. However, both verbal and visual information also seems to be remembered and recalled better when its conclusion is incomplete. The reader, listener, or viewer who has to fill in the blank seems, in the process, to commit a message more firmly to memory (Lewin 1947; MacLachlan 1984). This value of the incomplete message is one further reason not to overwork any particular communications medium.

An ad agency was asked to develop a marketing communication for a drug that could assist in controlling nervous symptoms (Caples 1974). The agency was undecided between two options. The first suggestion was a graphic listing a number of common nervous symptoms and a headline that read, "Thousands suffer from sick nerves and don't know it." The second suggestion was a photo of a neurologist with the headline, "Have you these symptoms of nerve exhaustion?" Both versions were tried out. The second was significantly more successful, for two principal reasons: The doctor was more interesting visually, and the question format of the headline aroused more reader curiosity and interest.

Health care consumers expect information in marketing communications, but it should be presented clearly and in a logical sequence.

Letters as Marketing Communications

Perhaps the importance of such a logical sequence is most apparent in the most common of all marketing communications: letter writing. Many letters are not written for marketing purposes. When someone does try to compose a marketing letter, he or she can therefore easily assume that the same approach used in other letters will be equally effective. However, the purpose of a marketing letter is different. Its goal is to motivate the reader to use a service. By comparison, most letters have different purposes: to share information, to communicate news, to give instructions, or perhaps just to stay in touch.

Because a marketing letter has a different purpose, it also has different implications for the recipient. He or she usually has a clear motive to read other types of letters (e.g., to hear news from a friend, to pay attention to the instructions of a boss, to be well informed, or to pay bills before the sender declares them delinquent). By comparison, the reading of a marketing letter is completely voluntary. The recipient who throws it away unread suffers no consequences; it is the sender who suffers by having his or her marketing message ignored. Physicians referring patients to a radiologist, for instance, must read the reports the radiologist sends them in order to carry on with their care of the patient, explain the results to the patient, avoid malpractice, and so on (McGraner 1987). The same physician is under no compulsion to read a letter from the same radiologist announcing a new service. He is free to read or to ignore it (Fisk and Brown 1987). The sender of a marketing letters thus faces a special challenge: to motivate the recipient to read it, to capture his or her attention and interest.

Because so many marketing communications are sent by letter, marketing scientists have carefully researched which types of letter seem to command the most attention. One of the most commonly followed approaches (Stone 1987) consists of seven steps:

1. Start (in a headline or first paragraph) with the most important benefit of the service to the reader

2. Next enlarge on that benefit

3. Be specific about what the reader will get

4. Offer proof that the offer is genuine

5. Say what the reader will miss if he or she does not reply

6. Restate the offer

7. Invite action and do so specifically.

Another common, but slightly different approach is to follow the *hierarchy-of-effects* sequence (Fisk and Brown 1987):

1. Write a headline or opening paragraph, or both, that captures the recipient's attention by offering an important benefit

2. Follow with a paragraph to create awareness by describing the offer

3. Follow with one or two paragraphs to create preference for the service, by citing two or three reasons why it is of value to the reader, and offering some proof

4. Conclude with a paragraph to motivate the recipient to respond.

A quick comparison of the seven-step model and the hierarchy-of-effects model will show that they have much in common, both in their content and sequence.

Here is the first draft of a letter that a radiology group intended to mail to local physicians. It was written without regard to the concepts described above:

Dear Colleague,

We are pleased to announce the opening of our third CT scanner. It operates 12 hours daily on weekdays, and on Saturday mornings.

The radiology service at Community General prides itself on the exceptional high quality of its imaging support to area physicians. The new scanner will be used for outpatient studies.

You may refer outpatients by calling 999-8888. We look forward to being of service to you.

Sincerely,

What is wrong with this draft? It fails to follow either the seven-step model or the hierarchy-of-effects model. As a result, its opening does not do a good job at capturing attention, the benefits to the recipient are left for him or her to determine, and it does not provide any strong incentive for the recipient to take action. Here is the longer, but more effective, letter as redrafted after applying the hierarchy-of-effects model. (Fisk and Brown 1987):

Dear Dr. Jones,

Your New CT Diagnostic Service

You may have been looking for an outpatient CT service that can schedule your patients quickly. Demand for in-patient CT has grown at area hospitals, and delays in scheduling outpatients have lengthened.

At Community General, a third CT scanner has been added. It will be devoted exclusively to outpatient studies.

This new service will shorten scheduling delays. It is also housed in a separate building at the hospital, closer to our patient parking, easier for them to access, and designed for their distinct needs. It operates from 7 a.m. to 9 p.m. on weekdays, plus Saturday mornings. It is staffed by radiologists and technicians from the Department of Radiology to assure you the same high professional quality. In most cases, you will receive a same-day telephone report on a patient's scan, followed by a written report the next working day.

You may refer a patient by calling 999-8888. Outside of working hours, you can leave a message at this number which will receive our priority attention the next day. We also invite you to visit the center to see for yourself how service to patients and referring doctors has been designed into it.

The emphasis of this new outpatient CT center will be on prompt response to referrers. We are, therefore, only, at this stage, informing established referrers about it. We will notify other possible referrers about the center two months from now, but those referring during this period will go on a priority list for future scheduling.

This redraft goes well beyond merely resequencing the first version to fit the hierarchy-of-effects model for such a letter. Further benefits for referrers are described, and further offers are made. Employing the hierarchy-of-effects model or the seven-step model to draft such letters compels the author to define the answers to several critical questions:

1. How, at the start, can the letter show that the service is really a solution to an important customer need?

2. What are the two or three key facts about the service of which the reader should be made aware in order to use it effectively?

3. What three or four arguments can be advanced to convince the reader that he or she should prefer this service over competitors? (If the service, as planned, does not contain three or four such competitive advantages, what further refinements should be incorporated in its design to provide such benefits?)

4. How does the service want the reader to respond? Can two or three different ways of responding be quoted? Can a reason be given for a prompt response?

Reread the final version of the letter with these four questions in mind, and try to identify what specific points were added to address each of them.

The precise wording of marketing letters can have a major impact on the level of response. A further step may therefore be worthwhile even when a final draft, like that quoted above, has been prepared. This extra step consists of trying to identify the one or two statements that might be most crucial to the reader. If there is any doubt that they have been worded in the best possible way, it may pay to develop two versions of the letter and to mail each to a small initial sample of the target audience. By tracking which version seems to draw the higher response, it may be possible to determine which version works best before a larger mailing is undertaken. Commercial enterprises that sell heavily by mail are often engaged in continuous testing and retesting of such alternative versions (Chase and Barasch 1977; Fisk 1986).

A company decided to advertise by mail, for a limited period, a half-price introductory offer for a new product. It developed three ways of stating this offer (Caples 1983): "Half Price!" or as "Buy One – Get One Free!" or as "50% Off!" It decided to test out three versions of the letter, one with each of these three variations. No other wording differed among the three drafts. It found that the version with "Buy One – Get One Free!" drew a 40% greater response than either of the alternatives.

Now re-consider the radiologists' letter. There seem to be two areas where the final draft might be still better worded. The first is the opening. The offer of more rapid scheduling than rival centers probably is of major value to the intended readers. However, as referring physicians they may place equal importance on fast feedback of results, a benefit only alluded to in the third paragraph. Why not add it to the introduction? The radiology practice involved realized that the competitive CT services also offered that benefit. It was important enough to allude to it, but it was not as much a distinguishing feature of their new outpatient CT center as its quick scheduling. Nevertheless, they might have tested an alternative version of the first two paragraphs:

> You need an outpatient CT service that both schedules your patients quickly and gives you rapid feedback on the results. Demand for inpatient CT has grown at area hospitals. They may give you same-day telephone results on your outpatients – once they manage to fit them into their schedules. However, those scheduling delays are often long – and growing even longer.

The new Outpatient CT Center at Community General is devoted exclusively to outpatient studies. It offers you both faster scheduling of your patients and same-day telephone reports.

The other crucial point in the radiologists' final draft is the ingenious idea that they have developed to encourage readers to try the new service quickly—qualifying to be included in the future priority referrer list. It might be worth giving this offer even more prominence by adding a new subheading immediately before that statement: "How To Get On Our Priority Referrer List." The radiologists may be concerned at possible reader reaction to emphasizing this point. Will it make the letter seem too blatant? Again, the solution to this dilemma might lie in testing two versions of the letter on small numbers of the intended audience.

The next consideration in all written marketing communications is the grade reading level of the wording. Most people in the health professions involved in drafting such letters, and other written material, are products of an educational system that rewarded them for mastering how to write, and read, complex prose. As a result, they tend to draft any written copy at an advanced-grade reading level.

As already noted, however, marketing communications are discretionary reading for their recipients (Fisk and Brown 1987). Decades of experimentation by enterprises that make heavy use of direct mail has shown that people are more likely to read material written at quite a low reading level. People whose education terminated with high school graduation seem to read most comfortably at about a sixth-grade level. People who have completed a college, postgraduate, or doctoral education read most comfortably at about a ninth- or tenth-grade level. They are, of course, used to reading at a much higher level when they have to (e.g., reading learned journals to stay up-to-date in their fields), but they usually prefer ninth- or tenth-grade material for copy they do not have to read. Discretionary reading material written above this level may, at first glance, seem to require more reading effort than they are willing to expend. If so, they are more likely to discard the material unread. This phenomenon has led one very successful marketing communicator to be wary of hiring anyone who has had a college education as a copywriter, even if specializing in material for professional audiences (Ogilvy, 1985). The effort involved in retraining them to write easily read prose is considerable.

One common method to assess the grade reading level of a draft marketing communication is the *fog index* (Fisk and Brown 1987). It consists of six steps:

1. Take the first 100 words of any copy.

2. Count the number of sentences. If the copy finishes with an incomplete sentence, count that as another whole sentence.

3. Divide 100 by the number of sentences to get the average sentence length.

4. Count the number of words with more than two syllables, but do not count verbs in which the third syllable is a common verb ending (such as -ed or -ing). Thus, *believing* would not count, because it only has two syllables without the -ing, but *demonstrating* would. Also do not count people and place names of more than two syllables. However, other polysyllabic words cannot be eliminated from the count just because the author chose to capitalize the first letter (e.g., *Hospital, Ultrasound,* or *Delivery*).

5. Add together the average sentence length and the polysyllabic word count.

6. Multiply that score by 0.4 (or divide it by 2.5) to yield the grade reading level.

To see the effect of applying this formula here are the first 100 words from an ad published by a Louisiana hospital. The polysyllabic words are shown in italics:

> Giving himself an *insulin* shot *every* morning isn't the *easiest* thing Greg does—but then it's not the hardest thing either. Living with *diabetes* can be challenging—maybe you need some help. That's why Marshall *Hospital* has developed its Center for *Diabetes*—a *specialized* treatment *facility dedicated* to the health, fitness and *emotional* needs of the diabetic. The Marshall *Hospital* Center for *Diabetes* offers a staff of three *registered dietitians* and a *Diabetes* Nurse

Educator to help you and your family do a better job of *understanding* and managing your *diabetes*. Through *outpatient* and *inpatient* services, the Marshall Center for . . . .

The extract contains five sentences, for an average sentence length of 20 words. It contains 21 polysyllabic words. Its grade reading level is 41 times 0.4, or roughly 16th grade. It is thus about twice as complex to read as most well-written marketing communications copy. How can it be easily simplified? It has several long sentences, which could be redrafted as two shorter sentences. It has some polysyllabic words that are unavoidable, but it has others for which shorter words could easily be substituted (e.g., *center* for *facility*, *diet experts* for *dieticians*). It has some polysyllabic words that could be omitted entirely (e.g., *specialized, registered*). It may take several redrafts to revise the text to an eight- or ninth-grade level, but it is not a major task, and none of the sense of the copy need be lost.

Does the length of a letter or other mailed piece matter? The best advice is to keep marketing communications brief, for two reasons: Busy readers may be more likely to read them in their entirety, and shorter documents are less costly. However, it may again be worth testing a shorter versus a longer version, if time and budget allow it. Some very successful mailings are very long and detailed (Caples 1973).

Written marketing communications work best when drafted and organized according to established successful models, when worded at an appropriate grade reading level, and when possible variations in the wording of their most crucial points are tested with small samples of the target audience.

Media Selection

As noted earlier, the four key questions in developing any marketing communication are: To *whom* shall we say *what*, using *which verbal and visual symbols* and through *which media?*" The number of media available for transmitting marketing communications is very large, and extending well beyond those most frequently considered as advertising.

Perhaps the most useful means of classifying these media is by the way in which each delivers a sponsor's message. The advantages, disadvantages, limitations, and special problems posed by each media option are made more obvious with this focus on how they deliver messages.

Marketing messages can be delivered by including them in forms of mass media (television, radio, newspapers, and magazines). It is this type of communication that is most commonly regarded as advertising. The distinguishing feature of the mass media is that they deliver marketing communications only as an ancillary task. Their ad content may make them financially viable, but their readers, viewers, or listeners primarily look at or listen to them for their non-advertising content. Because they have this other principal appeal to their audiences, they can be cost-effective ways of reaching either a very large number of people or a smaller one that shares a recognizable common interest (such as the readers of *Bride* or *Money*). As will be discussed shortly, however, the mass media vary considerably in their technical properties and value for different advertising tasks.

The second common way of delivering marketing messages is by mail. Here again, however, the options are quite varied, from a personal letter to distribution of a direct mail package. A direct mailing may itself range in content from an unaccompanied letter, to a catalog, to a multicomponent package, to an audio cassette or videotape.

The third common way of delivering marketing messages is by telemarketing. Once more, use of telephone for marketing can range from a personal call to a key client to "cold contact" mass canvassing.

The fourth common delivery mechanism for advertising is by display. This approach can range from billboards on major highways, to racks of information in selected locations through which large numbers of people may pass, to point-of-sale displays in locations to which customers actually come for products or services (e.g., a supermarket, bank, or hospital lobby).

A fifth delivery mechanism for advertising is reference sources, which people may consult if they identify a given need. The Yellow Pages are one common example, but there are many such sources available for different purposes. Their principal advantage lies in the fact that the people who consult them tend to be in need. Their principal disadvantage is that, if they are indeed well used by such people, one provider's ad is likely to be immediately surrounded by those of competitors.

Which medium is best for any given marketing communication depends on several critical questions:

1. What is the primary task of the communication?
2. Who constitutes the target audience for the communication?
3. What reach seems necessary among that target audience to secure the desired level of response?

The technical properties of different media tend to suit them more to some marketing communications tasks than others. For instance, newspaper ads work well to communicate quite detailed information and to produce an immediate response. By contrast, ads in the more upscale magazines tend to help build image better than do newspaper ads, but direct response is usually much lower.

The following list suggests what task or tasks each of the main marketing communications media performs best:

Mass Media

1. Newspaper ads allow the communication of quite detailed information and tend to draw good immediate response.

2. Magazine ads tend to be effective for image building messages that will benefit by being around for some time.

3. Radio ads are best suited to relatively simple image messages.

4. TV ads are well suited to relatively simple image messages, particularly where an important consumer benefit can best be demonstrated visually.

Mail Media

1. Letters, either personalized to a small number of recipients or mailed in bulk to large numbers of potential customers, are effective in communicating brief information and benefit statements calling for immediate response.

2. Direct mail packages, with a letter reinforced by a brochure or other materials, tend to be effective in communicating detailed information and in providing multiple response options (e.g., a reply card, plus a telephone number to call, plus some material to keep for future reference).

3. Both letters and direct mail packages can be effective in transformational advertising, to sustain and build the loyalty of past customers.

4. Mailing audio cassettes can be an effective way of conveying information, but it must usually extend beyond a simple marketing message to communicating facts of direct educational value to the listener.

5. To date, use of mailed videocassettes for marketing communications has been fairly limited and its effectiveness not well documented.

Telemarketing

1. Telephone sales calls to prospective customers can be effective in generating immediate response. They also, however, may be regarded as intrusive by some recipients. Their use tends therefore to be confined to enterprises who do not mind offending some of those called in the process of finding others who will buy.

2. Telemarketing can also be very effective in qualifying potential customers to assess whether they are worth more detailed follow-up (e.g., by mailing a package or by a personal visit). Such calls tend to take longer than the type of instant sales call described above, but are less frequently perceived as offensive.

Display

1. Point-of-sales displays (e.g., in waiting rooms) can be very effective in providing on-the-spot reinforcement of marketing messages to consumers who still have a residual doubt about the wisdom of their service selection.

2. Outdoor or billboard ads can be very effective at creating awareness of a service, its name, and one simple statement about it.

Reference Sources

1. Advertising in reference sources, like the Yellow Pages, can be very effective at getting a service's name, together with a simple statement about it, in front of some people active in searching for a possible supplier.

Reaching the Target Audience

Certain media may be read, listened to, or watched by the intended target audience. It may be important, however, to consider this issue in some detail. Superficial comparisons may be misleading. For instance, the radio station in the Philadelphia area with the highest average daily listening audience only outperforms other stations between 6 a.m. and 10 a.m. By lunchtime on weekdays it falls to eleventh place (Fisk 1986). The rating of a possible billboard location is sometimes stated in terms of gross circulation, which is merely a count of total traffic that passes it in either direction, not of the number of people who pass in a direction from which the ad is easily seen. A letter is less likely to be read if it arrives on a heavy mail day. One major reason why so many large-scale advertisers use ad agencies is not just to tap their creative skills but also because of the awareness of their media analysts of these subtleties in matching target audience and media.

The response rate, or the percentage of the target audience who can be reasonably expected to reply to a market communication, varies widely from medium to medium. For instance, finding 10 doctors to refer their physical rehabilitation patients to a particular center may be best accomplished by combining personal letters with personal visits. The number of respondents needed is small, and identifying the members of this target audience is quite easy. By contrast, attracting 1,000 patients with diabetes to self-refer to a treatment center may require communicating with at least 500,000 people. Not everyone has the disease, it may not be possible to find out who has it, and only a small percentage of people with the disease who receive the marketing communication are likely to try an alternative service. This effort may well, therefore, require a very large reach, which can usually be achieved at the lowest unit cost by mass media ads.

It is easy to be misled by generalizations about the relative value of different media in their reach to various types of target audience. As noted above, however, an effective media selection usually depends on a quite detailed examination of how many people, of what types, are likely to read, listen to, or watch particular media, at particular times, and in particular program or editorial environments. For instance, TV may be an effective way to reach middle-class parents of young children, but only in the late evenings, when they are likely not to be at work or tending to their children, and only if the ad runs during certain types of programming and not others.

An ad agency was asked to recommend a medium to reach middle- and upper-income men who might be potential patients for a sleep disorders program. The agency's first proposal was to run ads on TV in the early morning hours, when the station's charge for airing ads is very low and a high percentage of those watching may be insomniac. The doctor heading the sleep center then pointed out that insomnia as such was just one sleep disorder. The larger market consisted of men who regularly "woke up feeling tired." The agency therefore suggested the local Sunday paper. People who cannot get to sleep easily on a Saturday night might well buy an early edition of the Sunday paper to read. Those waking up feeling tired were highly likely, on a Sunday morning, to read the paper quite soon. Also, on a Sunday, people tend to read the paper more carefully than during the week. This case illustrates the process of asking detailed questions about the task of the marketing communication, the precise nature of the target audience, and the relative reach of different media to them at different times.

The best media selection for any marketing communication is one that is suited to the defined communication task, gets to the precise target audience, and does so with sufficient reach to produce the desired response.

Multimedia Approaches

Are two or more media — a *multimedia campaign* — always better than one medium alone? As a general rule, the answer to this question is yes. Some experimental research has strongly suggested that messages are more likely to be committed to memory and recalled if they have been received through more than just one medium (Moore and Reardon 1987). An empirical study comparing various ad campaigns suggests that adding a second medium to an advertising program increases average recall by about 33% (Schultz, Martin, and Brown 1984).

Although a second medium seems to improve the communication of marketing communication, in practice it may be necessary to make a choice between adding a second medium and increasing frequency in just one medium. As an example, a new dermatology center allocated $30,000 to its initial marketing communications. It defined its task as "informing adults — mainly women — that a new, convenient, and skilled option existed in the area for their primary dermatology care." It decided that the women's section of the local paper was an attractive medium. The paper was read by some 35% of the adult women in the area. Production of an ad for this medium would cost $5,000, and the paper charged $2,500 per appearance. This approach would therefore allow it to reach 35% of the target audience 10 times. The center was also attracted by the idea of ads on a local radio station popular with upper-class female listeners. Five spots scattered through the day on this station were likely to reach 20% of such women once each. Five percent of these women also read the local paper, while 15% did not. Production of a radio spot would cost $2,000, and the station charged $200 each time it was broadcast. If all of the $30,000 was allocated to radio, the center could afford 140 spots. On average, it would reach 20% of the target audience seven times each. Table 11-2 summarizes some of the center's options in combining these media.

Clearly, the radio-only option is not a good buy. It reaches fewer of the target audience than the paper-only option and with less frequency. However, the choice between the paper-only option and the 50/50 split is less clear. The paper achieves higher frequency (10 times) but lower reach (35%). The 50/50 split achieves higher reach (50%) but with lower frequency (3 for those only listening to radio, 5 for those only reading the paper, and 8 for those following both media). Which is the better option is a matter of judgment. In this case, the center elected to go with the 50/50 split. It did, however, track carefully which medium was responsible for each response that it received, so that it could later reassess the decision.

Table 11-2 Reach and Frequency of Local Media

Medium	Reach (%)	Frequency
Newspaper only	35	10
Radio only	20	7
50/50 split:		
Paper component	35	5
Radio component*	15	3

*Will also reach one in seven of those who read paper another 3 times.

Marketing communications programs that use more than one medium are usually more effective than one-medium campaigns. However, adding a second medium reduces the funds available for the first medium and the frequency of appearance in it. The added value of another medium has to be considered in comparison with the added value obtainable by greater frequency in one medium.

Getting Expert Help

Successful marketing communications are, as this chapter has shown, well planned, well budgeted, and well executed. At least some of the media options available to a health services provider require expert help to use effectively. Such expert help is more likely to be knowledgeable of, and experienced in, the detailed aspects of executing mass communications effectively. It is also much more likely to be knowledgeable about the full range of media options available, their respective reaches at different times, and how to assess multimedia versus one-medium strategies.

Enterprises that try a do-it-yourself approach to mass media advertising or to large-scale direct mail programs usually justify their action in one of four ways, each of which is very questionable (Fisk and Brown 1987).

It may appear that using expert help adds costs. However, ad agencies cover at least part of their cost in helping a client through media commissions. Many media pay an agency a percentage commission on ad space it reserves, but will not pay this commission directly to some organization doing its own advertising. Even if using an agency adds some cost, it should, if the agency is well chosen, also increase performance.

Some organizations claim that they have internal people who understand promotion. That may be true. Some very large advertisers have developed their own in-house agencies. Most health care providers, however, are much too small to replicate in-house the level of skills and knowledge of a good agency.

Some other organizations argue that they cannot afford an agency. However, in all probability, an organization that cannot afford an agency also cannot afford to use mass media advertising or large-scale direct mail campaigns. As already discussed, these media are only effective when used with reasonably high frequency, and that takes a sizeable budget. Within such a budget, the added cost of expert help is quite a minor item.

Still other organizations believe that no expert help is required in ad design and placement. As the preceding section showed, however, there is a great deal of expert judgment and knowledge involved in effective advertising. Also, many of the best advertising efforts come from the process of mutual dialogue and challenge of assumptions between a client and its agency. No agency can know a client's business as well as it does itself, but, equally, no client can be totally objective about how best to communicate that idea to the outside world.

These comments should not be taken to imply either that all agencies are created equal, or that any agency is better than none. Selecting the best agency with which to work is itself a very complicated decision. Among the issues that need to be considered are the agency's experience in health-related services, its willingness to avoid conflict of interest by not working for a competitor, whether it is more experienced in certain media than others and whether that "media bias" is a problem, and where the enterprise might rank among the agency's clients. (It may be wise to avoid being either among an agency's smaller accounts or by far its largest account.) Only after a candidate agency passes these tests is it even worth considering its creative ability and media analysis strengths (Fisk 1986).

Advertising in the mass media and large-scale direct mail programs are almost invariably best done by obtaining expert help outside the enterprise. Only in rare cases can an organiza-

tion match the skills and expertise of a good advertising agency, and even then it loses the extra level of critical dialogue between client and agency that lies behind most effective advertising.

Measuring and Monitoring the Results of Marketing Communication

There are three major reasons why experienced marketing communicators usually put a lot of effort into measuring and monitoring the effects of their efforts:

1. It enables them to correct mistaken judgments.

2. It allows them to reallocate resources from less effective to more effective forms of communication.

3. It provides a future basis for justifying their budgets, since they can show that they benefit the enterprise more than they cost it.

Two broad types of measurement and monitoring are most frequently conducted: *communication effect measurement* and *sales effect measurement* (Panda 1964). The first seeks to evaluate how widely and how well the message has reached the target audience. The second seeks to identify actual increased utilization and revenue attributable to the communications program.

The most common communications effects measured are (Fisk 1987):

1. Direct inquiries generated

2. Target audience recall of message

3. Before-and-after target audience attitudes

4. Increased loyalty of past customers.

The sales effects most commonly measured are:

1. Increased customers (e.g., patients) identifying themselves as ad respondents

2. Net revenue attributable to such extra sales.

Each of these approaches can take a large number of different forms, which are beyond the scope of this book to enumerate and explain. One illustrative example, however, is the so-called *triplex method*. Three samples of the target audience are called shortly after a campaign. The first is given the name and the type of enterprise (e.g., "You may have recently seen an ad by Plimstone, which is a hospital") and asked to summarize the central message of the communication. The second sample is given the type of organization and the central message (e.g., "You may have recently seen an ad from a hospital claiming it has good cardiac services") and asked to name the sponsor. The third is given the sponsor's name and the central message (e.g., "An organization called Plimstone has recently been advertising that it has good cardiac services") and asked to name the type of organization.

By averaging the percentages answering correctly and comparing the level of correct answer to each question, quote a lot of information can be obtained. A high score on the third question is to be expected, because many people can guess what type of organization might promote its cardiac care. The second question — naming the hospital — should be more difficult to answer, and the third question — summarizing the message — the most difficult of all. Thus, if 15% could recall the message, 18% the sponsor, and 20% the type of organization, the message has been well communicated, because the scores are closer than they should be purely randomly, and an average score of 17.5% is quite high. By contrast, if 15% could recall the message, and 20% the type of organization, but only 5% could name "Plimstone" correctly, the communication has failed to convey the sponsor's name effectively, even if the average 13.3% recall is reasonably good.

Effective marketing communicators usually put considerable effort into tracking the communications and sales effects of their campaigns, but in doing so they may use a wide variety of methods of monitoring and measurement.

As valuable as this process of monitoring and measurement is to the organization, there is no perfect method. Each approach has its limitations, but the better they are understood the more useful is the information that each yields.

Inquiries generated may not be a good measure of resultant sales or increased utilization. What matters more is how many of those inquiries are converted into actual service usage. This **conversion rate** can vary widely. Overreliance on inquiries as a measure of advertising performance can therefore actually lead to erroneous decisions of resource allocation. More dollars may be applied to types of communication that generate the greatest number of inquiries, rather than the greatest number of actual patients.

Recall — the ability of members of the target audience to remember the key point of a marketing communication — has been shown to be a poor measure of their subsequent use of the product or service (Ross, 1982). Thus, recall may be a useful measure of the success of an ad the purpose of which was solely image building, but a poor way of assessing the value of an ad intended to create actual service usage.

Before-and-after attitude surveys tend to take time to organize, execute, and analyze, and so they may not be much help in getting a rapid assessment of the effectiveness of a marketing communications campaign. In addition, some other factor may intervene to influence the result. If, for instance, the local media happens to give free publicity to a service while it is being advertised, can the specific role of the advertising be broken out? Some advanced research methods can do so, but using them adds further expense and perhaps delay to the survey. As with recall, changed attitudes among the target audience may not in any case correlate closely with changed level of use. For instance, Wendy's "Where's the Beef?" ads did seem to increase public doubts about the nutritional value of McDonald's fast food, but had no measurable impact on McDonald's sales.

Increased usage resulting from advertising may often not be easy to track. One hospital, for example, undertook some extensive advertising for its urology programs. The ads included mention of a referral service that readers could call for help in getting an appointment with a urologist. Through the 3 months of advertising, some 120 calls were received. The urologists had previously seen some 1,800 patients in a typical quarter. It therefore appeared that the ads had increased volume by about 6%. However, the urologists reported that their volume was up by 15% for that quarter. A survey was then conducted among that quarter's patients. It showed that 6% had seen the urologists after called the referral service, but another 9% reported that they had also consulted the doctors because of the ads. They had seen them and called the urologists directly. Since the urologists did not ask new patients how they heard of them, this additional 9% growth, attributable to the advertising, was almost missed in assessing its effectiveness.

The same difficulty can arise with *revenue generated*. If additional patients cannot all be tracked, the additional revenue cannot be calculated. Even if all the added patients can be identified, it is not always easy to quantify all the associated revenue. Consider the case of a hospital that advertised one of its neurology programs. The physicians interviewed each new patient during the next few months and identified some 100 who had come in response to the ads. They advised the hospital on the outpatient tests ordered on these patients and on the small number who were admitted. The hospital calculated that some $20,000 of marketing had produced $100,000 of added revenue, or $60,000 more net revenue after the cost of treating those patients had been taken into account. However, the neurologists pointed out that some 30 of these patients were found to have nonneurological problems and were referred to other physicians on the hospital's staff. The revenue identified did not allow for any use made of the hospital by these 30 patients. Tracking what had happened to those patients would, however, have meant pursuing some 20 different doctors, each of whom had received one or more of these 30 referrals. The hospital concluded that it had gathered enough data to show the profitability of this advertising and decided against mounting the extra research needed to pinpoint the value of these other 30 patients.

Each method of monitoring and measuring the results of marketing communications has its limitations. Even so, as long as these limitations are kept in mind, such tracking and qualification of ad effectiveness is very worthwhile.

References

Akaah, I., and Becherer. 1983. Integrating a consumer orientation into the planning of HMO programs. *Journal of Health Care Marketing* 3(2):9-18.

Bettman, J. 1979. *An information processing theory of consumer choice*. Reading, Mass.: Addison-Wesley.

Bradley, M., T. Fisk, and H. Owens. 1987. The finance/marketing interface in hospitals. *Health Care Strategic Management* 5(1):11-22.

Britton, B., B. Meyer, M. Hodge, and S. Glynn. 1980. Effects of the organization of text and memory. *Journal of Advertising Research* (July).

Caples, J. 1974. *Tested advertising methods*. Englewood Cliffs, N.J.: Prentice Hall.

Caples, J. 1983. *How to make your advertising make money*. Englewood Cliffs, N.J.: Prentice Hall.

Cermak, L., and F. Craik. 1979. *Levels of processing in human memory.* Hillsdale, N.Y.: Lawrence Erlbaum Associates.

Chase, C., and K. Barasch. 1977. *Marketing problem solver.* Radnor, Penn.: Chilton Books.

Cole, C., and M. Houston. 1987. Encoding and media effects on consumer learning deficiencies in the elderly. *Journal of Market Research* (February):55-63.

Cole, M., and B. Means. 1981. *A study of how people think.* Cambridge, Mass.: Harvard University Press.

Dean, J. 1951. *Managerial economics,* pp. 363-375. Englewood Cliffs, N.J.: Prentice Hall.

DeVito, J. 1971. *Communication: Concept and processes.* Englewood Cliffs, N.J.: Prentice Hall.

Dobrow, L. 1984. *When advertising tried harder.* New York: Friendly Press.

Durgee, J., and R. Stuart. 1987. Advertising symbols and brand names that best represent product meanings. *Journal of Consumer Marketing* 4(3):15-24.

Fisk, T. 1986. *Advertising health services: What works, what fails.* Chicago: Pluribus Press.

Fisk, T. 1987. Eight sure ways to raise your advertising pay-off. In *Proceedings of the 7th Annual Health Care Marketing Symposium.* Chicago: Teach'Em Books.

Fisk, T., and C. Brown. 1984. Hospital advertising: Rules for success. *Laubach and Rand Marketing Report* (March):63-65.

Fisk, T., and C. Brown. 1987. *Practice marketing: An introduction for radiologists.* Reston, Va.: American College of Radiology.

Health Care Advertising Review 1986. 2:5.

Heller, R. 1987. *The supermarketers.* New York: Macmillan.

Holbrook, M., and J. O'Shaughnessy. 1984. Emotion in advertising. *Psychology and Marketing* 1(2):45-61.

Hospital Product Line Report. 1987. Successful rehab program leads to formal product-line management. *Hospital Product Line Report* 2(2):1-4.

Hovland, C., and W. Mandell. 1953. An experimental comparison of conclusion-drawing by the communicator and the audience. *Journal of Abnormal and Social Psychology* 47:581-588.

Lavidge, R., and G. Steiner. 1961. A model for predictive measurement of advertising effectiveness. *Journal of Marketing* (October):59-62.

Lewin, K. 1947. Group decisions and social change. In *Readings in social psychology.* eds. T. Newcomb and E. Haltry. New York: Holt Press.

MacLachlan, J. 1984. Making a message memorable and persuasive. *Journal of Advertising Research* 23(6):51-59.

McGraner, R. 1987. Consumer research in radiology: Focus on physician relations. *Radiology Management* 9(1).

Mizerski, R., and J. White. 1986. Understanding and using emotions in advertising. *Journal of Consumer Marketing* 3(4):57-69.

Modern Healthcare. 1987. Treatment guarantees to proliferate despite claims that ads are misleading. *Modern Healthcare* (July 17)

Moore, J., and R. Reardon. 1987. Source magnification: The role of multiple sources in the processing of advertising appeals. *Journal of Market Research* (November):412-417.

Ogilvy, D. 1985. *Ogilvy on advertising.* New York: Random House.

Panda, K. 1964. *The measurement of cumulative advertising effect.* Englewood Cliffs, N.J.: Prentice Hall.

Plummer, J., and R. Holman. 1981. *Communication to the heart and/or the mind.* Chicago: American Psychological Association.

Reibstein, D. 1985. *Marketing: Concepts, strategies and decisions.* Englewood Cliffs, N.J.: Prentice Hall.

Ries, A., and J. Trout. 1981. *Positioning: The battle for your mind.* New York: McGraw-Hill.

Robertson, T., and L. Vortzel. 1977. Consumer behavior and health care change: The role of mass media. In *Advances in consumer research, Vol. 4.* Ann Arbor, Mich.: Association for Consumer Research.

Ross, H. 1982. Recall vs persuasion: An answer. *Journal of Advertising Research* 22(1):13-16.

Rubright, R., and D. MacDonald. 1981. *Marketing health and human services,* pp. 188-196. Rockville, Md.: Aspen Publications.

Schultz, D., D. Martin, and W. Brown. 1984. *Strategic advertising campaigns.* Chicago: Crain Books.

Shapiro, I., and R. Majewski. 1983. Should dentists advertise? *Journal of Advertising Research* 23(3):33-37.

Simon, J. 1965. Are there economies of scale in advertising? *Journal of Advertising Research* (June):15-20.

Stone, R. 1987. *Successful direct marketing methods*. 3d ed. Lincolnwood, Ill.: Crain Books.

Surmanek, J. 1980. *Media planning*. Chicago: Crain Books.

Vladimir, A., and D. Vladimir. 1984. *Fundamentals of advertising*. Chicago: Crain Books.

Wright, J., W. Winter, and S. Zeyler. 1982. *Advertising*, pp. 134-140. New York: McGraw Hill.

Review Questions

1. "Sometimes it makes sense in marketing communication to prioritize building the provider's image. Sometimes it makes sense to prioritize a specific service promotion." Comment.

2. What are reach and frequency, and why are they important considerations in marketing communication?

3. What are the five common approaches to deciding how much to budget for marketing communication?

4. In marketing communications, does a picture tell a thousand words?

5. Select some marketing letter that you have personally received recently, and review how closely it follows the recommendations in this chapter both for sequencing and for wording letters.

6. List the different ways in which the results of marketing communication can be monitored and measured.

Chapter 12

Reinforcing Marketing Communications

Reinforcing Advertising With Publicity

Free coverage of services by the mass media cannot be relied on as a means of creating increased use by customers. Any effort to interest the media in carrying a story about a service is uncertain in its results. The media may or may not decide that the story is worthwhile. They may or may not get distracted by other news breaking that day that they judge more important. Even if the media do report on a service, that coverage is likely to be nonrecurrent. They are unlikely to report on the same service frequently and consistently. Yet marketing communications, as already discussed, depend for their success on frequency. Effective marketing needs message repetition, yet by definition, "news" is a story that is original.

Even when the media do cover a health service, a good journalist usually looks beyond the one news release or interview. If a story seems to merit significant coverage, he or she will often research for other background. One common approach to such background research is to call competitive services for comment. The outcome, therefore, is often a report that promotes rivals as least as much as the enterprise that originated the story idea (Fisk 1986).

There are well-documented cases of the media "adopting" a product or service and giving it repetitive publicity support through time. The Trivial Pursuits game and Cabbage Patch Kids dolls were both "hyped" by the media for a considerable period, to such an extent that the maker could dispense with or minimize paid advertising. There are also a very few documented cases of this type relating to health services. One Houston journalist personally enrolled in a local fitness center and reported on his personal progress regularly through the following 12 months. One Philadelphia journalist followed a medical student with periodic stories on his 4 years at a prominent local university hospital. These examples, both in health care and in other fields, are, however, the very rare exceptions. To base the marketing strategy for any health service on the million-to-one chance of such major and sustained media coverage is not a sound approach.

> *The mass media report news, as they see it. Only in a few exceptional circumstances has such free publicity for a product or service been sustained with enough frequency to substitute for paid marketing communications. To depend on free publicity to generate customers is, thus, not a viable marketing communications strategy. However, seeking media coverage can be a useful adjunct to a marketing communications strategy.*

There are almost as many techniques to be mastered in managing media relations effectively as in managing successful marketing communications. A full explanation of these techniques lies beyond the scope of this book, and there are some excellent texts and manuals available (e.g., Adam, 1975; Stephenson 1976; Lesly 1980). However, several broad principles are worth bearing in mind:

1. An enterprise's relations with the media are best based on the basic marketing concept of creating an exchange (Kotler 1973). The enterprise can benefit from media coverage. The media, for their part, need news. They have an above-average need for health news, in fact, because health is one topic that commands high reader, listener, and viewer interest (Caples 1983). The media also need facts upon which to expand a story idea they already have developed (Banks 1987). As in other marketing activities, the enterprise that seeks to satisfy the needs of the media, as "customers" for news and facts, is most likely to satisfy its own need for media coverage.

2. Most opportunities that an enterprise has to secure free publicity are reactive rather than proactive. A journalist picks up a lead on a story from some other source and calls for facts and comment. An enterprise that makes itself available for such comment, and that responds well

when approached, will usually find it easier to place its own proactive news.

3. If a health provider sees that the media are already covering a health issue because of some national event (e.g., a Presidential illness), a rapid offer of local comment may arouse media interest (Peters and Tseng 1983).

4. The media seek out credible sources of comment and shun news from sources lacking such credibility. Consequently, an honest relationship with the media usually pays off. That does not necessarily mean being completely open with all information, but it does mean avoiding misleading comment. Johnson & Johnson's handling of the Tylenol scare is remembered with hindsight as an exemplary lesson in facing up to a problem openly. However, in the early days of the crisis, the company issued a statement that cyanide was "not used in the manufacture of Tylenol," only to have an employee leak shortly afterward that cyanide was used in testing Tylenol (Snyder 1983). This apparent lack of complete disclosure made the company's subsequent public relations challenge greater than it otherwise might have been. It was only after this initial false start that the organization's senior management took effective control the issue and did such an effective job at resolving it.

The best approach to media relations is a "marketing approach," trying, as far as is reasonable, to meet the media's needs for health news and facts. The enterprise that builds a reputation for credibility and responsiveness to media needs will usually find it easier to interest the media in its own stories, as long as they are really newsworthy.

One special form of media coverage that merits specific comment is the *public service announcement*. Some media set aside significant time for community announcements, including those of not-for-profit health care providers. It must be recognized, however, that competition among local community agencies for such free coverage is fierce, and most media want to remain impartial. They may well, therefore, ration the coverage given to any one organization to a fairly low frequency. In addition, the Federal Communications Commission (FCC) has, in recent years, eased the requirement that radio and TV stations devote a minimum amount of prime time to public service announcements. As a result, even when a not-for-profit health provider's announcements are aired, they may be at times when the listening or viewing audience is quite small. Public service announcements may be a helpful adjunct to other types of marketing communications, but they cannot be relied upon to achieve enough reach or frequency to have major impact.

Sales Promotion Efforts

Sales promotion consists of those marketing communication activities that are not strictly advertising, or publicity, or personal selling (Reibstein 1985). In a commercial context, sales promotion often takes two forms: *Consumer promotions* are aimed at the final customer; they include such things as free samples, price discounts, contests, sweepstakes, special premiums (e.g., "two-for-one" offers or free gifts with purchase), and coupons. *Trade promotions* are aimed at distributors, dealers, and storekeepers and may include discounts, free gifts, or cooperative advertising, whereby the manufacturer offers to share the costs of a retailer's own advertising as long as it features the manufacturer's products.

Many sales promotion ideas are proper and applicable to health services, while some others may raise ethical questions. One general rule to follow in considering all such activities is to give careful thought to the "psychology" of the intended recipient.

As an example, a hospital had a tradition of giving its medical staff members some token gift during the annual holiday season to thank them for their support over the past year. A great deal of effort each year went into choosing a suitable gift. However, the hospital had been disappointed to observe that its past choices had not remained long in evidence. Few of the calendars sent one year made it to the doctors' office walls. Few of the pen sets sent another year were visible in the doctors' hands at meetings or on their office desks. The hospital decided the following year, for the first time, to ask a few doctors for ideas of gifts that might be more appreciated. They replied that they were always oversupplied with calendars, pens, and the like, but, like other people, they never had enough sweaters to wear in the winter or T-shirts in the summer.

Two of the most common consumer promotions undertaken by health providers are health education programs and wellness programs. Two of the most common trade promotions undertaken by health providers are supplying printed materials to doctors' offices and seeking contractual arrangements with HMOs.

Public Law 94-317, the Health Promotion Act of 1976, encourages not-for-profit organizations to engage in programs to inform people about health, health protection and maintenance, and being more efficient users of health services. It is thus possible to undertake a fair amount of sales promotion through the vehicle of *public health education* (Dockery 1981).

For example, one hospital reported attendances of between 500 and 600 women at each of several educational sessions organized to promote its women's health center (Health Care Competition Week 1987). As long as there is a serious public health education content to such events, they appear to fall within the definition of the Health Promotion Act. It is probably important, however, to ensure that such a significant educational element is present. Without it, some third-party payers might have grounds to exclude the costs of such efforts from reimbursement for services.

The case cited above may also be misleading. A turnout of 500 people is exceptional for such events, unless they receive very heavy advance publicity and happen to address topics of high current interest among the target audience. It is also an open question how many attendees at such events are eventually converted into future patients. Consequently, the costs and benefits of such efforts should be measured and monitored as closely as those of other forms of promotion. Some level of loss may be supportable to underwrite the real health education role of such activities. However, there may be many health providers who maintain such programs at a loss well in excess of what they would otherwise devote to health education, out of an unproven belief that their efforts have an additional marketing value, which they may not.

The law encourages health providers to engage in public health education programs. Some such programs may also have incidental marketing value also, by introducing potential customers to a health service. That marketing value should, however, be as carefully measured and monitored as that of other types of marketing communication.

There is a fine distinction between public health education and *wellness programs*. Usually attendees at the former are not charged, while those who enroll in wellness programs are expected to pay. Often, therefore, the sponsoring health enterprise does not expect public health programs to break even. It is willing to invest a certain sum in these educational activities in the belief that the result will be increased future use of its services. By contrast, many organizations that sponsor wellness programs do so in the belief that they can break even or show a profit. Many hospitals have launched such wellness programs for sale to local companies, in the hope that they will eventually yield a profit, which can be used to subsidize other hospital activities.

There are, as yet, few if any well-documented cases of wellness programs that are truly profitable in their own right. Consider the case of a downtown hospital (Health Care Advisory Board 1987a) that in 1984 started a wellness program selling lunchtime health seminars to neighboring companies. The program started with four employees, start-up costs of $500,000 for marketing and for educational materials, and an annual budget of $180,000. It was projected that it would at least break even in its first year and recover its start-up costs within a few years. By the end of 1986, however, it had averaged only $70,000 in annual revenue. Accumulated losses now, therefore, exceeded $800,000. The hospital could not identify any positive impact that the program had on use of its other services.

There are other examples of wellness program sponsors who have started more modestly than this one, and probably have covered their more reasonable costs by increased utilization of their hospital services, but the above case illustrates an important point about such programs. The sponsoring organization must define for itself the purpose and goals of the program. Is it intended as a public health education initiative, with no direct return? Is it intended as a sales promotion activity, on which, like other forms of marketing, a certain expense will be allowed as long as it is more than matched by generated increases in service utilization? Is the program intended as a new service venture that is expected to show a profit within an acceptable period of time?

One program may, of course, be deliberately designed to achieve more than one of these three purposes, but it is important that its objectives be properly stated ahead of time. The downtown hospital's wellness program clearly failed as a new service venture. Since no resultant increase in hospital utilization could be identified, it also failed as a sales promotion program. If it was intended primarily as a public health education initiative, it should have been started with much less resources and not expected to generate any revenue.

It is important to distinguish programs primarily designed for public health education from those primarily designed as sales promotion, and from those expected to succeed as new ventures in their own right. Even if one initiative combines more than one of these objectives, their relative importance needs to be defined and allowed for in their revenue and expense projections.

Mailing of materials intended to serve as office aids for referral sources can serve as a valuable type of trade promotion. However, to serve their purpose, such aids must be designed and distributed with the intended user firmly in mind. Four important considerations, for instance, are (Fisk and Brown 1987):

1. Design the material to save referrers and their staffs time, not to add work.

2. Explain how the material can best be used to make their work easier.

3. Every office suffers from paper clutter, so health providers distributing such material may well be advised to distribute a holder, special file, or organizer, as well.

4. The distributor must also think out how the supply will be restocked once the referrer has used it up.

Health service providers seeking contracts with HMOs do so to gain access to patients whom those plans insure. Most HMOs expect a discount off the provider's standard fees in return for this volume. (A few plans only seek discounts from hospitals and are willing to pay normal fees to other health providers, but they are the exception.)

Even though the basis of contracting with HMOs is, therefore, a volume discount, these plans differ widely in their readiness to guarantee any given volume. Most will not provide any guarantee. All they offer any provider is a "fair share" of whatever health services are needed by those whom they succeed in enrolling. The major issues that confront the provider in seeking such a contract, in the absence of firm volume guarantees, are how successful the plan may be in its own marketing, how many people it may thus insure, and how many competitive providers the HMO may sign up and among whom its patients will be shared. HMOs vary widely in their market appeal, potential enrollment, and policy on having a large or small panel of providers. Consequently, not all HMOs are equally attractive contractual partners for any one health providers. The provider must investigate each plan's viability and policies to determine which are most worthwhile (Fisk and Somers 1987). Many health providers have entered into HMO contracts that yielded no worthwhile volume. Others have entered into contracts with HMOs that produced volume, but at too low a negotiated price. The most astute providers have chosen to contract with HMOs selectively, focusing on those with strong potential and acceptable policies.

National HMO was the first HMO to enter the market in the city where Lincoln University Hospital is located. Through several years, without a contract with Lincoln, National HMO grew until it was insuring 1 person in every 20 in the area. A second HMO, Liberty Health Plan, then started up, and within a year had 1% of the population enrolled. Lincoln's administration decided that the time had come to take the growth of HMOs seriously. It approached National HMO, as by far the larger of the two plans.

Twelve months and many meetings later, Lincoln was still a long way from concluding any agreement with National HMO. Why? National HMO marketed itself by offering two main appeals: It had lots of hospitals in the area under contract, to provide broad geographical coverage, and it provided a wide range of supplementary benefits to its members by requiring large discounts from hospitals and using the savings to pay for these extra features. They included free membership in Weight Watchers, prescription drug coverage, free membership in approved health clubs, and coverage for psychiatric services, all benefits not available under most traditional health insurance options in the area.

Lincoln assumed, as the area's only university hospital, that National HMO would see it as a prestigious addition to its list of hospitals, that the plan needed it for tertiary services not available at other hospitals, and that the plan would be willing to accept a smaller discount from Lincoln than from its other participating hospitals. None of these three assumptions were valid. National HMO was more concerned, as a matter of policy, with the geographic spread of its contracting hospitals than with subtle distinctions in their quality. As it mainly enrolled young families, its need for tertiary services not available at other area hospitals was very limited indeed. As another matter of policy, it was not prepared to accept lesser discounts from some hospitals than others. It told Lincoln that it would rather send the very few patients each year needing specialized services out of town to the Mayo Clinic at full charges, than potentially upset its existing hospitals by offering a better deal to Lincoln.

Liberty Health Plan then called the administrator at the university hospital. It had a very different policy from National HMO. It emphasized quality in its marketing and restricted itself to a few hospitals that had the best local reputations. It would like to add Lincoln as its "flagship hospital." It offered Lincoln a better price than National HMO and agreed to direct patients with a defined schedule of diagnoses exclusively to the university hospital. Even though it had only one-fifth as many members as National HMO, because of these policy differences, it anticipated referring twice as many patients a year to it as the rival plan would with its different business philosophy. This case illustrates that, for any one health provider, the prospects of reaching a mutually satisfactory sales promotion agreement differ widely with the policies of the various payers with which it might deal.

Sales promotion activities can be very effective means of maintaining or increasing the utilization of services, but they can also represent wasted effort and expense. The potential benefits of any such activity have to be realistically identified and weighed against the cost involved. Many U.S. enterprises rely on sound sales promotion as the key to their success. Others, however, avoid such activities and concentrate on other marketing methods.

Personal Selling as Marketing Communications

Despite the visibility of advertising in our society, most products and services are in fact sold in person. Personal selling can take three major forms:

1. *Cold canvassing*, or approaching potential customers in person who may not have been exposed to any other marketing communication from the enterprise

2. *Prospecting*, or using the telephone or some other method to prequalify potential customers as worth a personal visit (someone who is so identified is called a *hot lead*, to distinguish this approach from a cold canvass)

3. *Inquiry handling*, or processing telephone or mail responses to advertising.

The approaches recommended by experts in personal selling vary among these three situations.

With *cold canvassing*, the objective is actually to close a sale. To do so depends, as with all marketing processes, on creating an exchange of values — identifying with potential customers how a service meets some need of importance to them. The most commonly suggested way of structuring such discussions is in five steps: approach or introduction, presentation, handling objections, closing, and subsequent follow-up (Hanan 1987).

For the presentation step, it is advisable to follow four substeps, often referred to by the acronym *AIDA*: awareness, interest, demonstration, and action (Strong 1925). The first task in any presentation is briefly to create awareness of the service being offered. The second task is to arouse the potential customer's interest in the service. The third task is to demonstrate how the service meets one, or preferably more than one, of the customer's needs. The fourth task is to get the customer to take action, by, for instance, making a referral.

It will be noted that the AIDA model is similar to the *hierarchy-of-effects model* used in designing advertising, with the exception that, in a sales presentation, the potential customer's attention has already been captured prior to the presentation itself (in the initial approach). It will also be noted, however, that the presentation is just one step in the sales process. It is preceded by an approach, and followed by handling objections, closure, and follow-up. Personal selling, therefore, allows for a more extended marketing communications process than does advertising, because it permits the inviting and handling of questions and objections, as well as arranging actual use of the service.

One frequent error of inexperienced salespersons is their failure to take advantage of these other opportunities present in a face-to-face encounter. They may prepare, practice, and deliver a very good presentation, but the real skill of a good salesperson lies in knowing how to stimulate and manage the subsequent dialogue with the potential customer and how to close the deal.

An example is provided by a hospital that decided to set up a small sales team to go out and sell wellness programs to local companies. They persuaded two nurses to take on this new assignment. Both of the nurses knew the hospital well and were experienced at making well-structured and articulate presentations. They worked together to script the presentation that each would use in calling on local companies. They also developed a flip chart, to help illustrate their main points, and a "leave behind" summary. Both were well received on their visits, but 6 months later sales of wellness programs had not grown. What had gone wrong?

The nurses had defined personal selling as making a presentation and leaving behind a reminder for the potential customer to follow up. They had not realized that a good salesperson goes the two further steps of engaging the potential client in a structured dialogue and trying to close with a definite commitment. The experienced salesperson whose only "close" is to leave behind some reminder material sees that sales encounter as a probable failure, not as a success. Success is leaving the meeting with a signed order.

Prospecting, or contacting prospective customers by phone or other means to see if they are worth a more lengthy personal encounter, also often employs the AIDA model, but in a much more abbreviated form. The goal of prospecting is not to make a sale, but only to identify hot leads. The success of prospecting relies, therefore, upon setting a time limit to the initial conversation with a potential customer. If the person approached does not fairly rapidly seem really interested, it is usually far more productive to break off the conversation quickly and politely, and to approach another prospect. Effective prospecting is therefore an exercise in both salespersonship and time management. Time may be better invested in an approach to another possible customer than in repetitive attempts to win round a skeptical one (Fisk and Brown 1987).

Handling inquiries requires a modified approach. The respondent would not be calling or writing if not at least motivated by some prior marketing communication to make this effort. The first task in inquiry handling is therefore to discover, as rapidly as possible, how firmly interested the prospect may be. Is he or she calling for further information, or is he or she now ready to place an order or schedule an appointment?

The most efficient inquiry handling processes have several different offers predefined for respondents with varying levels of commitment. They may have further written information to mail to someone whose interest seems uncertain, an offer to talk directly with someone more senior (e.g., a director of a clinical program) if the respondent seems almost but not quite ready to make an appointment, or an on-line ability to make an appointment for the caller who is ready to do so. By comparison, the least efficient inquiry handling systems may just have one response available to callers. They may not even be able to handle the inquirer who is ready to make a purchase.

However effective other marketing communications may be in creating interest in a service, actual use of services usually depends, in the final analysis, on a well-managed process of personal selling.

Customer Service: "Follow-Up" Marketing Communications

The task of marketing communication should not stop with making the sale. In the most successful enterprises it continues through and after the actual delivery of service. It does so because, as noted earlier, transformational marketing—converting users into loyal customers—has two major advantages: It is less expensive to convert an established customer into a repeat customer than to find new customers, and their word-of-mouth marketing testimonials are the lowest cost but most effective of all marketing communications.

There are four critical areas of customer service:

1. *Guest relations* during a customer's service encounter

2. *Handling complaints* both during and after service

3. *Inviting feedback* both during and after service

4. *Follow-up communication* after service.

Guest relations focus on the treatment of the customer during service encounters as a "guest" of the enterprise as well as a consumer of its service. Sixty-one percent of all U.S. enterprises now formally train all their employees—not just some of them—in guest relations, or "customer relations," techniques; 36% of all U.S. companies maintain formal and ongoing programs in these areas (American Management Association 1987). These formal programs usually have four important elements:

1. Internal promotion of a formal set of rules or behaviors expected of all employees

2. Formal training in interpersonal skills needed to implement those behaviors

3. Formal translation of those rules into specific departmental goals and/or individual job requirements

4. Formal and well-publicized systems to identify and reward exemplary performance by employees in these job requirements.

The Scandinavian airline SAS employed 27,000 people worldwide, and was losing $8 million a year, when Jan Carlzon took over as its president. He introduced a program requiring every employee, including professional pilots, to undergo 2 days' training in "the service management concept." The program explained that there were some 50,000 interactions between SAS employees and the public daily, each of which was "a moment of truth," and for each of which service expectations could be defined. Two years later, SAS recorded a $71 million profit. Little else changed inside the company in that period other than its guest relations program. In fact, its competitive environment worsened during that period, with more excess capacity and price competition, making SAS's transition even more remarkable.

One hospital introduced a program similar to SAS's but had only limited success (Hafer and Joiner 1984). In comparison with SAS, its program had two shortcomings: It required the nurses to pay more attention to nonclinical aspects of their patients' needs just at a time when nursing morale in the hospital was low. The nurses felt that they were not being given sufficient professional recognition. Second, the hospital's physicians were exempt from the program, whereas Jan Carlzon deliberately included his pilots. (If doctors' behavior seems at times difficult to modify, consider the challenge represented by airline pilots. They see themselves as having not just one life in their hands at a time, but several hundred!) The exclusion of doctors from the program became a rallying point for the nurses and other employees, and an excuse for them to ignore it too.

A West Coast hospital also introduced its own guest relations program, but one much closer to the SAS example in scope and thoroughness (Health Care Advisory Board 1987b). Doctors were included in the program; all employees received 3 hours mandatory training; all 1,500 job descriptions were rewritten to include specific guest relations requirements; and a formal recognition program was introduced with cash bonuses and free parking for those selected as exemplary role models. The hospital even developed a "guest relations quotient test" to screen all new job applicants for their likelihood of good performance in this area. It consisted of showing them 10 situations on videotape and asking how they would personally handle each of them. The results of these rigorous efforts included reduced employee turnover, improved patient satisfaction, and a significant reduction in malpractice litigation.

> *Formalized guest relations programs are now becoming a common feature of service organizations, including those in health care. However, there seem to be important differences between those that succeed and those that fail to stimulate increased utilization. The successful programs are rigorous, include all associated professionals and other personnel, are ongoing, and are led from the top down.*

Successful service organizations also take the handling of complaints very seriously, for two main reasons:

1. They recognize that consumer complaints can be one useful source of information on quality control problems.

2. They recognize that complainants can still be transformed into loyal future customers if handled properly.

Quality problems among doctors, nurses, and other health professionals are traditionally managed by peer review processes. The most common sources from which they learn about possible quality problems are case review, internal or external utilization review, and accreditation and inspection visits. Patient complaints can be a valuable additional source of warning of possible quality control issues. They may highlight problems overlooked by these other review mechanisms or may suggest their presence before these other mechanisms reveal them.

Patient complaints may also draw attention to quality issues that "fall between the cracks" between various professional responsibilities. For example, a hospital noticed that it was getting complaints from inpatients about long delays in its ancillary service areas while waiting to be transported back to the nursing units. An investigation showed that most complaints were coming from patients with intravenous pumps and other ancillary equipment. Two people were required to move such patients back to their nursing floors: one to push the wheelchair or stretcher, and a second to manage the IV pole or other equipment. Because the second person was usually a nurse from the patients' units, with many other responsibilities to attend to, long delays often arose before both a patient escort and a nurse were simultaneously available.

In response, the hospital developed, with help from an outside equipment vendor, a system of clamps and supports that enable almost any conceivable piece of equipment to be attached to a wheelchair or stretcher for transportation. As a result, a patient escort now handles such movements unaided. Quality care has been improved in three ways: Patients with the types of problems necessitating IV lines, oxygen, or other equipment are away for shorter periods from the nursing units best able to care for them, nurses are no longer taken away from those units to aid in transport, and the less cumbersome "rolling stock" lowers the risk of accidents during transportation. The job satisfaction of patient escorts has also been improved by placing more responsibility in their hands.

Evidence exists that complaining customers can still be transformed into loyal future users of a service. A major federally sponsored consumer study (TARP 1986) found that 70% of consumers who had bought relatively low-cost items that they later found defective, and whose complaints had been well handled, reported that they would repurchase the product in the future. Even for very high priced products, 50% of well-handled complainants said they would buy the product again. In contrast, very few of those whose complaints had been poorly handled, and very few of those who bought a defective product, but did not bother to complain at all, would repurchase the product.

Faced with such evidence, many successful companies now treat customer complaints very seriously (American Management Association 1987). Forty-seven percent of enterprises have formal customer affairs departments, and many others, while lacking a distinct unit, assign responsibility for complaint management formally to some internal department. Seventy-three percent of companies keep regular counts of complaints and analyze them into their major categories; 66% of companies compile regular reports summarizing this information; and in 61% the circulation of these reports includes the top executive. Sixty-five percent of companies also measure and review how long it takes them to respond to complaints.

The administrators of one East Coast hospital, after reading these reports of modern corporate practice, decided to upgrade their own complaints handling process. The CEO issued a set of instructions to all the hospital's managers. Any complaint received by mail or phone was to be directed to the senior patient representative. That office was to acknowledge receipt of the complaint to the patient, by phone or postcard, within 2 working days. A note of the complaint would be sent to each department head and/or physician involved. They were each required to provide the patient representative with a draft reply within 5 working days. They were also required to provide a copy of their draft replies to their own superior, or, in the case of physicians, their chairman. He or she, in turn, was expected to give them feedback on inadequate responses. All such drafts would go in the manager's or physician's personal file and be formally reviewed as part of their subsequent annual performance appraisal or renewal of privileges. A quarterly statistical summary would go to the CEO, who would share it with the hospital's trustees.

Successful service organizations tend to take customer complaints very seriously, and to have formal systems to ensure rapid and appropriate response and to monitor and report on trends.

For every customer who complains, there are likely to be several more who have causes of dissatisfaction but do not pass them on. For this reason, some organizations go beyond systematic complaints management. They install various mechanisms to actively solicit customer feedback. They do so because they realize that complaints may not surface, and that it is easy for their managers and professional employees to overlook or get out of touch with issues that are irksome to their customers. One study, for instance, surveyed administrators, physicians, and patients at one hospital (Scammon and Kennard 1983) and found that neither the administrators nor the physicians had even a modestly accurate idea of how patients felt about their hospital experiences.

A contrasting example is that of the Benetton company begun in 1960 by a brother and sister in Treviso, Italy. She had designs for 18 sweaters. He had some business acumen and exactly $55. Benetton has since grown into an enterprise with 4,000 stores in 60 countries, and 11 factories in 5 countries, making casual clothing in 400 different styles and 500 colors. The Benettons attribute their success to one basic business practice. From the start they have demanded rapid feedback from each store on which designs customers liked and which were not selling. Every month they make strategic decisions, based on this information, to expand production of some items, reduce output of others, increase shipment of certain items to certain markets, and so on. In other words, they attribute their growth solely to automated and rapid feedback on customer preferences.

The Benettons illustrate one method of obtaining feedback: quick monitoring of what sells. Other methods commonly employed are calls to customers to inquire about their satisfaction, and formal customer surveys (Birsner and Balsley 1987). Another technique increasingly being employed is for senior managers just to walk about engaging in "naive listening" to customers during their service encounters (Peters and Waterman 1983).

Although some health services providers now employ these techniques, the majority do not. According to one survey, for instance, fewer than 1% of hospitals have a really effective patient satisfaction survey system in regular use (Palm 1987).

Many organizations now reach beyond just handling complaints into soliciting feedback from their customers, by talking to them or formally surveying them during or after a service encounter.

The fourth ingredient of comprehensive customer service is follow-up after the service encounter. Consider the following example: Sales of Saab autos have grown so rapidly in the United States because Saab's own marketing has been reinforced by positive word-of-mouth testimonials by existing Saab owners talking to their friends. The loyalty of many Saab owners to their car is, of course, partly a result of the product itself. However, it is also reinforced by Saab's extensive and systematic follow-up with its customers. Saab's dealers are required to brief customers at the time of sale on the fact that they will receive several follow-up calls from the dealer, and later from Saab itself. These calls from Saab include checking that the dealer performed all the steps prescribed by the company, and questioning buyers about their satisfaction. Yet other requirements are imposed by Saab on approved service centers. The company direct mails information about new models to customers in the knowledge that people change autos every several years and that the best prospect to buy a Saab is an existing, satisfied Saab owner.

The same concepts of follow-up customer relations can also be applied by health care providers (Fisk and Brown 1987). Indeed, health providers who do a good job at customer relations during the service encounter, but make no attempt at follow-up, may destroy much of the goodwill that they have created. The patient may feel "abandoned" and question the sincerity of the attentiveness he or she received at the hospital if there is no subsequent effort to check up on their progress.

One reason why so many apparently satisfied customers do not remain loyal to a service provider may well be the lack of any follow-up effort to stay in touch, invite their comments, and check into their progress. Those organizations that receive the most word-of-mouth marketing support from their past customers are often those that remain in contact with them through continuing marketing communications.

Summary

Effective marketing communications with potential customers are essential before, during, and after their service encounters. Marketing communications are inherently difficult because of the many barriers and impediments that exist between a supplier of a service and his or her potential customers.

Effective marketing communications, as Chapters 10, 11, and 12 have shown, are:

1. Carefully planned, with an awareness of the various technical and psychological challenges with which they must contend

2. Adequately budgeted, because persuasive communication with a target audience requires both reach and frequency

3. Well implemented

4. In the area of mass media communication, executed with expert help

5. Monitored and measured

6. Supported where possible by free publicity

7. Reinforced often by sales promotion methods

8. Backed by sound personal selling

9. Concluded with good customer service.

References

Adams, A. 1975. *Handbook of practical public relations.* New York: Crowell Books.

American Management Association. 1987. *Close to the customer.* New York: American Management Association.

Banks, L. 1987. Why the media look less fearsome. *Fortune* (August 17)

Birsner, E., and R. Balsley. 1987. *How to improve customer service.* New York: American Management Association.

Caples, J. 1983. *How to make your advertising make money.* Englewood Cliffs, N.J.: Prentice Hall.

Dockery, V. 1981. Health education as a marketing element. In *Marketing for hospitals in hard times.* ed. L. Block, pp. 137-148. Chicago: Teach'Em Books.

Fisk, T. 1986. *Advertising health services: What works, what fails.* Chicago: Pluribus Press.

Fisk, T., and C. Brown. 1987. *Practice marketing: An introduction for radiologists.* Reston, Va.: American College of Radiology.

Fisk, T., and E. Somers. 1987. HMOs: A negotiating strategy for university hospitals. *Journal of Health Care Marketing* 7(4):60-70.

Hafer, J., and C. Joiner. 1984. Nurses as image emissaries. *Journal of Health Care Marketing* 4(1):25-35.

Hanan, M. 1987. *Consultative selling.* New York: American Management Association.

Health Care Advisory Board. 1987a. *Hospital services targeted at the daytime population of downtown areas.* Washington, D.C.: Health Care Advisory Board.

Health Care Advisory Board. 1987b. *Profiles of guest relations programs.* Washington, D.C.: Health Care Advisory Board.

Healthcare Competition Week. 1987. Product line marketing: Does it work? *Healthcare Competition Week* (August 24).

Kotler, P. 1972. *Marketing management*. Englewood Cliffs, N.J.: Prentice Hall.

Lesly, P. 1980. *Public relations handbook*. Englewood Cliffs, N.J.: Prentice Hall.

Palm, K. 1987. Hospitals should devote more time, money to marketing before gauging results. *Modern Healthcare* (November 6).

Panda, K. 1964. *The measurement of cumulative advertising effect*. Englewood Cliffs, N.J.: Prentice Hall.

Peters, J., and S. Tseng. 1983. *Managing strategic change in hospitals: Ten success stories*. Chicago: American Hospital Association.

Peters, T., and J. Waterman. 1983. *In search of excellence*. New York: Warner Books.

Reibstein, D. 1985. *Marketing: Concepts, strategies and decisions*. Englewood Cliffs, N.J.: Prentice Hall.

Snyder, L. 1983. An anniversary review and critique: The Tylenol crisis. *Public Relations Review* (Fall)

Stephenson, H. 1976. *Handbook of public relations*. New York: McGraw-Hill.

Strong, E. 1925. *The psychology of selling*. New York: McGraw-Hill.

TARP (Technical Assistance Research Programs Institute). 1986. *Consumer complaint handling in America: An update study*. Consumer Affairs Council of the U.S. Office of Consumer Affairs. Washington, D.C.: Department of Health and Human Services.

Review Questions

1. What are the four main principles to remember in seeking free media coverage of a service?

2. "Public health education can be an effective type of sales promotion." Discuss.

3. "To promote a service effectively through person-to-person contact depends on careful planning." Comment.

4. "The most commonly neglected opportunity for marketing communication is follow-up contact with already established patients." Discuss some of the opportunities that nurses have to use this opportunity better.

Part V

Professional Applications of Marketing

Chapter 13

The Practice Arena—Customers, Consumers, and Competition

Today's competitive health care environment demands a success equation that features high-quality, low-cost patient care services. Health care organizations are challenged to develop new ways of thinking and to formulate new ways of doing business. A shift in perspective from one in which the provider establishes what is required to one that is consumer and customer oriented is essential. Hospitals, home health care agencies, physicians, administrators, social workers, and nurses are responding to these new demands. Proactive decision-making offers promise. Paralysis results in a diminishing market share, decreasing influence on the market, and financial implications unacceptable to boards of directors, administrators, staff, and the community.

Folger and Fee (1987) assert that health care professionals are moving from a marketing orientation that stresses "media madness" to one that emphasizes management of the clinical product. These authors state: "In actuality, the adaptation of marketing and product management principles is exponentially rapid compared with other service industries. It has to be. The free market has been thrust upon hospitals, and they have no choice. 'He who hesitates is not only lost, but miles beyond the next exit,' wrote one clever fellow." Nurses are uniquely qualified to play a key role in meeting the demand for and provision of marketing-oriented services.

The vignettes in this chapter feature nurses who are at the forefront of the marketing movement in health care, designing innovative, competitive consumer-sensitive health care services. "In the absence of competition, not much attention need be paid to the parts as long as the whole prospers. In the presence of competition and the concomitant complexity, the winners will be those who can

391

'think small,' at least in product terms" (Folger and Fee, 1987). Each of the case studies in this chapter corroborates this concept. These vignettes also demonstrate that nurses are close to the customer in the agencies and institutions that distribute health care products. Leadership opportunities in product design and distribution are therefore plentiful.

Rebecca Reynolds, R.N., M.S.N., used marketing principles and skills to successfully shape prenatal care services. Diane Mielcarek, R.N., identified a market opportunity and, in collaboration with other providers, championed its cause. In today's marketplace, efficient and effective patient care management takes on added significance, when considered within productivity and cost-containment analytical frameworks. Margo Neal, R.N., M.N., responded to the clinician's critical need for patient care planning tools.

Community health care services are also affected by competitive forces, as hospitals seek safe and effective inpatient care alternatives. Nancy Rhodes, R.N., B.S.N., demonstrates how management experience and clinical expertise are used in combination with marketing principles to achieve organizational goals and objectives. Consumer demand for health and wellness information provided Barbara Flewellyn, R.N., M.S.N., with a chance to participate in the corporate restructuring activities of the University Hospitals of Cleveland, through application of the marketing process. Finally, Mary Stinson, R.N., B.S., serves North Memorial Medical Center as product line manager for women's and children's services. Her strong clinical background and market sensitivity played a significant role in the creation of a "winner."

The factors that shaped these nurses' success continue to evolve, waiting for others to respond. Nursing can lead the way.

Marketing a Clinical Service

Nancy L. Rhodes, R.N., B.S.N.
Vice-President, Planning and Program Development
Visiting Nurse Association
West Allis, Wisconsin

The Visiting Nurse Association (VNA) of Milwaukee has been a home health care leader since 1906, responding to the many changes and challenges presented by the health care industry. "The transformation of the health care system not only applies to each link in the system, but also to the complexity of care each institution provides. Rapid growth, multiple agencies, earlier discharges, and changes in the reimbursement system," states Nancy Rhodes, "leave the health care consumer with difficult and confusing choices about home health care services."

"In 1984, our agency was confronted with competition. It was a new and strange experience for us all," Nancy reports. " 'Why market'? we asked. We've never done that. Referral sources know who we are and what we offer. It costs a lot of money. These statements had become topics of discussion, not only within the management group at Milwaukee VNA, but with similar providers across the country."

The agency turned to Nancy and her 19 years of experience in home health care. Leading the VNA marketing department was an opportunity and a challenge offered by the president. "My mind was flooded with questions. Was I really interested? What qualified me to lead our marketing effort? Was I ready to take a new career path away from involvement in operations and patient care? What skills and knowledge base did I have that could apply to marketing, and what additional skills and knowledge did I need?"

Nancy found that answers emerged through discussion with friends and her supervisor, and through self-appraisal. "Each phone call made and received, 12 years of supervision and management in all phases of VNA, working on community committees, and making presentations to multiple groups are all components of marketing. I accepted the position."

The Visiting Nurse Association's mission is threefold: (1) to grow through careful planning in response to identified community needs for home health care and related services; (2) to serve as an advocate for the disadvantaged and underserved; and (3) to develop related services and markets in response to changing community needs. Nancy welcomed the opportunity to educate the community about home health care and to assist consumers in making informed and knowledgeable choices. The time had come for the VNA to respond proactively in the marketplace.

"How should I begin?" Nancy wondered, "What did phrases like 'target group,' 'analyzing the competition,' and 'shotgun versus rifle approach' mean? It was clear that I needed to focus on rectifying my knowledge deficit." Nancy attended several continuing education courses at the Xerox Learning Center, where she mastered basic marketing theory and techniques and their application in the not-for-profit sector.

"I quickly learned that a benchmark market analysis was essential. We needed to measure awareness, attitudes, and opinion about home health and the VNA of Milwaukee. We did not have the in-house expertise to conduct such a study; thus, one of my first challenges was to retain the services of a market research firm." Developing a marketplace data base is as important to the development of a strategic marketing plan as assessment is to a patient care plan.

The VNA market analysis showed that the Milwaukee VNA enjoyed a positive image. However, the need to maintain and protect current market share and garner new target markets did not allow the agency to rest on its laurels. A strong reputation and tradition for quality services were precious assets that required proactive protection.

"I selected an advertising and communications firm to assist us in planning an effective promotional program. Selecting an agency is a critical step in ensuring a successful campaign," asserts Nancy. "I was fortunate to have met Dr. Philip Kotler, Professor of Marketing at the J.K. Kellogg School of Management, at a marketing conference, and he recommended a number of agencies. The program VNA implemented with the agencies' assistance reflects collaboration and creativity."

"Rich Roberson, Executive Director of the Kansas City VNA had shared an idea with me that I found very appealing. He used a Preferred Patient Card as a promotional technique. The card allows current and prospective VNA patients to enroll for home health care services. We took the card idea and combined it with a slogan developed by the advertising firm: 'Don't Stay Home Without It.' This became the cornerstone of our communication program, to create and maintain VNA visibility in the marketplace." Figures 13-1 and 13-2 illustrate how the promotion was used on billboards and city buses. Figure 13-3 details programmatic elements.

Three marketing objectives guided the Milwaukee VNA program. First, VNA strives to promote and increase public awareness and knowledge of home health care to assist consumers in making informed and knowledgeable decisions. Second, the program is directed at keeping the agency "top of mind" in the referral network and at reinforcing VNA's leadership image. The

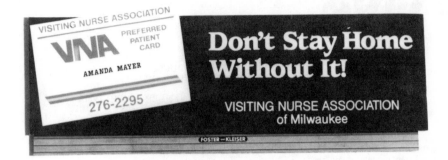

Figure 13-1 Billboard locations with high population interface were used to promote the program.

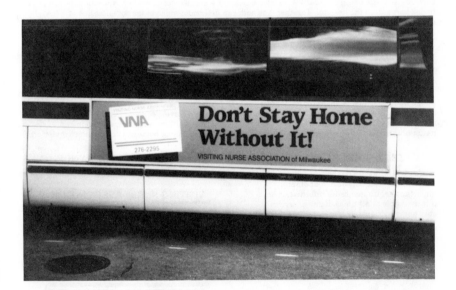

Figure 13-2 City buses took the VNA Preferred Patient Program message all over the Milwaukee metropolitan area.

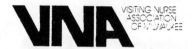

**VNA-MILWAUKEE INTRODUCES
"PREFERRED PATIENT PROGRAM"**

**CONGRATULATIONS! YOU ARE NOW A MEMBER OF THE VNA
PREFERRED PATIENT PROGRAM.**

To ensure that area residents receive the best in home health care, the Visiting Nurse Association of Milwaukee has a "Preferred Patient Program." This program will allow past, present, and future VNA patients to be pre-enrolled for comprehensive VNA home health care when it is needed. There are no enrollment or membership fees for VNA Preferred Patient Program members.

The Visiting Nurse Association has been in the forefront of the home health care field for such a long time that Visiting Nurse Association services have become almost a generic term for home health care. These days, to receive visiting nurse services from VNA, you have to ask for home health care from the Visiting Nurse Association of Milwaukee. The new Preferred Patient Program will help area residents get the real thing—genuine Visiting Nurse Association home health care.

HOW THE PROGRAM WORKS

As a Preferred Patient member when you are hospitalized and your physician orders home health care, you can receive VNA care by presenting the membership card and specifically requesting VNA care. A discharge planner, usually a registered nurse or a hospital social worker, will visit with you prior to discharge from the hospital. Together, you both can determine which of the complete line of VNA services will be needed once you return home. The membership card will make the entire discharge process easier for you and the discharge planner, plus help to ensure that you receive the best home health care possible. The VNA will bill Medicare or other insurance sources as required for services provided.

ADDED PROGRAM BENEFITS

Preferred Patient Program members will also realize other important benefits. Your card lists a phone number which is answered 24 hours a day, seven days a week. This number may be used by you to receive answers to any home health care question that you may have. Program members will also receive updated information about the rapid changes in home health care of local, statewide and national interest. Other information may also be sent to you including home health education materials.

KEEP YOUR CARD WITH OTHER IMPORTANT MEDICAL INFORMATION

You will want to keep your card in your wallet or purse, along with your other important health insurance information so it is available at all times. Remember, don't stay home without it.

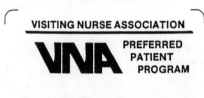

Figure 13-3 Clients received promotional literature describing program benefits with their own personal card.

third objective establishes a commitment to retain and increase current market share.

"Marketing," argues Nancy, "is not a quick-fix solution. Strategies must be continually defined and redefined, just as a patient's care plan is updated and revised in response to changing factors. Working with an advertising agency is a team effort, just as planning patient care involves multiple parties. The marketing team must be aware and knowledgeable about what is being planned, when and how the plan is executed, and how each individual's role facilitates achievement of marketing goals and objectives."

Where are Nancy and the VNA 4 years later? "The Milwaukee home health care arena is volatile. We are in a consumer-driven market where choices are available. We continually ask, 'What are our consumers' needs—patient, physician, HMO, insurance company? How are we perceived by our various publics? Who is the care decision-maker? How can we position ourselves to compete effectively? How can we deliver services in the most caring, yet cost-effective manner?' "

Nancy believes that nursing and marketing have much in common. "The skills of listening, caring, and evaluating how the patient responds are marketing assets. Learning to work within defined cost parameters while maintaining creativity, compassion, and quality are ever-challenging factors that nurses respond to effectively." The promotional program described above and others that the VNA has developed to market their clinical services are very successful. "We have been able to achieve our goals and in some cases exceed market share objectives. The work is satisfying, and I feel rewarded when services are shaped to enhance the quality of care and meet the perceived needs of the patient."

The Office Nurse as a Marketing Agent

Rebecca Reynolds, R.N., M.S.N.
President, Educational Consultants
Mt. Pleasant, South Carolina

"The office nurse is a market and a marketing agent," states Becki Reynolds, "one that is significantly underutilized. Office nurses can have a major effect on physician patient volumes."

In 1977, Charleston, South Carolina, had approximately 30 obstetricians and gynecologists in private practice. The majority of acute obstetrical care was provided by two private hospitals. "They offered," reports Becki, "very traditional care." Lamaze-prepared fathers were allowed in the delivery room, but the birthing experience did not allow for flexible consumer choices. The number of obstetricians and Charleston's demographics created a competitive environment for the private obstetrical patient.

"The interesting aspect," states Becki, "was that even though they were faced with competition, the physicians did not engage in activities designed to differentiate them in the marketplace. Patient movement was, for the most part, based on established colleague referral patterns, word of mouth, and mother-daughter care patterns.

"I see myself as an enlightened nurse and a women's advocate. When I had my baby, I felt that the experience was lacking from the hospital point of view. The physicians I selected for my obstetrical care were very interested in suggestions I made and very willing to make changes. Shortly after I delivered, a position opened up in their office."

Becki was reluctant to accept the position because of the stigma attached to the office nurse. "You hear phrases like, 'She's just an office nurse,' or, 'She isn't smart enough to work in a hospital.' Office work is not valued in our profession. In spite of my concerns, I was interested for several reasons.

"First and foremost, the physicians were genuinely interested in changing office systems to address patient preferences. The hours were right for me, and I liked the physicians. They sincerely wanted to respond to the market. We didn't call it marketing then — we called it responding to personal needs, improving the quality of care, and making our patients happier with their experience. In reality we were performing the first step in the marketing process: identifying patient needs and wants and making a decision to acknowledge and respond to opportunities in the marketplace."

In 1977, when Becki joined the practice, deliveries were 11 to 15 a month. Two years later, the same two obstetricians were delivering between 30 and 35 babies a month. "We listened to our patients, identified needs and wants, and established programs in response. Over a 2-year period of time we designed and implemented several programs which dramatically changed our visibility in the community and effectiveness with our patients."

The first step Becki took after joining the practice was to initiate a patient education program. The objective was to develop an informed consumer and improve outcomes. Not only did the office provide connections with traditional Lamaze and breastfeeding programs, but Becki met with each patient before her physician visit. "The patients had requested more attention and opportunities for questions and answers during their regular office visits. We designed and implemented a program which allowed me to spend time with each patient, reviewing topics such as nutrition, exercise, and the do's and don'ts of pregnancy. This increased personal contact enriched the office visit, enhanced the quality of patient care, and improved the educational effort."

The second aspect of the response program involved the hospital. "Continuity of care was a late-70s buzz phrase in nursing, and I felt a need to follow our patients into the hospital. The practice submitted a letter requesting hospital privileges, so that I could see our patients. After authorization was granted, I conducted pre- and post-op teaching, stayed with selected patients in labor and delivery, and made teaching rounds independent of the physicians. I positioned myself as a support person and focused on meeting the psychosocial needs of patients. The goal was to bond the patient to our practice."

Becki also planned, implemented, and serviced a home health care program for high-risk patients. "It can seem like a long time between office visits for a patient with a placenta previa or a patient on bed rest for complications. I developed a home care program for these patients and scheduled my visits between office appointments, so that the patient felt continuous support.

"In response to feedback, we also began to reshape our office hours to meet the needs of our patients. Many of our patients worked, so we extended office hours into the evening, to avoid conflict between keeping the boss happy and attending to health care needs."

One of the interesting changes Becki saw was an alteration in patient demographics. Socioeconomic status and educational background improved significantly. "This demographic shift provided us promotional avenues not previously accessed. Our new patient population was able to open the doors of television studios and the microphones of radio shows. They had media contacts and were willing to use their contacts to help educate the public. I spoke at community functions, appeared on local talk shows, and participated in radio spots directed at community service. These activities provided our practice meaningful exposure."

Becki also recalls the reaction of the other OB/GYN physicians in the Charleston area. "As our practice differentiation became more evident and patient referral patterns were affected, the initial response was resistance and objections. As time went on, however, competitive practices began to develop their own marketing programs. It was good for the patients, and it was good for competition. It meant that we couldn't rest on our laurels, but needed to keep moving forward.

"We responded to the changing marketplace and established a call-in program for our patients. I set aside two blocks of time during the week when I was available by phone. Any of our patients could call in and discuss their care. We developed an information brochure so that the patients had a calling-hours reminder. The program was based on a patient's suggestion and proved a very popular way of meeting a need."

Late in 1979, Becki made a decision to return to school and earn her certificate in nurse midwifery. While on leave, a third physician was added to the practice. When she returned, her role expanded to include prenatal patient care, well-women gynecology, chart screening, and development of individual patient care plans.

"The thing that I want to emphasize," states Becki, "is that, for the most part, our marketing program was incorporated in my salary. The informational and educational materials were done in a basic fashion at minimal cost. We did not invest large sums in advertising — indeed, we did not spend a dime on any type of media. Our efforts weren't flashy, but they were responsive and oriented to psychosocial need.

"All I needed was physician support and the sensitivity to respond in new and different ways to our patients. After I returned from graduate school, the physicians and I put together our own marketing/consulting firm to develop educational and promotional materials for office practices. The market was changing rapidly, and increased resources and expertise were obviously required. Since we were ahead, this allowed us the opportunity to offer our vision to others."

The patients and physicians that Becki worked with during her 8 years as an office nurse continue to enjoy her unique and creative programs. She left her position in 1986 and joined St. Francis Xavier Hospital in Charleston, where she served as Assistant Vice-President for Service Development and Director of Women's Health Services. Today, in addition to her own consulting service, Becki is the

Assistant Administrator for Resource Development and an Instructor at the Medical University of South Carolina, Department of Psychiatry and Behavioral Sciences, and in the College of Nursing. Her experiences in marketing and her contributions to health care continue to enrich the Charleston marketplace and enhance its products.

The Clinical Nurse as a Product Line Manager

Mary Stinson, R.N., B.S.
Manager, Consumer Marketing and Business Development
North Memorial Medical Center
Robinsdale, Minnesota

Mary Stinson began her professional nursing career with North Memorial Medical Center in 1968, shortly after completing her program of study at Swedish Hospital School of Nursing. "I had decided that I wanted to be a pediatric nurse, and after interviewing at four area hospitals I selected North Memorial. It had a new 40-bed unit that was exciting to a new graduate. I wanted to be part of its development." Mary remained with North Memorial and the pediatric unit for 7 years, until her husband's job took them to Illinois for 3 years.

"When we got to Illinois, I couldn't find a pediatric position and ended up working on an adult oncology unit. I found that I liked big people, so when I returned to North Memorial I worked on the oncology unit." In 1981, 5 years after returning from Illinois, Mary was asked to accept an administrative position. For the next 2 years she served as an evening supervisor at North.

"In 1983, I moved to the nursing office as staffing coordinator, and I was still there when the Minneapolis nursing strike hit in 1984. Our community was overbedded, occupancy rates had fallen dramatically, and job security was a real issue." During the strike, Mary worked in the neonatal intensive care unit. After the strike, she returned to her role as staffing coordinator.

"Part of the strike settlement involved a recall process for nurses. There wasn't anyone who had participated in such an exercise. The process of recovering from the strike totally burned me out. I was ready for something new. When the position of Perinatal Manager/Marketing opened up, I applied."

North Memorial Hospital is a 582-bed tertiary hospital located in the greater Minneapolis area. During the years 1982 to 1984, a highly competitive marketplace developed in response to implementation of the prospective payment system and heavy HMO market penetration. Hospitals found themselves competing for HMO contracts and dealing with reduced length of stay almost simultaneously. In response, North established a marketing department, hired a Senior Director, and retained its first product manager for outpatient surgery.

"When I interviewed for the perinatal job, the Senior Director was impressed with my clinical credentials, but admitted he was reluctant to hire a nurse. He really got my dander up," states Mary, "and I wanted to know why." Mary found that he was concerned that she would take on the "I-know-what's-best-for-you" attitude that health care providers typically display when dealing with patients. What he needed, he said, were marketing skills, not clinical skills.

"I knew that I could talk the product, and I challenged him to teach someone with marketing skills my 17 years of clinical experience. It was easier and more effective to teach me marketing skills than to try and teach clinical skills to someone with marketing skills. My arguments must have been effective—I was hired as the Perinatal Product Line Manager for Women's and Children's Services in December 1984."

Two weeks after Mary reported for her new job, her boss left. She found herself alone for the next 4 months. "I decided I just couldn't wait for direction. I looked at my area as if it were a business. I started by comparing our program with those of the other hospitals.

"The Twin Cities obstetrical programs were structured around the labor-delivery-recovery [LDR] care distribution concept, or LDRP, which adds the postpartum course. Because of structural limitations, we had an LDR delivery system. With that basic decision made for us, I began to critically examine amenity packages."

Mary found that Minneapolis had its share of champagne dinners, baskets of food, and baby supplies for the new parents to take home. "I thought baby supplies were great, but they were gone within a short period of time. What seemed to be missing in the marketplace was something permanent—something that stayed with the baby and its parents after the hospital experience." Mary had an idea. She approached a local manufacturing firm and developed a diaper bag as a patient amenity. The bag's unique feature is a changing pad on the front, so that mom can lay her baby down anywhere and change a diaper. "The bag has gone over like hotcakes," reports Mary. "It's a traveling advertisement for North Memorial. I have actually had patients change doctors so that they can get our bag. It's a visual status symbol."

Another factor that came to Mary's attention as a result of North Memorial's market research was the postpartum unit's care delivery system. "We had conducted focus groups, and participants expressed concern about our care delivery system. They felt as if they were thrown back and forth between the nurse who was taking care of mom and the nurse caring for the baby. If they couldn't distinguish between the nurses and happened to ask the baby nurse a question about breast care, they were apt to get referred back to the 'mother nurse.' "

The next major change in North's obstetrical program was based on their market research analysis. "A mother-baby delivery system concept was ideal," reports Mary. "It made good sense from a nursing care perspective and focus group feedback as well. In 1984 we renovated, and 1985 was devoted to changing our delivery system to mother-baby care."

Over the years since Mary Stinson became the women's and children's product line manager, a number of changes have taken place in North's marketing department, in the perinatal program, and in Mary's position. Currently, Mary Stinson is Manager, Consumer Marketing and Business Development. As such, the coordinators of four consumer marketing programs report to her (Figure 13-4).

The marketing department at North includes two major divisions. The first division is concerned with medical markets. It includes a position for a Medical Markets Business Development Manager and four account managers, two of which target senior citizen and oncology services. Two other positions are authorized but not yet staffed. The second major division is headed by Mary Stinson. She is responsible for the Birthday Advisor Program, North Women's Center, North Physician Referral Service, and the Cosmetic Surgery Center Program. A description of each of these programs follows.

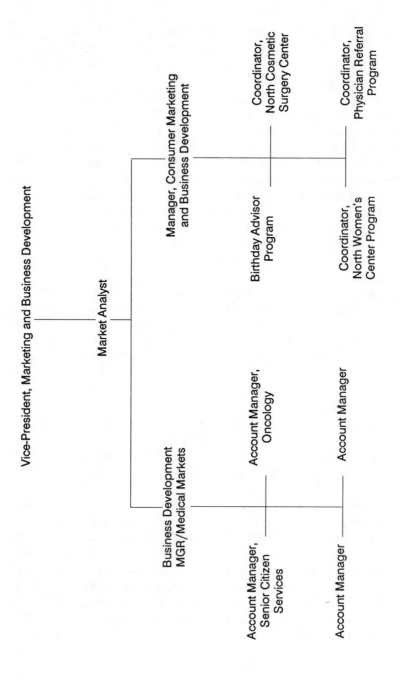

Figure 13-4 Marketing department organizational chart, North Memorial Medical Center.

The Birthday Advisor Program

The purpose of this program is to provide women with access to information about North's obstetrical program and physicians. All educational programs related to the maternity program are housed here, so that couples in Lamaze, grandparents interested in grandparenting, or parents interested in sibling education can inquire and register for classes through the advisor. The Birthday Advisor also handles any special processing problem that a patient may require. For example, the Birthday Advisor may receive a call from a woman who is dissatisfied with some aspect of care she is receiving. The Advisor contacts the physician, and they work together to effectively manage the problem.

Physician Referral Program

Mary also has responsibility for North's Physician Referral Program. This service offers consumers an opportunity to call the hospital, review their health care needs and preferences, and receive a referral that meets their needs. The coordinator will even make an appointment for the caller, if requested.

Cosmetic Surgery Center

Plastic surgery is a particularly sensitive consumer market, and has experienced dramatic growth over the last few years. The coordinator of this program deals directly with patients interested in plastic surgery, answers questions about procedures and their cost, offers information about the physicians who perform the work at North, and provides referrals that meet their needs.

Women's Center

This program focuses on education and topics of interest for women. North has two large one-day programs a year directed at women. They feature such topics as "Recent Advances in the Treatment of Breast Cancer" and "Menopause: What Does It Mean to Me?" The center also plans an annual 2-day retreat for women where topics such as stress, single parenting, financial planning, and working women and family demands are discussed.

As a product line manager, Mary Stinson has access to marketing information and a perspective that may be somewhat different from that of the nurse at the bedside. She analyzes and plans to meet the needs and wants of a consumer group, but she does not have the direct authority to act on the information. Mary works through the Vice-President of Nursing, the clinical nursing director, the medical staff, the head nurse, and all members of the nursing staff to achieve marketing objectives.

"One way I work with the patient care staff is by being visible on the units and meeting biweekly with the maternal-child leadership group. I provide them with survey feedback, marketing statistics, and general information on competitive forces in the marketplace. There is one factor that has helped me a great deal: The staff know me. I've been around North a long time and have earned my clinical stripes. My background provides me with credibility. When I go to the floors I wear my lab coat, so that I am seen as close to the clinical setting. I have never been perceived as 'one of those marketing people.' In order to raise consciousness, I spend a lot of time educating the staff about the philosophy and science of marketing.

"When I receive feedback affecting other departments, I contact the appropriate department heads and make them aware. If, for example, I receive information from a postdischarge survey that moms are expressing concern about the admitting office, I review the data with the admitting manager and we problem-solve together. Not infrequently, the department requests more information to help them address systems alterations. I collect the data and return it to them. I am fortunate—I get full cooperation."

As indicated earlier, Mary Stinson recognized that while she brought a comprehensive understanding of the product to her first marketing position, she needed to acquire marketing knowledge and skills. Over the years, Mary has completed her baccalaureate degree and attended marketing workshops offered by Richard Ireland at the Snowmass Institute. She now participates as faculty in these programs on a regular basis. Mary is a member of the American Marketing Association and the American College of Healthcare Marketing. By participating in community organizations such as Nannyfinders, Inc., Twin West Chamber of Commerce, the Business and Professional Women's Group, and the Minnesota Women's Network, Mary meets marketplace assessment objectives.

Mary was asked to share one of her most satisfying experiences as a product line manager. She chose her experience at North in marketing to the first-time mom.

"When we initially analyzed our obstetrical data, it became quite obvious we were losing first-time moms. This market segment is critical, particularly in relation to repeat customers. The idea is to attract them and then provide the kind of experience that will bring them back for other deliveries. We decided to target this group with a media promotion campaign coordinated through our Birthday Advisor Program.

"I worked closely with our media people and with our advertising agency. We developed an ad directed at the beginning family and tracked its success through the advisor. During the first year we ran the ad, we saw a 17% increase in our first-time mother population—a most gratifying response. Our tracking data demonstrated that the ad had been effective" (Figure 13-5).

Mary Stinson's experience demonstrates the value of the nurse as product line manager. Nurses can acquire marketing skills and successfully integrate their broad clinical knowledge to achieve marketing objectives and improve clinical care. In 1983, North Memorial Hospital delivered 2,055 babies. In 1987, they delivered 3,165—a remarkable 54% increase in 4 years. That's clinical marketing!

Marketing to Meet Clinician Needs

Margo C. Neal, R.N., M.N.
Vice President and Editor for Nursing
Williams and Wilkins
Pacifici Palisades, CA

Not-for-profit organizations, particularly hospitals, rarely had market presence before 1982. The sweeping changes that followed the enactment of prospective payment systems are responsible, at least in part, for market share competition among hospitals. It has created untold opportunity for new and nontraditional nursing roles. The challenge and opportunity Margo Neal identified and actualized is one example of a successful response. "I learned," begins Margo, "that one of the basic principles of marketing is the difference between needs and wants for a specific group.

"Hi Honey, are you sitting down?"

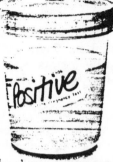

"Sure thing, Sally. What's up?"
"I've, uh, got something to tell you."
"Uh huh, shoot."
"I'm pregnant."
"Great. How about Chinese tonight?"
"Honey, did you hear me?"
"Yup, you said you're...ohmygod!"
"There's no easy way to tell your husband you're pregnant. Especially when you didn't expect to be expecting. Once Bill got over the initial shock, though, he was terrific. Indulging me with backrubs, practicing our breathing, whipping up liver health shakes (remember, I said he was terrific, not a gourmet).

Fact is, Bill was the one who found out about North Memorial's Birth Day Program. And after we talked with Becky, North's Birth Day advisor, we were delighted with options like early and late prenatal classes, family involvement and specialized care that enabled us to really personalize our baby's delivery.

The day (or should I say very early morning) of the big event, I felt scared but confident. Our private birthing room at North Memorial was cheerful and homey. The nurses were wonderfully supportive.

I felt extra safe because of North Memorial's great reputation for being able to care for very sick babies. And because Bill coached, coaxed and congratulated me every step of the way, having a baby turned out to be as beautiful as making one."

To find out about The Birth Day Program at North Memorial, call Becky at 520-5830. THE **BIRTH DAY** PROGRAM.
At North Memorial Medical Center

Figure 13-5 An illustration of advertising targeted at first-time mothers.

"At the time my opportunity presented itself, I was an in-service education instructor in a community hospital. Together with my department head, I developed a series of classes for nurses in the intensive care unit. My associate and I felt that we knew what the nurses needed. Did we ever ask if they *wanted* the information? No. You can guess the result: Very few nurses attended the classes. Then and there I realized the difference between needs and wants, and I learned to develop plans to provide what people wanted first and what they needed second."

Margo recognized that nurses wanted information on nursing care plans and the nursing process. She did not conduct market research to see if her product was viable; she simply acted on her idea. "I remember sending out my first workshop flyer on nursing care plans. To my great surprise, 200 people responded!"

Based on her initial success, Margo expanded product development and the promotion of nursing care plans. "I decided to present the workshop on a national basis. The response rate continued to grow, so much so that I had to hire other nurses to present the content in different geographical settings. The more workshops we gave, the more I realized we were not only responding to a want, but filling a need at one and the same time."

Margo worked with another tested marketing principle: She asked herself what other service, product, or entity related to the nursing care plans and the nursing process could she develop and promote. "It didn't come to me like a bolt out of the blue. In fact, it was more than 2 years before I made a firm decision. I wrote and published a book called *Nursing Care Planning Guides*. The content was directed at helping nurses write nursing care plans. The workshop participants told me they wanted and needed such an instrument." Margo's first book was very successful, and she later brought out additional volumes in the series. Collectively, her books have sold nearly 1 million copies.

"In the process of readying my first book for publication, I utilized another fundamental marketing principle. I offered buyers a special prepublication price. Consequently, I had enough orders to pay for the entire cost of producing the book. Needless to say, the results realized from this promotional approach were very rewarding."

Margo Neal achieved a high degree of success with her first publication. While the business was relatively small, she was able to run it on the basis of her best judgment, but as it grew, she identified a need for more sophisticated business techniques. "I knew I needed to enhance my skills and expertise in the marketing process and marketing techniques." Margo read extensively, earned continuing education credits, and developed a network of colleagues who could offer expert counsel and advice.

"The results were impressive. The business expanded and I began to get nibbles from larger companies regarding acquisition." The result: The company Margo started in 1970, NURSECO, was acquired by Williams & Wilkins of Baltimore, which has published medical books and journals since the turn of the century. Williams & Wilkins wanted to initiate a nursing product line and felt it would be more efficient and effective to acquire a small publishing house than build one from scratch.

"We made a good fit," states Margo. "They had in-depth experience in all phases of publishing, and I had an excellent track record for developing and publishing high-quality books for nurses. Now each of us does what we do best. Williams & Wilkins provides the expertise in marketing and production; together we develop nursing editorial policy, focus, and long-range plans. I am responsible for acquisitions: strategy, projects, and development. The result is that the small line of nursing books I published under the NURSECO label has been expanded in both quality and quantity."

The experience of Margo Neal in responding to the needs and wants of clinicians is gratifying. She cautions the novice not to get too mired in the science of marketing, however. Formal market research is extremely helpful, but it is not foolproof or the last word. Consider the example of the Polaroid camera. Market research said there would be no demand for such a camera, because it was too expensive and more of a toy than a camera. Fortunately, Dr. Land's intuition and persistence prevailed—and so did Margo's.

Marketing Clinical Programs

Diane Mielcarek, R.N.
Medical/Surgical Clinician
Mercy Hospital
Toledo, Ohio

Diane Mielcarek's marketing experience began early in 1985. Dr. Steven Sutton, an attending urologist at Mercy Hospital in Toledo, had not been successful in getting a positive response to an idea from hospital administration. When the dilemma reached Diane's ears, things began to happen.

Dr. Sutton was caring for a patient who developed impotence as a complication of diabetes mellitus. The patient had read about a self-help group for impotent males in a Detroit, Michigan, newspaper. He attended one of the programs at Grace Hospital, in Detroit. The emotional and educational support he received at the meeting encouraged him to ask his physician to form a group in Toledo.

Dr. Sutton turned to the nursing staff on the urology unit for assistance. He asked what they thought about the idea of having a Recovery of Male Potency (ROMP) group at Mercy. "I was really interested in the idea of helping this group of patients deal with a very difficult problem," states Diane. "I must confess that I didn't think it would have a positive effect on the hospital's bottom line, but now I know a little more about marketing, return on investment, and the effects of promotion. It's really nice to know that you can meet the educational and emotional needs of patients and have a positive business outcome as well."

Diane discussed the program with her immediate supervisor, Janet Gardner, R.N., B.S.N., Director of Nursing, who in turn presented the matter to Sister Kathleen Mary Moross, Vice-President. "Sister gave us the OK to find out more about the program. Janet called Grace Hospital and talked with the program's founder and coordinator, Cindy Meredith, R.N., M.S.N. Cindy sent us information and offered to meet with us and clarify concerns or questions."

ROMP is a self-help program that addresses the emotional and educational needs of impotent men. It was started at Grace Hospital by Cindy Meredith with two penile implant patients in 1983. Today, the program is known across the country and is franchised by Grace Hospital. "With this basic information in hand, and with the assistance and persistence of Sister Kathleen Mary, Dr. Sutton, and our nurses, Mercy Hospital's administration gave approval to purchase the program and begin its implementation. Needless to say, we are all thrilled with our success."

Following purchase of the franchise, several members of the nursing staff and Mercy's Planning Coordinator, Doug Funsett, traveled to Detroit and spent a full day learning about ROMP. "When we returned," states Diane, "we knew we needed to designate a coordinator. Confidentiality is a critical factor in making the program work. We learned that the same person must talk with potential participants and coordinate the program on a monthly basis. With these requirements in mind, we felt that Marlene Reynolds, R.N., B.Ed., Patient Education Coordinator, was the perfect person. Fortunately, she was interested in the project, too.

"We purchased the program for $1,350 in July 1985. It included a license to use the ROMP trademark and the educational and promotional materials developed for the program. Dr. Sutton and another Mercy physician, Dr. Steve Ariss, agreed to serve as physician program advisors. Dr. Hy Kissen, a psychologist, Sister Kathleen Mary, Doug Funsett, Janet Gardner, and myself rounded out the program steering committee. At our first meeting we decided to move fast. The competition between hospitals was severe in our market, and our physician advisors had picked up news that another facility was interested in a similar program. We set an objective to have the first group meeting in August."

Over the next month, the steering committee placed newspaper advertisements, prepared brochure materials supplied by Grace Hospital, oriented the medical and nursing staffs to the program, and arranged for impotence testing equipment and penile implants for demonstration purposes.

"We found little support among the members of the medical staff for the program. They were particularly offended by the title of the program — ROMP — and expressed the opinion that it was particularly troublesome when associated with a Catholic-affiliated institution. There were many meetings and discussions about not using the title. We knew, however, that if we didn't use ROMP, we could not be part of the overall program. After multiple meetings we were asked to proceed with implementation by the hospital administration."

Marlene Reynolds, ROMP Program Coordinator, held a press conference to announce the program in July, and Cindy Meredith attended to answer questions regarding program development at Grace Hospital. Following the announcement, resistance, in the form of written expressions on concern, continued. One physician wrote to the Bishop of the Diocese of Toledo. Sister Kathleen Mary handled these situations personally, writing the Bishop herself. "If it hadn't been for the support of our Vice-President," argues Diane, "I doubt that we would have gotten the program off the ground.

"We held our first meeting in August, 1985. Twenty-seven people attended. By December, attendance was 40." The ROMP group continues to meet monthly at Mercy Hospital. The number of physicians on the advisory team has doubled. They are featured speakers each month, and self-referral commonly follows for those who attend. Media promotion continues through the newspapers, listings with local support groups, direct mailings to ROMP members, and speaking engagements at area civic and professional group meetings.

Urological admissions have increased at Mercy since the initiation of the program, as have transurethral resection surgical cases. Increases are related to problems identified during the urological workup for sexual dysfunction. "One of the most distressing things about the impotent patient," states Diane, "is that they don't see any hope. The one comment we hear over and over again since we have offered ROMP, is that the participants feel a sense of relief. They have a place to go — a place where they are not alone and where they can find some answers to their problems. It's comments like this that have made marketing this clinical program satisfying to everyone associated with its development and implementation."

A marketing program requires time, money, and expertise. Many institutions do not have the resources to build a successful program from the ground up. The route followed by Mercy Hospital demonstrates another avenue that nursing departments have available: to acquire well-developed, tried-and-true programs that are "transplanted" to achieve marketing objectives. As health care marketing grows and develops, program acquisition should be considered as a possible alternative to internal development.

The Nurse as a Health Promotion Agent

Barbara J. Flewellyn, R.N., M.S.N.
Director, Health Enhancement Center
University Hospitals of Cleveland
Cleveland, Ohio

University Hospitals of Cleveland is an 874-bed facility located in the heart of Cleveland, Ohio, on the main campus of Case Western Reserve University. Within a 2-mile radius of the hospitals are six other acute care facilities, one of which is the 900-bed Cleveland Clinic. The medical care provided by University Hospitals is widely recognized, drawing patients from local, national, and international markets. In 1984, University Hospitals, like many other facilities, began to analyze how it could organizationally cope with the implications of prospective payment and other forces reshaping the health care marketplace. Although the hospital's occupancy rates exceed 90%, the board of directors and hospital administration wanted to plan ahead and anticipate need.

Early in 1984, the board and the administration decided to restructure and diversify over a 16-month period. First, a home health care service was established. Second, a health promotion program, now known as the Health Enhancement Center, was developed, and finally the hospital established an HMO. The HMO was completed in June 1985 as a joint venture with the Metropolitan Life Insurance Company.

Barbara Flewellyn is the founding director of University Hospitals' Health Enhancement Center. "The center has three primary goals," Barbara reports. "Our first goal is to establish a health care link with the Cleveland business community. When I was employed, in December 1984, University Hospitals did not have a marketing department. In essence, we became the marketing department for the hospital. Our target market is the business community. Second, the center serves University Hospitals' two large suburban centers, located within a 10-mile radius of the main facility. The suburban centers house selected health care services and private physician offices. Health Enhancement provides classes to attract a well population for potential physician referral. Finally, we serve as a referral source for physicians at University Hospitals, and they in turn refer patients to us."

During the first six months, Barbara contracted with outside professionals to teach two programs. "Smoke cessation and weight control are standard in any wellness program. These programs enable us to promote the center and earn revenue, while going through the important exercise of deciding what business we are in — our target markets, operational concepts, and how we would structure the center."

Some important groundwork had already been laid. When the board and the administration made a strategic planning commitment, they retained outside consultants to assist. The consultants helped the administrators verify the need and select staff for home health, wellness programs, and an HMO. "While we promoted our first two programs, I worked closely with the consultant. I wanted to know what aspect of the industrial sector to target. Certainly, the literature and research indicated a need for and interest in health promotion, but we didn't know if the corporate leaders in Cleveland saw health promotion as a priority.

"We began by putting together an information base on corporate Cleveland. The type of business, size, product, and number of employees were identified. We called on selected business leaders and talked with them about priorities and health care needs. During this same period of time, I completed a thorough literature review on wellness and the development of health promotion programs. I also made site visits to other hospital-based wellness centers that had been in business 3 to 5 years, to learn about growth rates, programmatic development, and leader perceptions of positives and negatives. Visits with individuals who are well published in the area and considered experts in the health promotion field concluded our initial assessment.

"The data established a consumer need for health promotion services. The data also indicated that establishing our business wouldn't be easy. The executives appreciated and understood the need to allocate resources for health promotion, but it was an area foreign to them and not a high priority. It was evident that employer education was essential, as well as instruction on provider selection.

"Our mission statement was formulated on the basis of our market research. Initially, we served as the marketing arm of University Hospitals to provide a link with the corporate community. Today, our mission has expanded and includes health promotion for University Hospitals' employees, in addition to contractual arrangements with nine other hospitals beyond our immediate service area. The most significant change, however, is our status as revenue center. Now, we are self-reliant."

Barbara utilizes the nursing process as a framework for developing health promotion product lines. Assessment includes an analysis of the employees' environment. The appraisal takes several forms. First, it considers the physical structure in which the employees work. Second, from a human resource perspective, the appraisal considers health care costs related to compensation, injuries, and disabilities. This information, in addition to employee-specific health risk appraisal data, is used to generate a corporate employee health profile of problems and priority programming to address identified needs.

"When we completed our research, developed our initial product lines, and confirmed our strategy, we were ready to hire staff and implement our programs," Barbara reports. Over the past

3 years our staff has grown to 15. It includes seven full-time independent contractors, who teach the smoke cessation and weight control programs, and six full-time staff, in addition to myself and my secretary."

The center employs a salesperson, a nurse counselor, a project coordinator, a program assistant, and an administrative assistant. One position is shared by a nutritionist and a fitness instructor. "The idea of hiring people who were not acute care providers was really an unusual experience for the hospital. We were one of the first departments to hire employees on the basis of skills not directly related to acute care services. We hired the first salesperson in the history of University Hospitals. The group is highly skilled, academically well prepared, and varied in their employment background. They include nurses, respiratory therapists, nutritionists, and clinicians, who have experience in public speaking and curriculum development."

University Hospitals inaugurated its Health Enhancement Center with the tag line "Just for the Health of It." Barbara recalls, "In October 1986 we had six corporate clients and six different community health promotion classes. Today we offer a total of 12 programs and have 24 corporate clients. Our sales promotion needs have declined significantly—the corporations we serve are our referral agents. We use other hospital professional resources when we develop new programs. It is gratifying to know that our service excellence sells itself. Our success is based on sound research, good planning, and strategy development. Because we are in such a new area of service, the implementation process is not always smooth, but we are learning as we go along. Our limited staffing complement has been an advantage—flexibility is key.

"The evaluation component was built in on the front end, so that we could go back in, after the implementation phase was completed, and measure change. This process helps the employer understand how improvement translates into cost savings, and meets our need for measurable outcome data.

"Another way of evaluating our effectiveness has been corporation-to-corporation referral by current and former customers. When we complete a service contract with a corporate client, we establish outcome criteria. They collect and provide some of the data—did we represent ourselves well, did we meet the needs, and are they pleased with the outcome? Some programs are provided to enhance morale, so we measure against this criteria. Frequently outcome criteria are related to productivity. Written feedback is always provided to each client on the predetermined criteria.

"I am often asked to discuss our strengths and weaknesses —why do corporations buy from us? First and foremost, the name and image of University Hospital work in our favor. On the other hand, it's a double-edged sword, because it generates high expectations we must meet to achieve customer satisfaction.

"Second, our medical staff leadership speaks to current developments in all aspects of health care and assists the staff in developing response programs, This means we can short-cut some of the laborious data gathering and developmental aspects by working directly with the experts. Third, and most important, we are client oriented, market driven, and service sensitive. The staff keeps in touch with the customer and focuses on individual needs. We tailor every program to the specific setting in which it is offered.

"Our weaknesses are twofold. First, we are hospital based, and the mindset is acute care and illness. Because wellness is perceived to be at the other end of the continuum, it creates mission variation problems. The challenge of separating our needs and activities from the acute care focus is constantly on our minds. Second, the customers we serve do not want to come to a hospital for wellness programs, particularly one located in the middle of a large city. It takes additional resources and efficient planning to coordinate a business which services clients in outlying areas. Our instructors work from 12 noon to 1 p.m. in one location, 3 to 4 p.m. in another location, and may have a weight control session for another corporate client in a third setting at 5 p.m."

During 1988, Barbara and her staff plan to make a thorough assessment of the total program. The outcomes will be new programs and redevelopment of existing ones. "In our fast-paced environment, you must be aware of what the competition is doing and respond."

Some information sheets on some of the Health Enhancement Center's major product lines are presented on the pages that follow. Given the success that Barbara and her staff have achieved to date, the attainment of future objectives is assured.

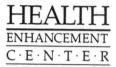

JUST FOR THE HEALTH OF IT

• • • • • • • • • • • •

More than five million Americans now living have a history of cancer; approximately three million of them were diagnosed five or more years ago. Because of early detection and treatment, more people are surviving cancer and living longer lives.

Early detection is the key to preventing and treating cancer. The Health Enhancement Center can teach your employees several detection techniques that will give them an added advantage in fighting cancer.

Cancer Overview
University Hospitals Ireland Cancer Center specialists are available to give your employees a general overview of cancer. During this one-hour presentation, your employees will learn:
• The seven safeguards against cancer
• Methods of detection
• Proper nutrition for preventing cancer.

Colorectal kits that enable employees to screen themselves at home for signs of colorectal cancer are available for distribution at the worksite.

Breast Self-Examination Instruction
Nurses from Univeristy Hospitals Ireland Cancer Center will teach your female employees how to check themselves monthly for breast abnormalities. Employees view a slide and film presentation about breast self-exams and are taught the proper techniques on plastic models.

Testicular Self-Examination Instruction
Ireland Cancer Center healthcare professionals are available to teach your male employees how to check for early warning signs of testicular cancer. Male employees see a slide and film presentation and are taught the proper techniques on a plastic model.

Fee
Fee depends on the number of sessions and participants. Corporate rates are available.

University Hospitals
of Cleveland

Figure 13-6 Health Enhancement Center program information.

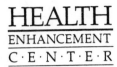

HEALTH
ENHANCEMENT
C·E·N·T·E·R

JUST FOR THE HEALTH OF IT

Personal Health
Appraisals

. . . .

These medically designed computer appraisals let employees know what their current health status is and identify risk factors that are precursors to disease, premature death and disability. Health Enhancement Center professionals use the computer results to develop personalized programs that help employees get back on the path to good health. Each employee receives a summary of the results, and employers receive a group profile that quantifies the major health risks of their employees.

All appraisals are confidential and may be performed at the worksite or in other group settings. There are two types of appraisals available: Health Age and RISKO Appraisal.

Health Age Appraisals
By answering questions about one's health and lifestyle, employees receive computer results that determine their health risks and "health age" as compared to one's actual age. The computer also calculates an "achievable age" that can be reached by changing lifestyle habits. A smoker, for example, may be able to add seven years to his or her life by quitting smoking.

The Health Age Appraisal is a good tool for motivating employees to change their lifestyle and improve their health. Employers receive a group profile with suggestions for improving employees' general health.

RISKO
RISKO is an appraisal system specifically designed to assess cardiovascular risk and is best used after screening with the Health Age Appraisal.

By answering questions related to health, heredity, diet and stress, employees receive personalized appraisals that are produced by a computer. The computer identifies health risks and risk patterns and makes recommendations for preventing heart disease.

Fee
Fee depends on the type of appraisal used and the number of participants. Corporate rates are available.

University Hospitals
of Cleveland

Figure 13-6, continued.

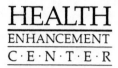

HEALTH
ENHANCEMENT
C·E·N·T·E·R

JUST FOR THE HEALTH OF IT

Nutrition Education —
Eating Right for Life

• • • • • • • • • • • •

Poor nutrition is linked to many chronic diseases, such as cancer, heart disease, hypertension and diabetes. "Eating Right for Life" can help your employees increase their nutritional awareness and encourage them to develop good eating habits that will help them maintain and improve their health.

The program is divided into eight, 30-minute sessions that are conducted twice a week for four weeks. The sessions are led by a registered dietitian on staff at University Hospitals of Cleveland.

Session I: Why All The Talk About Nutrition?
Session II: Keeping Calories Under Control
Session III: Eating Well With Less
Session IV: Carbohydrates — You Need More Than You Think
Session V: Supplemental Vitamins and Minerals — Are They Necessary?
Session VI: Salt — Are We Eating Too Much?
Session VII: Healthy Eating Away From Home
Session VIII: Changes for Life — A Look at Changes Made and Those Planned For the Future

Fee
Fee depends on number of sessions and participants. Corporate rates are available.

University Hospitals
of Cleveland

Figure 13-6, continued.

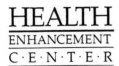

HEALTH
ENHANCEMENT
C·E·N·T·E·R

JUST FOR THE HEALTH OF IT

**Blood Pressure
Screening**

Employees with high blood pressure miss work 17 percent more often than other employees due to illness and disability. High blood pressure not only causes absenteeism, it also increases insurance costs $400 per year for employees with hypertension. If left untreated, high blood pressure [hypertension] can cause strokes, heart attacks, kidney problems and premature death or disability.

Detection is the first step in preventing high blood pressure. The Health Enhancement Center can screen all your employees for high blood pressure at the worksite. If an employee is found to have high blood pressure, we will direct them to their personal physician or a University Hospitals of Cleveland physician who will help them reduce their blood pressure level to an acceptable range.

Fee
The fee depends on the number of participants. Corporate rates are available.

University Hospitals
of Cleveland

Figure 13-6, continued.

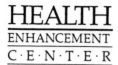

HEALTH
ENHANCEMENT
C·E·N·T·E·R

JUST FOR THE HEALTH OF IT

By surveying your employees, we can learn their health needs and areas of concern. Once these are identified, our health professionals are available for brown bag seminars during employee lunch breaks. The lunch hour provides an informal atmosphere for employees to learn more about good health and preventive measures that can be used at work or in the home.

Brown Bag Seminars

University Hospitals of Cleveland professionals, including physicians, nurses, nutritionists and clinical psychologists are available to discuss any of your employees' health and lifestyle concerns. Some topic examples include:

- Nutrition Education
- Stress Management
- Heart Disease
- Women's Health
- Men's Health
- Parenting
- Cancer Detection
- Prevention of Sports Injuries
- Fitness

Brown Bag Seminars are tailored to fit the needs of your employees.

Fee
Fees depend upon the frequency of the program and the number of participants. Corporate rates are available.

University Hospitals
of Cleveland

Figure 13-6, continued.

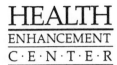

HEALTH
ENHANCEMENT
C·E·N·T·E·R

JUST FOR THE HEALTH OF IT

• • • • • • • • • • • •

Be Trim is a sensible approach to weight loss. Through changes in lifestyle, Be Trim can help your employees lose weight permanently. Participants learn how to lose weight steadily over time rather than through endless diet/weight-gain cycles. They'll also learn about the pyschology and physiology of eating and how to make positive food choices based on sound nutritional information.

Be Trim

Be Trim is a seven-week, 10-session program, which can be modified for each worksite.

Staff
Be Trim instructors are University Hospitals health professionals specially trained in conducting weight control programs.

Results
Studies show that a year after completing Be Trim, between 58 and 64 percent of the participants are either maintaining their weight loss or are continuing to lose weight.

Fee
Phase I: Introductory session — free
Program fee: $95 to $150

University Hospitals
of Cleveland

Figure 13-6, continued.

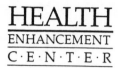

JUST FOR THE HEALTH OF IT

• • • • • • • • • • •

Smoke Stoppers is a multi-component, three-phase program that helps smokers put out their cigarettes for good. Phase I prepares individuals psychologically and physically for smoke cessation. Phase II provides participants with the actual techniques, guidance and structure necessary for quitting smoking. Phase III is a support forum that addresses transition needs and facilitates other lifestyle changes that make quitting smoking easier.

Smoke Stoppers is a five-week, nine-session program, which can be modified for each worksite.

Smoke Stoppers

Program Staff
Smoke Stopper instructors are University Hospitals of Cleveland health professionals who are former smokers and are specially trained in conducting Smoke Stoppers.

Results
Smoke Stoppers is a nationally proven program with up to a 70 percent success rate in smoking abstinence at the end of one year.

Fee
Phase I — Introductory Session: Free
Program fee: Corporate rates available.

University Hospitals
of Cleveland

Figure 13-6, continued.

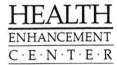

HEALTH
ENHANCEMENT
C·E·N·T·E·R

JUST FOR THE HEALTH OF IT

• • • • • • • • • • •

I. Health Information Center
The Health Information Center is a bulletin board that can be displayed in high traffic areas in the worksite. Cafeteria, time clock areas and company information centers are ideal locations for the Health Information Center. Each Center contains:
• Health posters
• Health and wellness program schedules
• Health information bulletins
• Brochures

Posters, schedules and brochures are changed at regular intervals. Employees become accustomed to checking the colorful Health Information Center for health information and health tips. The give-away brochures and program schedules help stimulate participation in community and worksite programs.

Employee Communications

II. Payroll Stuffers
Payroll stuffers are an easy and inexpensive way to provide your employees with health tips and information about Health Enhancement Center programs. These payroll stuffers are available for distribution by calling the Health Enhancement Center at **844-3850**.

Fee
Fee depends on the number of employees. Corporate rates are available.

University Hospitals
of Cleveland

Figure 13-6, continued.

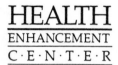

HEALTH
ENHANCEMENT
C·E·N·T·E·R

JUST FOR THE HEALTH OF IT

• • • • • • • • • • •

Aching backs are often the result of using the wrong muscles at the wrong times. Preventive measures can help keep your employees walking tall.

The Health Enhancement Center's Back Injury Prevention Program can help your employees prevent back injuries, thereby reducing medical costs, worker's compensation claims and lost productivity time.

The program consists of three sessions that are conducted at the worksite by University Hospitals of Cleveland health professionals.

Session I: A one-hour session that consists of a pretest, an audio-visual presentation titled "Understanding Your Back," and an explanation of the back's anatomy and biomechanics.

Session II: A one-hour session that includes a review of Session I; instruction in lifting techniques; instruction in proper sleeping, posture, sitting and standing positions; and a slide presentation that identifies ways to avoid back injury at work.

Session III: A one-hour practice session of preventive back exercises.

Session IV: [For supervisors only] A one-hour session that teaches supervisors how to reinforce proper posture and lifting techniques to their employees.

Back Injury Prevention

Written material is included in the program, i.e. exercise booklets, back injury prevention booklets, industrial workbooks and reinforcement posters.

Fee
Fee depends on the number of sessions requested and the number of participants.

University Hospitals
of Cleveland

Figure 13-6, continued.

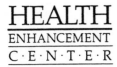

JUST FOR THE HEALTH OF IT

Background Documentation

Video display terminals [VDTs] are now an integral part of automated office environments. There are an estimated five to 10 million VDTs in use and seven million VDT operators in the United States. According to projections for 1990, more than three-fourths of all office employees will do jobs that call for work on some types of computors or VDTs.

Alleged health risks associated with VDTs are of primary concern to VDT operators and union leaders. These risks include reproductive changes, vision changes, radiation exposure, musculoskeletal problems, headaches and stress.

The Health Enhancement Center's VDT program is designed to meet the needs of VDT operators. Staff from the Health Enhancement Center draw from University Hospitals Departments of Psychology, Occupational Therapy and Ophthalmology to work together to address the unique concerns of VDT operators.

The program offers an opportunity to provide risk reduction activities to VDT operators and assess the effects of these activities on the productivity, morale, number of health-related complaints and absenteeism.

The VDT program consists of seven sessions over a nine-week period.

Fee

Fee depends on the number of participants. Corporate rates are available.

**Health Program
for Video Display
Terminal Operators**

University Hospitals
of Cleveland

Figure 13-6, continued.

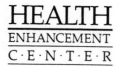

HEALTH
ENHANCEMENT
C·E·N·T·E·R

JUST FOR THE HEALTH OF IT

We all experience stress in some form or another. But too much stress can lead to physical disabilities, such as heart attacks and depression. Since stress affects one's attitude and productivity, it's important for your employees to not only have sound bodies, but sound minds as well. Clinical psychologists and nurses from University Hospitals of Cleveland can help your employees overcome their stresses. After identifying your employees' stresses, our health professionals develop personalized stress management programs tailored to fit their needs. An employee who is laid off and an employee who has too much work to do both have different stresses that need to be managed in different ways.

Fee
Fee depends on the number of sessions and participants. Corporate rates are available.

Stress Management

University Hospitals
of Cleveland

Figure 13-6, continued.

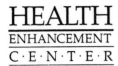

HEALTH
ENHANCEMENT
C·E·N·T·E·R

JUST FOR THE HEALTH OF IT

• • • • • • • • • • • •

The range of work-related health problems and concerns has grown tremendously in recent years due to the vast array of exposures and ever-changing industrial processes. In addition, the Hazard Communication laws have provided both employers and employees with much more information on exposures than was previously available. Many questions and concerns are now being raised about the health effects of workplace exposures.

The University Hospitals of Cleveland Occupational Health Center brings together various specialists to address these questions and concerns. The center provides consultations based on firm scientific and medical evidence to address work-related health problems. Our multidisciplinary team includes board-certified Occupational Medicine physicians, industrial hygienists, epidemiologists, toxicologists, pulmonologists, dermatologists and other healthcare professionals. The type of problem will determine the composition of the evaluation team that provides any or all of the following:

• Worksite evaluations
• Consultations on workable remedies
• In-depth assessments of individual cases

The depth of the assessment depends on your needs; some problems can be resolved solely through discussion with an expert over the phone. Worksite visits involve an initial plant walk-through and discussion to pinpoint the issues. Special environmental or worker screening tests may be needed.

Fees depend on the extent of the evaluation, types of testing, number of workers, sites involved and the on-site team staffing.

For more information about Occupational Health Services, call the Health Enhancement Center at 844-3850.

Occupational Health Services

University Hospitals
of Cleveland

Figure 13-6, continued.

Reference

Folger, James C., and Fee, E. Preston. 1987. *Product management for hospitals: organizing for profitability,* Chicago: American Hospital Publishing, pp. 11-12.

Review Questions

1. Select three of the vignettes presented in this chapter. Compare and contrast the means by which the market opportunity was identified and a program implemented. Why did one approach "work" in one situation as opposed to another?

2. "To market successfully, you must be in a market-sensitive organization." Identify and discuss how the nurses in this chapter were supported in their marketing efforts by those with whom they work.

3. How did each of the nurses involved in the marketing programs in this chapter evaluate the effectiveness of their efforts?

4. Discuss the advantages and disadvantages of utilizing a franchised marketing program. What circumstances, organizationally and market wise, might lend themselves to such an approach?

Chapter 14

The Nursing Education Marketplace: Challenge and Opportunity

The philosophy and science of marketing are indispensable in today's educational marketplace. Two major factors are responsible for education's enhanced interest in marketing. First, the competitive health care arena requires the development of skills previously foreign to clinicians, educators, and administrators. The programmatic and curriculum implications that flow from this circumstance are profound. Second, the education industry is dealing with its own unique set of marketplace forces in the form of enrollment patterns. Nursing education is and will continue to be affected by these factors.

Now as never before, nursing education is operating in a volatile environment. The problem of attracting and retaining a sufficient number of consumer-conscious students is a matter of national concern. Against this backdrop, higher education strives to address the problem of diminishing economic resources through greater cost-effectiveness, while the health care system itself undergoes fundamental change. These circumstances offer powerful incentives for education to utilize the marketing process. The single most important challenge facing nursing faculty today is to turn enrollments around (Figure 14-1).

This chapter reviews the factors shaping the educational marketplace, briefly explores the effect of health care system transition on nursing education, and illustrates marketing concepts and principles by highlighting creative, responsive, and applicable faculty activities and research.

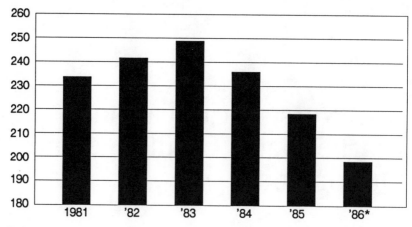

*Preliminary

Source: American Nurses' Association

Figure 14-1.

The Educational Environment

Admissions to generic nursing programs have fallen dramatically since 1984. Gothler and Rosenfeld (1986) conducted a retrospective study of admission, graduation, and enrollment data from National League for Nursing annual surveys. Their findings illustrate the challenge and opportunity open to nursing educators and nursing education.

In 1985, 118,200 students entered basic nursing programs. In 1986, admissions fell to approximately 83,000, an 8.8% decrease in the space of one calendar year. This reduction followed an equally dramatic 9% decline between 1984 and 1985. As yet, enrollment trends do not show signs of turning around.

Diploma schools of nursing are the hardest hit. Over the past 22 years these schools have experienced a steep decline in admissions, enrollments, and graduations. Between 1961 and 1971, enrollment fell from 95,983 to 70,990, and during the next 10-year period it went to 41,009. Since 1981, graduations have fallen by 30,000 — a 26.4% drop through 1986. Of the 209 diploma programs currently accredited by the National League for Nursing, 45 (21%) are in the process of closing (National League for Nursing, 1987).

Associate degree programs are also experiencing difficulty in attracting and retaining students. Between academic years 1984 and 1985 they sustained an 8% decline in enrollment. On the other hand, whereas hospital-based diploma program graduations have declined over the years, associate degree production has steadily increased. In 1985, 45,000 students completed associate degrees in nursing, a 1.5% increase over the previous year. Overall, however, the trend in associate degree program admissions across the nation is down (Gothler and Rosenfeld, 1986).

Generic baccalaureate program graduations have grown from 19,195 in 1958 to a 1977 peak of 101,430. These programs experienced a 4% decline in enrollment between 1984 and 1985, and graduations decreased 3% between 1979 and 1984. Although the admissions, graduation, and enrollment picture is less dramatic in baccalaureate schools of nursing, the pattern is not evenly distributed. Some programs report dramatic decreases in their admission and enrollment patterns, while others have achieved increases (Gothler and Rosenfeld, 1986).

The factors shaping admission, enrollment, and graduation patterns are many. The number of traditional college-age students is declining; hence competition for them across all of nursing education, as well as from other collegiate programs is increasing. In addition, factors such as the women's movement have resulted in significant social change. Women of all ages have numerous options available, in addition to the traditional careers of nurse, teacher, social worker, secretary, and librarian. A 1986 nationwide survey of college freshmen showed that almost five times as many women plan business careers as nursing careers (*Wall Street Journal*, 1987). Evidence also suggests that registered nurse mothers are steering their children away from a career in nursing. *Nursing Life* (1987) conducted a reader poll of almost 1,000 nurses and asked if they would encourage their children to seek a career in nursing. Respondents were also asked to give three reasons for their choice.

Seventy-seven percent of the respondents reported that they would not encourage their child to consider a career in nursing. The most frequent reasons cited were poor pay, overwork, stress, no respect, no thanks, poor hours, infrequent and unfair promotions, divided professional leadership, lack of power, and an educational system that does not adequately prepare its graduates for the real world.

Eighteen percent of those surveyed stated that they would encourage a nursing career. Their primary reasons centered on the personal rewards realized in nursing, the multiple career track options available, and the transference of nursing skills and competencies to other aspects of life such as motherhood, marriage, and community activities. Finally, when respondents were asked if they would enter nursing again, 57% reported they would not. Only 27% of those surveyed stated that they would select nursing as a career the second time around.

Amid declining enrollments and an image crisis, nursing education faces increased pressure to improve productivity and cost-effectiveness. These factors operated in decisions to discontinue basic nursing programs at Duke University, American University in Washington, D.C., and Boston University. Other universities, such as the University of Nebraska/Lincoln, have waged vigorous and successful campaigns to save their nursing schools. All of these programs experienced enrollment problems, but fiscal pressures in conjunction with negative enrollment patterns have made and will continue to make nursing a convenient target when reduction, retrenchment, and reallocation decisions are mandated.

The Health Care System in Transition

As the system continues to respond to economic, social, political, and technological factors, the demand for registered nurses will intensify. According to the U.S. Department of Labor, the need for nurses will increase 49% between 1982 and 1995. This means that 650,000 additional registered nurses will be needed, making nursing one of the professions providing the highest number of job opportunities through the mid-1990s (*The New York Times*, 1987).

The increasing complexity of technology and hospital-based care; the rapid growth of clinics, free-standing emergency and ambulatory surgery centers, and corporate wellness programs; and the staffing needs of long-term care and home health programs are the major factors affecting the demand for registered nurses. In addition, the knowledge, skills, and experience registered nurses have are attractive, for a variety of reasons, to law firms, insurance companies, health maintenance organizations, and utilization review and risk management services, as well as occupational health and other private industries. The utility of the registered nurse is remarkable.

Demographic trends, social change, an image crisis, constrained educational economic resources, and the restructuring of the health care system have all combined to dramatically affect the demand for and supply of registered nurses in the marketplace. In order to respond, nursing educators and nursing education must utilize the marketing process to identify and design educational products for traditional and nontraditional student target markets; to enhance the desirability of existing programs; to develop effective mechanisms to retain those recruited; and to address the programmatic, curriculum, and continuing education implications generated by the changing health care marketplace.

Marketing incorporates a philosophy and a science. The marketing process provides a framework through which goals and objectives are achieved. Assessment includes gathering background data on the marketplace, its products, the competition, and product distribution. This exercise promotes the identification of opportunities, threats, strengths, weaknesses, and issues that must be addressed.

The marketing plan is defined by establishing measurable objectives related to market share and enrollment targets. Marketing strategies, programs, or activities are used to achieve objectives by outlining what will be done, when it will be done, who will do it, and how much it will cost. Finally, parameters are established to monitor success of the marketing plan.

Utilization of marketing science and philosophy by educators is influenced by many factors. Experts may be retained to formulate a strategic marketing plan, or application of the process may be limited to the judgment of key individuals. Comprehensive application is to be encouraged whenever possible, but one must recognize that multiple factors shape the sophistication of educational marketing activities. The vignettes that follow illustrate how nursing education and educators are responding to these circumstances. Consider the example of the University of Maryland School of Nursing.

Market-Driven Strategic Educational Planning

Susan Bond Chambers, M.B.A.
Marketing Specialist
Office of Evaluation
University of Maryland
School of Nursing
Baltimore, Maryland

Ten years of rapid growth and development, reports Susan Chambers, and constrained economic resources resulted in a need to prioritize educational programs. In essence, states Susan, administration recognized that the School of Nursing could not be all things to all people.

To accurately identify priorities, Dean Nan Hechenberger initiated a strategic planning process. One goal of the planning process was to maintain the school's competitive position in the marketplace. Susan reports that a modified strategic marketing process was utilized as a framework to design and implement a marketing program.

The strategic marketing process at the University of Maryland School of Nursing not only focused on attracting students, but also incorporated the school's various markets and publics such as potential students, current students, alumni, legislators, and health care providers. In addition, the changing nursing education marketplace, the health care environment, competitors, and the school's own strengths and weaknesses were analyzed.

One of the more useful primary data collection methods designed and implemented at Maryland is an applicant survey. It includes information on factors that influence program selection as well as on how the prospective student views the school in specified areas. This instrument is an efficient and effective way to collect ongoing data about the school's image and useful demographics to keep abreast of needs and wants in particular student market segments. Other primary data sources included a marketing survey of graduating students, interviews with administrators and faculty, a retrospective analysis which compared enrollment and program cost and perceptions held by selected market segments. Secondary information was also used extensively in the development of the plan. A review of the nursing literature and of existing school documents was undertaken. The University of Maryland Office of Evaluation conducts numerous investigations on an ongoing basis. The results of these studies provide critical data.

The synthesis process, states Susan, resulted in the specification of market opportunities and threats, organizational strengths and weaknesses, and competitor strengths and weaknesses. From this information, detailed short- and long-range marketing strategies and action plans were developed. The formulation of comprehensive strategic marketing plans is always a time-consuming and costly process, and that established by the University of Maryland was no different. Susan reports, however, that with a developmental framework and strategic marketing plan in place, a periodic update based on monitoring of data is all that is required. Once marketing activities become an ongoing part of operations, efficiency is realized. The major benefit, however, at least from Susan Chambers' perspective, is the acceptance of the marketing process by the faculty and the recognition of market factors in tailoring programs and developing teaching and learning strategies.

Customer-Oriented Educational Programming

Kathryn Wood, Ph.D., R.N.
Associate Professor
Department of Nursing
State University of New York/Brockport
Brockport, New York

A less sophisticated but equally effective example of educational marketing can be found in Brockport, New York. While this effort may be short on marketing science, it is strong on marketing philosophy and is included to illustrate that effective initiatives can be developed without big budgets and formal analytical activities.

Kay Wood begins discussing the "customer orientation" of the SUNY/Brockport School of Nursing faculty by asserting that she wants to share how the faculty got involved in "bringing education to R.N.s." The SUNY/Brockport marketing story begins in 1971. At that time, the graduating class consisted of three students, one of whom was an R.N.-to-B.S.N. student. By 1975 the number of R.N.-to-B.S.N. students had substantially increased, and a full-time coordinator was hired.

Contact between the generic and R.N. students began to decline when the coordinator was employed, and today, Kay states, they seldom see one another. "We believe that these students need to have classes by themselves, because they are a unique group, and educational instruction must be modified to meet their needs."

When you place nurses with 5, 10, 20 and more years of nursing experience, Kay argues, with those whose clinical and life experiences are limited, the R.N. student is understandably threatened — or perhaps it is better to say embarrassed, demeaned, and angered by the ego message that such a practice sends. The sensitive, consumer-oriented practice adopted at SUNY/Brockport provides an instructional approach that recognizes and responds to who the students are, what they are, and what they need. This approach brought almost 150 students to the SUNY/Brockport program by 1975. Such practices continue to attract students today.

The faculty's approach to the R.N. market, Kay reports, was modified again in 1979 when a new program director came to the Brockport campus. Increased service to the R.N. student became an academic goal. Programmatic initiatives resulted in meetings between faculty and nurse executives in the community. The purpose of the meetings was to establish how SUNY faculty could better meet the educational needs of working registered nurses. These meetings resulted in the establishment of a community advisory committee and in curriculum revision.

The curriculum revision process took the better part of 2 years to complete and implement. Its key feature was a modular framework, which offered students the option of either testing out of or challenging entire components of the curriculum. "Even with the introduction of a curriculum which was much more acceptable to the R.N. student, and in many respects shaped by their feedback," states Kay, "we really did not think that we were doing enough for the R.N. student."

Meetings were scheduled at a local hospital, and a decision was made to offer introductory statistics on site. This course was selected in order to support the next course offering: nursing research. Needless to say, the acquisition of analytical skills and an understanding of the research process promoted staff development — a win/win scenario for all parties.

The mix of hospital-based classes includes not only nursing courses but general education credits as well. Lower division credit courses are offered by a community college. This practice, Kay reports, is consistent with the policy of using local educational institutions to teach satellite courses where demand exists. Because of the overwhelming success and acceptance of on-site courses, Kay has begun to work with other hospitals to develop similar programs.

Meeting the needs of student consumers is an integral aspect of the faculty's objectives at SUNY/Brockport. This value was established prior to any concerns or incentives created by declining enrollments. The faculty, Kay states, is committed to providing professional education to nurses prepared at the associate and diploma levels. There are times, Kay admits, when she has asked herself why the faculty has such an outward and flexible orientation. She believes it is related to their strong belief in baccalaureate education as the professional-level credential and the fact that many faculty members began their careers as nursing assistants, licensed practical nurses, and diploma graduates.

Self-awareness, enriched by an application and projection of need and responsiveness, serves this faculty well. Feeling tones and human sensitivity are valid marketing ingredients.

Curriculum alterations and programmatic initiatives are appropriate marketplace responses, but faculty members are understandably cautious when they believe that educational objectives are in jeopardy. The next vignettes summarize how two professors conducted educational research in order to validate program changes and instructional design. Neither of these research projects was directly motivated by marketing objectives. They are presented here for two reasons: First, they represent a commitment to quality, and second, the need for research will grow as educational experimentation increases in response to the competitive environment.

Nursing Education Research and Student-Oriented Marketing

Sharon Bea Cannon, Ed.D., R.N.
Director of Nursing Staff Development
University of Alabama Hospital
Birmingham, Alabama

Sharon Cannon admits that she was not primarily motivated by marketing objectives, declining enrollment, cost containment, or the changing health care marketplace when she began her research on instructional methods and R.N. students. She was, however, bothered by an attitude she repeatedly encountered in this student group, which she describes as the "What are you going to teach me" posture. Further, she was searching for a dissertation topic, one that interested her and one that would make a contribution to the nursing education knowledge base. Interest in her students formed the basis on which she built her research.

"During a span of several academic years, I kept meeting students with the same feelings. They didn't want to be treated like generic, basic students, and they thought that their clinical nursing experience was worthy of recognition. At the same time, the University of Missouri School of Nursing faculty, where I was employed, had embraced the fundamental philosophy of adult learning—that adults are self-directed, motivated, and that they have a repository of knowledge to share."

Sharon Cannon's research was designed to compare the effects of the lecture and discussion method of instruction, rather traditional in its approach, with the effects of an individualized method of instruction for R.N. students. The individual instruction method emphasized the concepts and principles of adult learning. The formal hypothesis of Sharon's study was that R.N. students taught by an individualized method of instruction would master more of eight selected communication constructs than R.N. students taught by a lecture-and-discussion method.

Sharon's subjects were readily available—they were R.N. students at the University of Missouri School of Nursing. She prepared a course syllabus for the experimental group which included a self-learning package for each of the eight communication constructs taught in the course. The eight modules contained the learning objectives, all the lecture material available to the traditional student group, a list of learning-related activities, and a self-administered guide for assessing progress. The entire package was introduced with information on self-instruction and usage directions.

At the time each student was given the learning package, an individual contract was developed. The process of establishing the contract involved a review of the course objectives, identification by the student of those objectives previously mastered, and where and how the student had acquired the knowledge. The student was then asked to develop individually specific objectives within the scope of the course constructs.

The experimental group also developed a clinical contract. It identified their learning objectives, the resources they would use in meeting the objectives, and the learning strategy. Sharon also required each student to identify what factors would signal achievement and what criteria she would use in evaluating performance. Finally, the group was asked to indicate what helped or hindered learning and any course content areas requiring further development.

Two instruments measured student perceptions about instructional methods and actual mastery of course content. A statistically significant difference was found between the two groups regarding the instructional methods. In other words, the two instructional methods used were seen as fundamentally different by the students. An evaluation of the relationship between the instructional methods and student mastery could not be undertaken, since students in both sections mastered all eight of the course constructs.

The key marketing question becomes one related to student satisfaction with course instructional methodology. In other words, from a marketing perspective, which instructional method yielded the most significant degree of student satisfaction? One of Sharon's research tools did gather information regarding student satisfaction with instructional methodology. The analysis of this item demonstrated that the course based on adult learning principles resulted in a more satisfied customer. Perhaps more important, again from a marketing framework, the study verified that different methods can yield a similar product — an educated student.

Market-Driven Faculty Research

Helen F. Marsh, R.N., Ed.D.
Retired from University of Wisconsin-Madison
School of Nursing
Madison, Wisconsin

In many respects the philosophical essence of marketing is responsiveness to perceived need — the engineering of satisfaction. Dr. Helen Marsh and two of her colleagues at the University of Wisconsin-Madison — Dr. Patricia Lasky, R.N., and Marilynn D. Jenkins, B.A. — tested the educational impact of the programmatic modifications designed to respond to the learning needs of registered nurses.

Registered nurses, as cited above, bring diverse backgrounds to baccalaureate education. They not infrequently express concern that R.N.-to-B.S.N. programs do not acknowledge the rich and varied backgrounds of these students. By increasing the educational options available to these students, this faculty responded to student need.

In the late 1970s, a study group made up of School of Nursing faculty at the University of Wisconsin-Madison closely examined the concerns of R.N.-to-B.S.N. students and faculty. As a result, recommendations for increased program planning flexibility were developed. This, Dr. Marsh states, was the beginning of a process that resulted in substantial modification of the R.N.-to-B.S.N. curriculum and provided an opportunity for evaluation.

The study group reported that R.N. students expressed dissatisfaction about instructional methodologies specifically designed for generic students; they felt a need for new content and educational experiences that would expand their knowledge and skill as clinicians. Also, as a group of adult learners they felt that their educational needs varied from those of the traditional learner.

In response, the faculty developed three curriculum options. First, exemptions from selected course requirements were offered where evidence of prior learning existed. These courses included such introductory sciences as anatomy, bacteriology, and chemistry. Pharmacology, under specific circumstances, was also exempted. Dr. Marsh reports that the decision to allow these exemptions was based on faculty assessment of an adequate knowledge base achieved in science courses taught in a noncollegiate setting. They judged that learning experiences beyond graduation and professional practice had enabled the students to master the course content.

The second choice was an expansion of opportunities for credit based on prior learning. When that learning had taken place in a comparable institution, transcript review and course equivalency tables were used as convenient and expeditious mechanisms for transfer of credit. Nursing courses taken by students in other baccalaureate programs were reviewed by faculty on an individual basis, and comparable credit was transferred. Credit by examination, using standardized or teacher-made tests, was also made available for selected courses.

A portfolio option was also offered as a credit mechanism for selected courses. The portfolio provided a means by which students could validate learning outcomes consistent with collegiate expectations. In essence, it served as an alternative to a paper-and-pencil test. Portfolio preparation methods and requirements were included in the baccalaureate program orientation course. The third and final option was substitution for selected courses required in the generic curriculum. This alternative provided the students with an opportunity to address their individual needs.

These curriculum alternatives generated questions about their impact on programs of study. Helen Marsh and her colleagues developed three questions to guide their research on R.N. student groups before and after the curriculum options were introduced:

1. How are the R.N. student's total program and nursing credits affected by exercising one or more options?

2. What differences can be identified between the programs of R.N. students admitted prior to 1980 and those admitted after?

3. What patterns of option use can be identified?

Dr. Marsh reports no change in credits granted on the basis of transcript review. Credits based on examination, however, did increase. The difference was explained by the portfolio option. In fact, Dr. Marsh states, all R.N. students used this method when it became available. The portfolio accounted for 16% of total program credits and 41% of credits related to nursing courses. A dramatic change occurred in the number of course substitutions. Almost half of the students took advantage of this option, compared to 13% before the program modifications.

The time required to complete degrees decreased slightly, although precise statistics are not available because part-time study complicated the issue. Attrition in the new program increased over time. Dr. Marsh and her colleagues are examining this area to identify the cause. A small increase in advanced-standing course credits did occur, and academic achievement, as measured by grade point average, was not adversely affected.

In an environment of declining enrollments, faculty should examine current academic requirements in relation to study perceptions. This early work by the Wisconsin faculty serves as an example of how educational objectives can be met without compromising quality. One of the challenges ahead is to develop creative and responsive program options that will make the educational product more competitive in the academic marketplace.

Pam Maraldo, Ph.D., R.N., Executive Director of the National League for Nursing, states that in order to successfully recruit students, educators must attend to the demands of the marketplace. She argues that nursing education must acknowledge that the marketplace defines the product. Faculty, she states, must engage in an emotional transition to offer nontraditional educational experiences. Dr. Maraldo argues that there is nothing more powerful in the marketplace than customer satisfaction — in this case students who feel that their needs have been met and that they are well prepared for the working world (Maraldo, 1987).

Drs. Pam Baj and Marcia Bradley of the University of San Francisco and the University of Wyoming, respectively, share their nontraditional marketplace responses in the following vignettes.

Educational Market Segmentation

Pamela A. Baj, R.N., D.N.Sc.
Associate Professor
University of San Francisco
San Francisco, California

The University of San Francisco, founded in 1855, was the first institution of higher education established in San Francisco and the third in California. The Jesuit tradition of scholarship and dedication to the humanities is the foundation for all academic programs. This aspect of the educational mission is reflected in the School of Nursing program. Since its establishment in 1957, states Dr. Pam Baj, over 3,000 students from diverse backgrounds have received their baccalaureate degrees in nursing from the university.

Despite this background of tradition and pride in service to the community, the School of Nursing found its enrollment declining. Besides the general impact of this phenomenon across the entire country, the University of San Francisco, Pam says, experienced competition for students from other area schools, principally two other Bay Area baccalaureate programs at Samuel Merritt and Dominican. Thus, the challenge was how the school could position itself in the undergraduate marketplace, meet community obligations, and recruit a sufficient number of students.

The faculty recognized that, as society moves from an industrial base to a service base, markets develop for educational programs that recognize prior academic achievement. One strategy developed by this faculty is designed to attract individuals with baccalaureate degrees in other fields who for one reason or another want to make a career change. The dean, administration, and faculty wanted to seize the opportunity, by presenting professional nursing as one viable option to these prospective students. In addition, says Pam, "we knew that the U.S. Department of Labor estimated that registered nurse demand would increase by 49% between 1982 and 1995." The critical market factors were present, and faculty and administration wanted to position the school competitively in the educational marketplace. Today, states Pam, the market assessment and planning have paid off. She credits the dean's vision for the program's success.

The Accelerated Second Baccalaureate Program in Nursing at the University of San Francisco School of Nursing is an option for the individual who wants to make a career change to the nursing profession. Eligible candidates can complete the course work in a period of 15 months, once prerequisite courses in human anatomy, human physiology, microbiology, chemistry, statistics, and sociology are completed. Some candidates who come from other health care occupations such as medical technology already meet many of these requirements.

The program's academic content mirrors the traditional 4-year program, but the timing is accelerated. Applicants must have a baccalaureate degree from an accredited institution and an overall grade point average of at least 3.0 on a 4.0 scale. Clinical courses begin in the first academic period and comprise nearly half of the total credits. A wide variety of community health and acute care agencies are used as clinical practice sites. Graduates of the program, states Pam, accept positions in ambulatory care centers, home health agencies, hospitals, and nursing homes. Upon completion, they are eligible for licensure by examination.

"As a group," states Dr. Baj, "these students demonstrate high academic achievement and success on state board examinations. Although formal mechanisms for longitudinal follow-up are not yet developed, informal feedback from graduates indicates that their new careers are satisfying and rewarding." The dean and the faculty are developing mechanisms — surveys and interviews — to further analyze this target educational market. "Programmatic promotion is," Pam reports, "under development and directed at increasing our visibility. With additional promotion and the good word that our graduates are spreading, we believe the program has a bright future."

Graduate Education Innovation and Creativity

Marcia Bradley Dale, Ed.D., R.N.
Professor, University of Wyoming
School of Nursing
Laramie, Wyoming

The University of Wyoming is located in a sparsely populated rural state. It is the only public higher education institution in the state and has responsibility for meeting the educational needs of approximately 3,000 Wyoming registered nurses. This is the way that Dr. Marcia Dale sets the stage to tell her story about how an innovative and responsive graduate program was developed. The faculty, Dr. Dale reports, found by analyzing demographic data and through informal networks that there was an opportunity to help baccalaureate-prepared nurses in the state move ahead educationally. Because of job and family responsibilities, however, they could not leave their communities and move to Laramie.

To address the needs of these nurses, the faculty began working on a weekend master's program, which was first offered in 1982. Graduate school enrollment increased from 4 students in 1980 and 2 in 1981, to 9 in 1982, 14 in 1983, and 17 in 1985.

At Wyoming the weekend format is defined as Friday evenings from 7 to 10 p.m., Saturday from 8 a.m. to 5 p.m., and Sunday from 8 a.m. to 1 p.m. According to the contract hour formula, a three-credit course meets 48 hours during the semester. The class schedule in planned so that students complete three credits by attending two full weekends and two partial weekends, or six credits in six full weekends a semester.

The graduate program curriculum in rural health nursing is divided into five major components. Sixteen credits involve core courses, which provide a foundation in rural health nursing and the advanced knowledge and specialization necessary for practice. Six credits in clinical practicum are required, and an equal number in role preparation as a clinical specialist, educator, or administrator. The remaining 12 credits are for electives and cognates outside nursing.

When Marcia Dale completed a program evaluation study, a total of 48 students were enrolled. Forty-five completed the questionnaire. She found that 70% of the students were employed full-time in nursing, 76% were married, and 67% had one or more children living at home. Twenty-nine percent commuted between 51 and 150 miles to attend class.

The data verified that the program meets student needs in several ways. Seventy-one percent of the students reported that they enrolled in the master's program because of its scheduling options. It allows them to work while advancing educationally, without relocating. In addition, the physical separation from home is viewed as facilitating learning because it fosters total immersion in the educational process.

Fifty-eight percent stated that they found the weekend format stimulating and challenging. They also viewed course content as meeting perceived learning needs. In particular, the students placed high value on the group's interaction and the network that developed across the state as a result of the program.

The students' written comments highlighted the program's flexibility and the faculty's availability as primary strengths. The data also provided faculty with information about areas needing attention. The students requested extended library hours, better bookstore services, a more consumer-friendly application process for parking permits, and enhanced weekend food services. The class scheduling patterns of other academic departments caused concern. The students experienced difficulty in meeting their elective and cognate requirements because of traditional class times. Intervention across departments by academic administrators is addressing this need.

The impact of this program is being felt across the state of Wyoming. Five of the state's seven community colleges, Marcia Dale reports, have faculty enrolled in the program, and students are making significant changes in nursing service delivery patterns. Some of the student projects involving designing patient care programs are being implemented in communities and various agencies. The program's first four graduates are nurse practitioners; two are employed as school health nurses, and one is employed as a nurse epidemiologist. The program was fully accredited by the National League for Nursing in 1985.

The authors see this program as an example of how the mission of an educational institution and market needs can be skillfully combined to move nursing ahead and better meet the health care needs of Wyoming's citizens. The potential, however, could never have been realized without the efforts of Marcia Dale and the University of Wyoming School of Nursing faculty.

The development of these two educational programs represents only a fraction of the response effort under way. For example, Dr. Dora Eldridge, Dean at the University of South Alabama, has implemented a weekend program for the R.N.-to-B.S.N. student, and she reports that students are coming to Mobile from as far away as New Orleans and Tallahassee, Florida, to attend. The program is also primarily responsible for maintaining current faculty employment levels.

In Arizona and in Rochester, New York, educational leaders are addressing other areas of opportunity. Dr. Claire Parsons, University of Arizona's Dean of Nursing, is designing marketing strategies directed at undergraduates undecided about their major, minorities, and students needing remediation. The future nursing student will require more assistance, she believes, in the form of remediation. Minorities offer nursing programs a target market that can maintain enrollment and not compromise quality. Many of these students, Dr. Parsons asserts, have significant academic potential if deficits are remedied.

Dr. Kay Charron, Program Director, and Dr. Mary Pat Pennell, Dean of Allied Health Sciences at Monroe Community College in Rochester, New York, are developing what they call the S.O.S. Program (Save Our Students). These academic leaders found a high correlation between failure on the first clinical course examination and student dropout. Student recruitment is important, they argue, but student retention must also be addressed. "The program we are developing at Monroe Community College," Kay states, "is designed to address this area of need."

Other academics, such as Doris Lippman and Karen Ponton, are conducting research that is aimed at better understanding nursing's perceived image problem. Their study is included here to facilitate research networking and to communicate that perception is not necessarily reality.

Image as a Promotional Concept

Doris T. Lippman, R.N., Ed.D.
Associate Professor
Fairfield University
School of Nursing
Fairfield, Connecticut

Karen S. Ponton, R.N., M.A.
Executive Director
Connecticut Nurses'
  Association
Meriden, Connecticut

What can be more important to professionals than their image? Although the answer seems rather obvious, it is only recently that nursing has concentrated, in a proactive sense, on this all-important area. As enrollments continue to decline and practicing nurses move away from acute care into other career paths, image issues are paramount. The image of nursing—that held by nurses and by others—has much to do with promoting nursing as a worthy career. Studies that examine nursing's image provide information that separates fact from fiction. Doris Lippman and Karen Ponton conducted such a study. The results of these studies can assist in strategic planning designed to enhance nursing's image.

Doris and Karen tested the image of nursing portrayed in the mass media. While media influence on nursing's image cannot be underestimated, little research has been done on whether the public actually agrees with the image created by the mass media. This study asked the question: What is the image of nursing held by university faculty?

The mass media image of nursing is stereotypic, sexist, and derogatory. Television, motion pictures, and trade publications also present a highly negative nursing image. Television is the medium with the greatest impact today. Ninety-eight percent of American households own at least one television set, and Americans average 30.6 hours of television viewing per week. Beatrice and Philip Kalisch (1982a) reported that television nurse characters score highest on the characteristics of obedience, permissiveness, conformity, flexibility, and serenity. On the other hand, they found that nurses were seen as equal to physicians on efficiency, organization, and discipline.

Motion pictures also affect nursing's public image. During 1984 and 1985, 234.2 million Americans attended the movies and spent $7.9 billion on tickets. The Kalisches (1982b) reviewed 204 motion pictures and found that nurses were portrayed in them as passive and subordinate.

Books also help shape public opinion and values. The Kalisches (1982c) reviewed 207 novels and found that they pictured nurses as characters who served men as mother, companion, and childbearer. The sexually promiscuous nurse was introduced into novels during the 1960s. This image persists today, particularly in extremely popular romance novels.

Doris and Karen believed that such perceptions if held by university faculty might dramatically affect the socialization of nursing students. They asked their subjects questions directed at better understanding the contact faculty had with media portraying nursing, what contact nonnursing faculty had with nurses and nursing, and how faculty image measured up against the media's image of nursing.

The survey was conducted among 1,000 faculty members in departments other than nursing, who were randomly selected from 19 northeastern universities offering baccalaureate degree nursing programs. They were mailed a questionnaire, developed by Karen and Doris expressly for the study, which contained 42 statements about nursing. The questions were developed from the literature and their experience. The final product was reviewed by a panel of experts for face validity.

A total of 539 faculty members completed and returned the questionnaire, for a 55.1% response rate. The respondents were predominantly white males between the ages of 30 and 59 years. Sixty-six percent (66%) held doctoral degrees, earned between $31,000 and $50,000 a year, and held the rank of associate or full professor.

Overall, the study found that university faculty held a positive image of nursing rather than the negative image portrayed in the mass media. One of the most significant findings was that faculty held nursing in high esteem. More than 80% of the sample agreed or strongly agreed that skilled and knowledgeable nursing care is essential to recovery from an illness. The respondents also reported that they felt nurses were valuable sources of health care information. Seventy percent did not see nurses as physician handmaidens, nor did they feel that nurses practicing without physician supervision were operating in unsafe circumstances. Not only did the sample see nursing as a vital component of the health care system, but they valued nursing's contribution to health-related matters as separate and distinct from that of medicine.

Another group of questions focused on the caring dimension of nursing and its related stereotypes. Respondents did not report a strong bias toward nurses as "angels of mercy," nor did they reinforce the idea that motherhood and nursing are strongly related. Some of the long-held stereotypes about nurses, at least in this group, are beginning to break down.

Nursing and nurses, argue Doris and Karen, must also recognize and respond to the attitude that, "You don't need any brains to be a nurse." This sample held its strongest opinion on this point, with more than 92% expressing disagreement. Further, the sample strongly agreed that nursing education belongs in higher education, as opposed to the apprentice-type programs of the hospital-based era.

Another sexist belief called into question by the study was that nursing is a "female-only" career. Only 10% of the sample agreed with the statement that they never wanted their son to be a nurse, compared to 7% who agreed with the parallel item, "I'd never want my daughter to be a nurse." Even though it appears that faculty would not object to their children becoming nurses, only 42% disagreed that, "Bright young women should study medicine, not nursing." This finding supports the current trend that women are being encouraged to pursue more prestigious careers than nursing.

In summary, this study found that university faculty held a different and more positive view of nursing than that currently presented by the mass media. Nurses are perceived as educated, autonomous, and compassionate individuals, whose role is vital to health care. The findings were influenced, state the researchers, by the high degree of contact the sample reported having with nurses — on the average, 70% reported direct contact with nurses. The implications derived from this finding for every public encounter with nurses is significant.

We are only beginning to understand nursing's image, how it is formed, and how we can affect its formation. Image research forms the basis for marketing plans directed at turning things around. Karen and Doris are ready to assist.

Educators and educational institutions also have a responsibility to transmit nursing's professional culture — its values, attitudes, and beliefs. Generic, graduate, and continuing education students must have an opportunity to learn more about marketing concepts and principles. As stated earlier, Pam Maraldo, Executive Director of the National League for Nursing, has called for an emotional transition in nursing, in order to concentrate energies on marketplace opportunities.

The University of Wisconsin School of Nursing in Milwaukee is one school that has accepted the challenge of emotional transition, by including marketing in their curriculum. According to Super

(1987), "The University of Wisconsin healthcare marketing course is a collaboration between the business community and the nursing school. Richard E. McDonald, President of McDonald Davis and Associates, a Milwaukee healthcare marketing firm, conducts the course with co-instructor Florence Selder, Ph.D., an Associate Professor in the Nursing School." Between 30 and 40 students — graduate, undergraduate, and nurses in continuing education — are enrolled. One of the course objectives is to develop the knowledge and skills required to produce marketing plans. In addition, the course graphically illustrates how marketing concepts and principles interface with nursing services. Although marketing courses are traditionally found in business schools rather than nursing schools, Barbara Redman, Executive Director of the American Association of Colleges of Nursing, reports that nursing schools are increasing marketing course content through collaboration with business school faculty. "We do know marketing is terribly critical in today's marketplace," said Redman (Super, 1987).

At George Mason University School of Nursing in Fairfax, Virginia, Dr. Rita Carty, Dean and Professor, is leading the development of a dynamic curriculum based on marketplace opportunities, which offers new and restructured programs at the baccalaureate, master's, and doctoral levels. The options offered at George Mason now include:

Accelerated B.S.N. pathway for college graduates

Accelerated special pathway for registered nurses

R.N.-M.S.N. pathway

R.N.-nonnursing baccalaureate-M.S.N. pathway

Advanced clinical nursing in chronic care, gerontology, and oncology

Adult and gerontological practitioner in primary care

B.S.N.-nonnursing master's-D.N.Sc.

The educational leadership exercised by the University of Wisconsin and George Mason University schools of nursing supports a positive emotional transition in nursing education. Their leadership, and that of other educators cited herein, is essential in today's health care marketplace and vital to the development of a contemporary professional culture.

References

Fowler, E.M. 1987. Careers: nation's nursing shortage. *The New York Times*, p. 52, December 1.

Gothler, A.M., and P. Rosenfeld. 1986. Nursing education update: enrollments and admission trends. *Nursing & Health Care*, December, pp. 555-559.

Kalisch, P.A., and B.J. Kalisch, 1982a. Nurses on prime-time television. *American Journal of Nursing* 82 (February):265.

Kalisch, P.A., and B.J. Kalisch. 1982b. The image of the nurse in motion pictures. *American Journal of Nursing* 82 (April):611.

Kalisch, P.A., and B.J. Kalisch. 1982c. The image of nurses in novels. *American Journal of Nursing* 82 (August):1220-1221.

Maraldo, P. 1987. Address at the American Organization of Nurse Executives meeting, Anaheim, Calif., September 13.

National League for Nursing. 1987-88. Diploma programs in nursing. *Nursing and Health Care* 8(7):428-429.

Super, K.E. 1987. Many nurses taking a new course: how to take care of hospital's image. *Modern Healthcare* 17(4):100.

Tobin, B.K. 1987. Would you encourage your child to be a nurse? *Nursing Life*, May/June, pp. 42-45.

Tregarthen, T. 1987. This nursing shortage is different. *The Wall Street Journal*, p. 9, November 11.

Waltz, S., S. Bond Chambers, and N.B. Hechenberger. 1988. *Strategically planning marketing and evaluating nursing education and service*. New York: National League of Nursing, in press.

Review Questions

1. After reviewing this chapter and the advice on presentations in Chapter 12, prepare an outline of a brief talk to high school juniors and seniors on the reasons for considering a nursing career.

2. Nurse educators in this chapter identified marketplace opportunities and designed programs to meet identified needs. Select a target market and describe how you would evaluate if the development of an educational program is appropriate.

3. To what extent does the professional autonomy of an educator to design curriculum and program requirements conflict with a student-focused market-driven approach to the development of educational programs at the undergraduate level? the graduate level? Discuss.

4. Compare and contrast nursing education products/ services before and after the enrollment crisis in a nursing school in your area. Identify the alterations and discuss their impact from your perspective.

Chapter 15

Marketing and the Nurse Administrator

The need for knowledgeable and skilled nursing service administrators has never been greater. Health care is in a period of dramatic and fundamental change, driven by the implementation of Medicare's prospective payment system and the growth of alternative delivery systems. The role implications generated by this process are substantial. Change, challenge, and opportunity are the order of the day.

Nurse administrators occupy key leadership positions in the evolving health care system. They can capitalize on the potential their office offers by incorporating marketing philosophy and theory in their practice. The opportunities are plentiful and limitless in scope.

Service excellence is defined by the consumer rather than the provider. Leadership groups identify customers and use the marketing process to assess need, develop and implement responsive products, and evaluate effectiveness. Organizational performance and nursing's professionalization will be shaped by the degree to which nurse administrators embrace this aspect of the cultural change mandated by a health care system in transition.

Nursing administration's customers are many and varied. Patients, families, and physicians can be readily identified as consumers of nursing administration services. The nursing staff and the public at large are less often acknowledged as administrative customers. Recognition of these groups, however, is pivotal if nursing executives are to profit from the opportunities currently available. Administrators, regardless of where they practice, must carry the "close to the customer" banner, by personal example and by incor-

455

porating marketing in every aspect of professional and organizational life.

This chapter presents six examples of how nursing administrators utilize the marketing process. Administrative marketing is as simple as practicing exemplary guest relations or leaving a business card when dealing with patients, families, and physicians. It is as complex as formulating marketing plans or developing policies and procedures to guide patient teaching materials. While one activity may require more knowledge and skill than another, in marketing terms all effort on behalf of excellence is valued and its utilization should be encouraged by those in leadership positions.

The Physician as Customer

Barbara Parrish, R.N., M.S.
Director of Professional Relations
Ingham Medical Center
Lansing, Michigan

In July 1985, Barbara Parrish assumed the position of Director of Professional Relations at Ingham Medical Center (IMC). Hospital administration acknowledged the impact of prospective payment and the competitive environment. They could no longer assume they were meeting consumer needs and concerns. One objective was quite clear: The hospital needed to focus on physicians as customers.

The unique feature of Barbara's position is her target market. She acts as the professional liaison among Ingham, referring physicians, and their office management staff. "I learn about the care patients feel they are receiving, physician perceptions about the quality of service Ingham offers, such as nursing services, and, for example, whether clinical reports are being returned to physicians in a timely fashion." In other words, Barbara is the contact point for any concern involving the relationship between Ingham Medical Center and referring physicians.

"As with any new venture," she reports, "program development was paramount." Role confusion and a lack of understanding were problems Barbara encountered. "It took time," Barbara confides, "before I was consistently seen as a support—a valuable source of customer information. I work closely with the vice-presidents and department heads most directly affected."

When Barbara first began her new job, she visited with administrators of selected hospitals in Ingham's 11-county service area. The purpose of the visit was to introduce herself, explain her position, and communicate Ingham's interest in promoting services that were not available in their facilities. "The administrators were receptive and appreciated that I had taken time to contact them before calling on members of their medical staff." She also found referral physicians pleased by their first office visit, but, "they didn't know quite how to take me, because they had never had anyone ask them what they would like." Barbara travels the hospital's catchment area 3 days a week, visiting physicians, office staff, and hospital personnel. She maintains regular contact, learns about area developments, and identifies market implications. The information is used to develop marketplace responses.

"When I started visiting physicians, I identified problems that made access to IMC difficult. I suggested a number of options, and the hospital decided to implement an 800 number, or referral physician line. This aspect of our program has been very well received by office staff and physicians in our region. They express confidence in our ability to respond and deliver professional service."

When physicians identified transfer resources as a concern, Barbara coordinated a helicopter service between Ingham and referral facilities. "Management was surprised that I could respond to a need so quickly, but I gathered information about existing helicopter services, other resources available to us, comparatively displayed the data for administration, and made my recommendation." The hospital, the medical staff, and referring physicians report a high level of satisfaction with the helicopter service.

To further enhance relationships, Barbara participated in the production of a quarterly magazine. It highlights specific Ingham Medical Center services, features selected referring physicians, and provides information on changing conditions in the marketplace. The magazine is an excellent vehicle through which to promote services and programs. Each edition also highlights a member of Ingham's medical staff and provides information about the associated program. "Also in *Colleagues*, we profile a referring physician. The article is entitled, "Partners in Medical Excellence," and I select the individual who is featured. I work closely with public relations, who actually write the articles, and I provide direction on content, in collaboration with our product line managers."

In addition to marketing Ingham's primary product lines, called "centers of excellence" — cardiology, orthopedics, oncology, and pulmonary services — Barbara supports outlying hospitals by cooperatively developing programs that enhance and promote local health care resources. Ingham cardiologists, for example, staff a cardiovascular van that visits participating area hospitals. It offers echography and peripheral vascular diagnostic services. This service is currently used by seven area hospitals. "I do a lot of follow-up with the clinics and mobile van services we offer, to make sure that reports are returned in a timely fashion."

Barbara has organized two seminars on physician marketing and office management by Greg Korneluk, a nationally recognized expert in this area. This service represents one more effort by the hospital and Barbara to assist IMC medical staff and the referring physician. As Barbara points out, "Our success depends on their success. Many small community hospitals do not have the resources to offer such valuable and timely presentations."

Ingham Medical Center is the first facility in its geographical area to offer external physician marketing. It has provided them with a 2-year marketplace advantage. "It's been interesting," says Barbara, "because I'm approached by other hospitals in our immediate service area about working with them. They are feeling the effects of our marketing program, particularly in relation to our primary product lines. Two of our competitors have recently hired personnel and developed external marketing programs."

The scope of Ingham's external physician marketing program continues to expand. As new product lines develop, and as new physicians enter the referral area, Barbara adds physicians to her roster, so as to constantly update her information system. They are selected because of their past patterns of association with Ingham, current hospital affiliation, and referral pattern. Particular emphasis is placed on developing strong relationships with general practice, family practice, orthopedic, pediatric, and internal medicine physicians in the service area.

The formal description of Barbara's position that follows gives some idea of the scope of her responsibilities.

Position Description
Director of Professional Relations

Summary:

To provide a professional liaison with referring physicians for the purpose of encouraging and facilitating the use of Hospital services and the professional services of the Hospital medical staff.

Responsible for:

1. Visiting the offices of referring physicians on a regular and routine basis for the purpose of:

   a. introducing new Hospital programs or services.
   b. establishing and maintaining a communication link with each physician.
   c. providing feedback to the Hospital on problems, concerns, or suggestions made by the referring physician or his office staff.
   d. assisting referral physicians in resolving Ingham Medical Center-related problems.

2. Planning both strategies and tactics to achieve the goals and objectives of the position.

3. Conducting ongoing analyses and needs assessments for Hospital services for the purpose of suggesting additions, deletions, or modifications.

4. Recommending methods of promoting Hospital programs and services to the referring physicians:

   a. plans the promotion strategy and materials, taking into account the promotion strategies of the Product Line Manager.
   b. suggests, on a yearly schedule, the specific content of regular publications (e.g., *Colleagues*).
   c. works with Public Relations to plan the scheduling and production of routine and extraordinary publications.
   d. reviews and recommends approval for all promotional materials targeted at referring physicians, other than product line information.

e. submits a marketing plan for referring physicians on a yearly basis.

5. Keeping current regarding Hospital programs and services, medical staff programs and services, and the content of the various Hospital product lines.

6. Developing and implementing a monitoring system for physician contacts, physician referrals to Hospital services, physician satisfaction with services, and the appropriateness of referral programs in the service area.

7. Assisting in the promotion of services provided by Ingham Medical Center medical staff.

8. Providing liaison with hospital departments regarding information received from, or forwarded to, referring physicians.

9. Promoting the hospital's continuing education program, seminars, and consultative relationships.

10. Implementing, promoting, and reinforcing the Ingham Medical Center *Code for Caring*.

11. Related duties as defined and determined by the Executive Vice-President and the Associate Vice-President for Planning.

The Community as Customer

Sydney D. Krampitz, R.N., Ph.D.
Associate Dean and Director of Graduate Studies
The University of Kansas Medical Center
School of Nursing
Kansas City, Kansas

Sydney Krampitz's marketing philosophy and its relationship to her profession are best reflected in her community activities. As an educational administrator, she recognizes that broad community support for a professional group is vital to its advancement. "The impact of public support and subsequent funding for the profession," asserts Sydney, "clearly enhance the profession's image and impact the recruitment of well-qualified students to professional schools."

As a new faculty member, in 1981, with major administrative responsibilities, Sydney was increasingly exposed to situations that made her feel that nursing and nurses should more aggressively market their services. She believed that nursing's visibility in the community ultimately affects employment opportunities and shapes student recruitment efforts at both the undergraduate and the graduate level. An effort was needed to change the community stereotype of the nurse as a "handmaiden in white."

Sydney acted on her concern and became involved in a wide range of community activities. She became a board member of the Johnson County Mental Health Center, a member of the American Red Cross Disaster Committee, and Chairman of the Crisis Intervention Committee of the American Red Cross.

"As I became increasingly involved in community mental health programs, it was apparent that psychiatric nurse clinical specialists and other professional nursing personnel were either not utilized or, in the case of the staff nurse, underutilized." An opportunity developed, however, for Sydney to demonstrate how nursing expertise could be used to advance the goals and objectives of the Johnson County Mental Health Center. She led the development of policies that expanded the patient care role of nursing personnel and changed the social worker/nurse staffing mix caring for the chronically mentally ill.

As time went by, she found increased opportunities to make a positive impact on long-standing patient care management problems. Suggestions she made were readily accepted by key staff and members of the board. "The support I received from other members of the board, as well as staff, reinforced by commitment to engage in an ever-increasing range of community activities."

Sydney's American Red Cross volunteer work provided her with a very special community service opportunity in 1987. The situation and her involvement later received media coverage. The following passage from the September 30, 1987, *Kansas City Star* describes background information regarding the incident and how Sydney approached the assigned task.

Counseling Offered to Witnesses of Fire

A few have had nightmares about what they saw. Others have had trouble sleeping or have felt frustration or anger about how their lives have been disrupted.

Most of the people who were in Lucille's Restaurant on the night of September 19th, when former employee Christopher O'Crowley doused himself with gasoline and set himself on fire, have been affected in some way by the incident.

On Tuesday night, the American Red Cross sponsored a counseling session to help some of them understand and deal with feelings that are common to those who have experienced a disaster or traumatic situation.

About 10 employees of the restaurant attended the session conducted by Sydney Krampitz, a psychiatric nurse and clinical specialist at Kansas Medical Center.

Krampitz, who worked with rescue workers and health-care providers after the Hyatt Regency disaster, said it was important for people involved in a traumatic situation to talk about it with others who had shared the experience.

"It's an opportunity for them to share the horror," she said and "It provides them with less of a sense of aloneness. It makes them realize that the things they are experiencing are not unique."

A common thread for many disaster victims is a feeling of loss or a sense of vulnerability, she said.

"They get a sense that anything can happen to you at any time," she said.

Employees of Lucille's lost their jobs because of the fire, which destroyed the restaurant's interior, but most have now found other jobs, one employee said.

The employee, who did not want to be identified, said a Red Cross volunteer talked to employees on the night of the fire but most didn't think they would need counseling.

"It didn't hit us right there," she said. "A few days later we started thinking she was right."

The employee, who said she suffered severe headaches and sleeplessness after the fire, said the incident had changed the way she looked at other people.

"I may not be quite so trusting of my fellow man from now on," she said.

The Red Cross was able to reach only restaurant employees about Tuesday's meeting but has scheduled a session on this Sunday for the estimated 85 patrons who were in the restaurant during the incident. That meeting will be at 7 a.m. at the Red Cross headquarters building, 211 W. Armour Blvd.

The employees who attended Tuesday's meeting also will meet again a week from Sunday, Krampitz said.

It is difficult to measure the impact of Sydney's professional contribution in this community crisis. Certainly, however, the image of nursing was enhanced by her participation. "Marketing a wide range of nursing services to client populations has become the challenge of the 90s. It is only through our efforts as nurses that we can demonstrate to the public our expertise, commitment, and value as a health care provider. Recruitment of highly motivated individuals, retention of committed and skilled practitioners, and continued satisfaction of the public and a positive image of nursing are all goals to be achieved by a concerted marketing effort."

Sydney Krampitz's efforts on behalf of her community and her profession reflect the commitment of one educational administrator to advance nursing practice and enhance nursing's image. Imagine the effect if every nurse in an administrative position emulated her involvement. That's administrative marketing!

The Registered Nurse as Customer

Patricia J. Graham, M.S.N.
Assistant Administrator/Director of Nursing
Mount Vernon Hospital
Alexandria, Virginia

Pat Graham assumed her responsibilities as chief nurse executive just as the impact of the nursing shortage was being felt in Alexandria and the surrounding Washington, D.C., area. In response, she began to work directly with the nursing department's Retention and Recruitment Committee. Committee members included staff nurses and public relations and personnel department representatives.

The group, Pat reports, was looking for a way to promote their department. They felt strongly that the Sunday display ads in Washington's major newspaper were overwhelming to the reader and thus would be relatively ineffective in achieving the goal. The group was looking for a more personal promotion technique.

Since the majority of Mount Vernon's current nursing employees lived in the primary and secondary service areas of the hospital, a decision was made to communicate directly with licensed registered nurses in that geographical area. Access was gained by contacting the Virginia State Board of Nursing and obtaining mailing labels for registered nurses in the primary and secondary service area zip codes.

In the meantime, efforts were directed at developing promotional materials that would be mailed to the registered nurses. A decision was made to personalize the communication and have it come directly from Pat (Figure 15-1). Thus, the Mount Vernon Nursing Department introduced their new director to the nurses who lived in the immediate service area and highlighted the unique departmental features that they offered the R.N. "customer."

Particular emphasis was placed on the hospital's child care facilities, primary nursing, and all-R.N. staff. Included with the letter was additional information on benefits, from health care insurance to preretirement counseling, and how the availability of these benefits was affected by full-time, part-time, or temporary employment status.

Other materials included in the mailing were a map locating the hospital and a self-addressed, postage-paid card for requesting fol-

The Mount Vernon Hospital

2501 Parker's Lane, Alexandria, Virginia 22306

STEPHEN C. RUPP
Administrator

Dear Colleague:

As a nurse working in today's changing healthcare industry, you have many professional opportunities available to you. If you have not already done so, I would like for you to consider working at Mount Vernon Hospital, a stimulating nursing environment near your home.

As a neighbor of Mount Vernon Hospital, you are perhaps aware of the tremendous growth that we have been experiencing. Our average daily census has shown a 20% increase since last year. This growth has occurred in all areas: psychiatry, medicine, surgery and rehabilitation.

As a result of this increase in patient volume, challenging nursing opportunities now exist in both full-time and part-time positions. Besides the satisfaction of working in a friendly environment that appreciates nursing, we are confident that you will also enjoy being associated with us. We offer a wide range of benefits, including an award winning on-site child care center for children aged six weeks to 5 years.

Mount Vernon is a 235-bed hospital founded in 1976. We offer all the services of a community hospital, except for obstetrics, and have an all-RN staff which practices primary nursing. We have an excellent working environment which allows us to provide high quality care to our patients.

If you would be interested in learning more about Mount Vernon Hospital, please call me at 664-7200 for an appointment to see our beautiful facility. Find out what nursing at Mount Vernon Hospital is all about. I look forward to meeting you and sharing with you some of the plans for our future growth and expansion.

Sincerely yours,

Patricia J. Graham

Patricia J. Graham, R.N.
Assistant Administrator

FAIRFAX HOSPITAL ASSOCIATION
A voluntary, not-for-profit corporation
Commonwealth Hospital — The Fairfax Hospital — The Mount Vernon Hospital

Figure 15-1 Promotional letter to registered nurses.

low-up information. This card also contained a checkoff box for inactive nurses interested in a refresher program offered by the hospital. This mechanism gave the hospital an opportunity to evaluate whether there was sufficient demand to warrant implementation of the refresher program.

Pat reports that the response to her letter and the other enclosures has been brisk. There is equal distribution between card return and use of the dedicated telephone line for further information. Most important, this method of promotion was far more cost efficient, states Pat, than newspaper display ads. It is certainly a creative and personal method of communicating with nurses established in the community.

In the future, Pat plans to expand the program by promoting changes and developments that are taking place within the agency and the department of nursing. Also, programs are being formulated for marketing segments that include both new graduates and experienced nurses moving into the area. The staff has expressed satisfaction with the personal nature of the communication and the efforts made by administration to promote the facility.

While this campaign was primarily pointed at recruitment, it also represents a creative technique for introducing a new nursing executive to the registered nurses in the hospital's immediate service area.

An Association as Customer

Phyllis Clancy Sippel, M.A., R.N., C.N.A.A.
Vice President for Nursing Services
Holy Cross Hospital
Fort Lauderdale, Florida

Phyllis Sippel had her first experience with administrative marketing in 1980. Her experience is just as relevant today as it was then.

In 1980, hospitals in Pinellas County, Florida, which includes Tampa and St. Petersburg, were faced with an acute shortage of registered nurses. Seventeen of the 22 facilities in the county participated in a survey to determine the severity of the shortage. Analysis of data revealed 300 full-time equivalent R.N. positions vacant.

The Bay Area Hospital Council (BAHC), whose members included the chief executive officers and chief operating officers of the affected facilities, felt an obligation to respond proactively to the crisis. They retained the services of Arlene Rak, R.N., Vice-President of the Illinois Hospital Association, as a consultant to complete a feasibility study for the council. She had developed a registry in response to similar problems, and published accounts of her experience indicated great success in recruiting registered nurses back into the acute care field. BAHC hoped that the program could be successfully transplanted to Pinellas County. Upon completion of the study, which was enthusiastically supported by the area directors of nursing, Rak recommended implementation of a registry program.

Phyllis was hired by BAHC as the project's Director of Nursing, in July 1980, to develop and implement a not-for-profit registry. "My immediate assignment," states Phyllis, "was to develop a budget, select an office location, formulate policies and procedures, design a logo, obtain the necessary licenses, develop a promotional marketing plan, recruit staff, and determine how to evaluate the program's effectiveness. We managed to accomplish all of these tasks between July 7th and September 8th, when the first registered nurse was assigned to a facility."

The hospitals that supported the program ranged in size from 99 to 745 beds. There were for-profit and not-for-profit hospitals among them, with a variety of nursing care delivery systems as well as of types of units and medical staff support. The program Phyllis developed matched nursing skills, geographic location, and clinician availability with hospital characteristics.

Financial support was provided by the BAHC. "I was the council's second staff member. My salary and benefits and those of my secretary were assumed by the council. Start-up funds were provided by 'taxing' each hospital that intended to utilize registry resources. Fourteen of the 22 facilities in the county initially agreed to participate in the registry project."

The major budgetary item, other than telephone, utilities, licenses, salaries, advertising, and paper goods, was the hourly wage offered registered nurses. In the county, the average R.N. was earning $6.32 an hour, almost $2.00 less than the national average. For-profit registries, Phyllis reports, were just beginning to move into the county. Most of them offered the R.N. between $6.95 and $7.50 an hour. Phyllis settled on $7.25.

The goal, as Phyllis saw it, was to recruit registered nurses back into the field, and simultaneously to ascertain the needs of nurses from an overall perspective, so as to influence wage and benefit packages for all registered nurses. With all these factors in mind, she submitted a $100,000 budget. It was approved by the BAHC.

After finding an office centrally located in Largo, Phyllis set about developing the registry's operating standards. "My goal was to develop a 'Blue Ribbon' agency. As a matter of fact, a blue ribbon became one of the media symbols used in our promotional materials (Figure 15-2)."

Three standards guided the agency's basic operation. First, an agreement with participating hospitals provided a paid orientation period for each agency nurse. Second, experience as a registered nurse and excellent references formed the basic requirements for employment. The agency matched the interests, skills, and experience of the nurses to the hospitals. For example, if a nurse had experience in a teaching hospital and was interested in reentering the teaching environment, the assignment process was almost complete. Finally, written evaluations for each of the first 10 nursing assignments and a summary evaluation every 3 months thereafter were required of each participating facility.

Phyllis designed the agency's logo — an outline of Florida with a star locating Pinellas County (Figure 15-3) — and then turned to promotional activities and staff recruitment. "With a limited budget and an aim to attract nurses from a variety of settings, my marketing activities were basic and demonstrated practicality and common sense.

"I knew that nurses were part of the high tourist concentration in the county and might be interested in creative employment opportunities. They could visit Pinellas County, work three or four shifts a week, and enjoy all that Florida had to offer thereafter." A copy of the letter Phyllis sent to each candidate interested in a working vacation is shown in Figure 15-3. This aspect of the overall program grew, and resulted in many nurses being employed full-time by the hospitals in which they worked.

"I appeared on public television and radio several times. Our not-for-profit status was a major advantage in getting the business community to support promotional activities. I solicited free ads for the agency on radio, television, and in the area newspapers. One local bank agreed to put fliers in their monthly checking account statements, but only after several inquiries and 'sit-ins' outside the

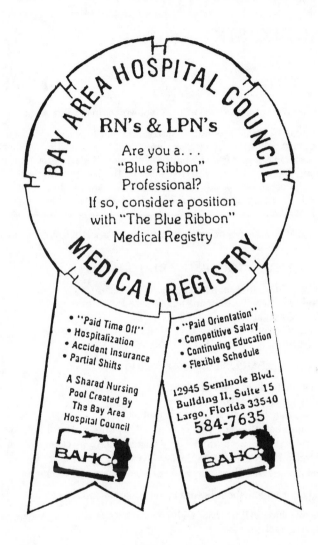

Figure 15-2 Media symbol used in promotional material.

BAY AREA HOSPITAL COUNCIL
MEDICAL REGISTRY

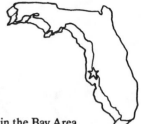

Dear

Thank you for your recent inquiry regarding employment in the Bay Area.

Bay Area Hospital Council, Medical Registry is a not-for-profit Medical registry created by hospitals in Pinellas County. We provide full time and supplemental staff for 14 hospitals ranging in size from 99 beds to 745 beds. We also provide staffing for 2 nursing homes. You may schedule partial shifts or 10 hour and 12 hour shifts. You will be matched geographically and skill-wise to a hospital of your choice. A paid orientation has been designed to meet the needs of a supplemental nurse, and our salaries are competitive.

Our idea is to give you an opportunity to explore all available nursing possibilities before relocating to the area.

MEDICAL REGISTRY RESPONSIBILITIES:

1. Provide information re; hospitals, housing, licensing
2. Interview - Hire - Placement Assignment - Evaluation
3. Provide Orientation
4. Provide Worker's Compensation, Malpractice insurance
5. Deduct FICA & Federal Tax

EMPLOYEE RESPONSIBILITIES:

1. Be eligible for licensing in Florida
2. Qualify for employment
   A. A graduate of an approved school
   B. Have had at least 1 year of acceptable performance of hospital clinical experience within the last 4 years, or have successfully completed a refresher course within the last 4 years
3. Schedule at least 3 shifts per week for a minimum of 2 weeks

I have enclosed information about licensing, our program and the county.

After your review please call or write with particular questions and indicate your interest in a "working vacation."

Enclosed for your convenience is an application and a self-addressed envelope.

Looking forward to hearing from you in the near future.

Sincerely,

Phyllis M. Clancy, RN
Director of Nurses

Figure 15-3 Promotional letter.

president's office. Fast-food establishments allowed us free advertising on menus, napkins, and bulletin boards. I used them all!"

Recruiting staff involved continuing personal contacts, letter writing, and telephone calls, but the major payoff, Phyllis reports, came from the program itself. It emphasized flexible schedules, partial shifts, and job sharing. "It's important to note that the shortage problem was directly related to the rigid scheduling practices of the area facilities. If you didn't work full-time, you didn't work as a registered nurse in a Pinellas County hospital." There were no pools established and none of the flexible options so familiar in today's marketplace. The registry targeted nurses going to school full-time, mothers at home with small children, single parents, and those otherwise occupied with personal goals, offering them an opportunity to practice their profession.

"I spent a lot of time interviewing, screening, and making certain that each assignment was appropriate. We matched skill, clinical interest, geographical location, and desired shift to the participating facilities. A special feature allowed student nurses to work as advanced nursing assistants. This helped them supplement college expenses and at the same time develop nursing skills. Most of the students came from an associate degree nursing program where clinical opportunities were somewhat limited."

Phyllis personally visited each nurse during the first two assignments, regardless of the hour, to determine how things were going and to offer support and guidance. "They were elite," states Phyllis, "they were blue ribbon, and I felt they needed to know that they belonged to a good company and were supported in their association with us."

In addition to ongoing personal contact on the job, Phyllis planned social functions for the nurses, which were underwritten by the hospital administrators. Nurses' Day was a special day for the BAHC Nurses' Registry. Phyllis visited all 14 participating hospitals and personally pinned a "blue ribbon" carnation on each nurse. Christmas banquets, spring picnics, and luncheons were also held. On one occasion, BAHC registry nurses spent 7 hours accepting phone calls on a public television channel soliciting funds for public television.

During the 18 months that Phyllis directed agency activities the number of participating hospitals grew from 14 to 17. Over 100 nurses were recruited back into the acute care setting, and hospitals began to implement flexible schedules.

Phyllis Sippel's role in the development and implementation of a not-for-profit registry was successful, not only because of her skill and dedication to the project, but because she utilized marketing concepts and principles. These skills are more in demand today than when Phyllis first used them.

The Learner as Customer

Loretta C. Spittle, R.N., M.S., C.C.R.N., C.N.A.
Director, Critical Care Nursing
Fairfax Hospital
Falls Church, Virginia

Loretta Spittle's nursing career includes leadership positions in nursing administration, education, and clinical practice. One of her favorite activities is teaching review courses for registered nurses who want to earn critical care nurse certification. While teaching a review course for her critical care staff, she found group members repeatedly expressing concern about maintaining their certification. Loretta admits, "Not only did I want to keep their credentials current, for their own sense of self-worth, but as an administrator, I understood the effect on unit morale if a nurse let it lapse. I also felt pressure and wanted to respond when staff approached me at the eleventh hour for recertification assistance."

Loretta reviewed the recertification requirements and the variety of professional and educational activities that could earn continuing education recognition points (CERPs). It became apparent to her that diligent planning and recordkeeping are required of each certified clinician in order to maintain certification.

The American Association of Critical Care Nurses (AACN) accepts CERP credit in six different categories: clinical programs that offer CERPs or continuing education units; academic courses for credit; professional publications; critical care presentations; individualized continuing education activities; and quality assurance activities. "I thought that if I labeled a folder for each credit category, CERPs could be conveniently filed away for future reference. As long as the system is simple and straightforward," Loretta states, "compliance is enhanced."

The first "CERPs Keeper" consisted of no more than six file pocket folders. Loretta copied the requirements for each credit category and affixed them to the file pocket. A cover note from

Loretta offered suggestions on how to earn the required 100 CERPs over the 3-year recertification period. She finished off the folder with a cover featuring the AACN logo. Loretta presented a complimentary copy to each staff member earning certification.

The CERPs Keeper was so well received by the staff that Loretta decided to write AACN's certification headquarters and make them aware of the idea. AACN asked Loretta to forward a copy of the Keeper. "Then," states Loretta, "I promptly forgot about it, because I really did not believe it had much promise." Several months later, Loretta was contacted by AACN officials, who informed her they would like to produce a sophisticated version of the Keeper and offer it to the membership.

AACN announced the development of the CERPs Keeper in May 1987, at their annual meeting in New Orleans, Louisiana. "The idea has really caught on," reports Loretta. "Many CCRNs purchase them for personal use, as well as congratulatory gifts for friends." Indeed, Loretta reports, the chairman of her local AACN chapter recently told her that she is purchasing the Keeper to use as a door prize.

The Patient as Customer

Joan Bretschneider, R.N., M.S.N.
Assistant Director of Nursing
Women and Children Care Program
Psychiatry Care Program
Thomas Jefferson University
 Hospital
Philadelphia, Pennsylvania

Madeline P. Albanese, R.N.,
 M.S.N.
Clinical Nurse Specialist,
 Neurosensory
Thomas Jefferson University
 Hospital
Philadelphia, Pennsylvania

In 1985, Mary Ann McGinley, R.N., M.S.N., Associate Executive Director and Director of Nursing at Thomas Jefferson University Hospital in Philadelphia, appointed a Patient Education Committee to critique materials used in patient education at Thomas Jefferson Hospital. This action was based not only on her knowledge that patient teaching is a vital part of nursing's professional role, but also on her understanding of the relationship between patient education and client satisfaction.

Since its inception, the committee's mission has grown and developed. It now occupies a strategically important position within the nursing department, involved in both the production and evaluation of patient education materials.

Joan Bretschneider serves as administrative advisor to the Patient Education Committee. Madeline Albanese has been committee chairperson since its formation. The group, composed primarily of clinical specialists and staff development educators, reviewed the administrative charge and decided to conduct an extensive review of the literature. The committee felt confident that they could serve as content experts, but recognized they had little knowledge of or experience with the science of developing promotional materials. When the literature review was completed, the committee developed criteria to guide the production and evaluation of patient education materials.

The document developed by the committee has standardized production of patient education materials at Thomas Jefferson University Hospital. The standards are not only directed at achieving the goal of customer satisfaction, but address critical patient care goals as well. The following excerpts from the committee's manual (consisting of the Introduction and sections II, III, and IV) demonstrate nursing's commitment to content and presentation excellence in all patient education publications.

Introduction

The Patient Education Committee has formulated Policies, Procedures and Guidelines for the Development and Evaluation of Patient Education Materials. The standards contribute to the creation of effective teaching tools and materials which are valuable adjuncts in patient teaching.

The manual includes five sections: (1) Content Guidelines, (2) Readability Guidelines, (3) SMOG Readability Formula, (4) Appearance and Format Guidelines, and (5) Guidelines for Pretesting Patient Education Materials.

Material in the first section helps clinicians structure and organize information during early stages of development. The appearance and format section offers assistance on print type size, color, and layout best suited to patient teaching materials. Guidelines on the use of illustrations are also included in this section.

Tips on readability in sections II and III, from the U.S. Department of Health and Human Services, are included to structure the use of language. Content can reflect a high level of knowledge and expertise by the author, but it must be presented in such a way that the consumer can understand it. Finally, guidelines for pretesting patient education materials are included so that the author(s) can gather valuable data on how the target audience responds. This step allows for revision prior to final printing.

During the development of patient teaching materials, a member of the Patient Education Committee is available to provide assistance in all aspects of production. A typed draft of the material must be submitted to the Patient Education Committee for review of content, readability, structure, and format before final production. Sections III and IV are included for information and utilization in the production of patient education materials.

References

Doak, C., L. Doak, and J. Root. 1985. *Teaching patients with low literacy skills*. Philadelphia: J.B. Lippincott.

Falvo, D. 1985. *Effective patient education*. Rockville, MD: Aspen Systems.

Health Education Center. 1981. *A guide to evaluating and using patient education materials*. Pittsburgh: Health and Welfare Planning Association.

National Institutes of Health. 1984. *Pretesting in health communications* (NIH Publication No. 84-1493). Bethesda, MD: National Cancer Institute.

Pichert, J.W., and P. Elam. 1985. Readability formulas may mislead you. *Patient Education and Counseling*, 1:181-191.

Review Questions

1. Identify and discuss marketing opportunities that nursing administrators have with ancillary departments in acute care settings. Formulate a marketing plan for one area.

2. After reviewing the comments on customer service in Chapter 12, make a list of how each of the nurses discussed in this chapter provides such a customer service and follow-up.

3. Select a piece of promotional material from your agency and evaluate it following the principles illustrated in this chapter.

4. Staff development activities offer a key opportunity to utilize marketing principles and techniques to increase morale and enhance human resource development. Identify products that you might develop in your agency to take advantage of such opportunities.

SMOG Readibility Formula (Doak, Doak, Root, 1985; Falvo, 1985; Health Care
Education Center, 1981; National Institute of Health, 1984; Pichert, Elam,
1985)

II. READABILITY

GUIDELINES   EXAMPLES

A. GRADE LEVEL

Material should address the
6-8 grade reading levels as
determined by use of the SMOG
Readability Formula as follows:

SMOG FORMULA FOR MATERIAL CON-
TAINING 30 OR MORE SENTENCES.

Step 1: Count off 10 consecu-   BEGINNING EXCERPT (10 CONSECUTIVE
tive sentences near the   SENTENCES)
beginning, middle and end of
handout/booklet.   What is Diabetes?

Note: A sentence is a string of   If you have diabetes your body does
words punctuated with a period,
exclamation point or question   not have enough insulin to use.
mark.
                                      Insulin helps your body use the food
Step 2: Circle & count all words
with three or more syllables.   you eat for energy. There are several

Note: • Include repetitions of   ways to take care of this problem.
        same word.
      • Hyphenated words are   Keeping your weight at normal or near
        considered one word.
      • Numbers written as   normal will help the small amount of
        numerals should be
        pronounced to determine   usable insulin do the job. Your
        number of syllables.
      • Proper nouns should be   doctor or nurse will tell you what
        counted.
      • Abbreviations should be   your normal weight is. If you need
        read as unabbreviated
        to determine the number   more insulin, it can be made ready
        of syllables.
                                      for your body with the use of oral

                                      diabetes pills or by injecting

                                      insulin.

                                          Who gets Diabetes?

                                      Anyone may get diabetes at any time.

                                      Diabetes is found most often in

                                      three types of people.
                                          TOTAL WORDS = 15

Figure 15-4 SMOG readibility formula.

MIDDLE EXCERPT (10 CONSECUTIVE
SENTENCES)

Take special care of your feet!

You should take care of your feet to
avoid infections.

- Look all over your feet daily for
  red areas, sores, cuts, scratches,
  blisters, or bruises.
- Tell your doctor about any changes
  you see in your feet.
- Wash your feet daily with mild
  soap and lukewarm water.
- Carefully pat (don't rub) your
  feet dry with a soft towel,
  especially between your toes.
- Use hand cream lanolin-based
  cream, or petroleum jelly to
  soften dry skin.
- Be careful not to hurt your legs,
  feet and toes.
- File your nails straight across.
- Wear shoes that fit well (not too
  tight or too loose).

                    TOTAL WORDS = 4

Figure 15-4, continued

END EXCERPT (10 CONSECUTIVE
SENTENCES)

Working with your doctor and nurse
is important !

- You should do what your doctor
  and nurse tell you to do. They
  are trying to help you.
- You should take care of yourself
  everyday.
- You should eat the right foods.
- Tell your doctor if you feel a
  change from usual .
- Always tell your doctor or nurse
  of changes in your living habits.
- Ask questions if you don't
  understand something.
- Keep your doctor appointments .

This way you can control the diabetes
and lead a more normal, active,
full life.

Step 3: Estimate square root of
the grand total:

Step 4: Add 3 to square root to
determine the SMOG reading grade
level.* This will indicate the
grade level the person must have
reached to fully understand your
handout.

*See following conversion table.

TOTAL WORDS = 6

GRAND TOTAL = 25

SQUARE ROOT = 5

SQUARE ROOT + 3 = 8th GRADE
            READING LEVEL

Figure 15-4, continued

* SMOG CONVERSION TABLE

Total # of Polysyllabic Words	Square Root of Total	Approximate Grade Level
5	2.2	5-6
10	3.1	6-7
15	3.8	6-7
20	4.4	7-8
25	5	8
30	5.4	8-9
35	5.9	8-9
40	6.3	8-9
45	6.7	9-10
50	7	10
55	7.4	10-11
60	7.7	10-11
65	8	11
70	8.3	11-12
75	8.6	11-12
80	8.9	11-12
85	9.2	12-13
90	9.4	12-13
95	9.7	12-13
100	10	13

*Developed by: Harold C. McGraw, Office of Educational Research, Baltimore County Schools, Towson, Maryland.

Figure 15-4, continued

SMOG FORUMLA FOR MATERIAL CONTAINING
<u>LESS THAN</u> 30 SENTENCES)

<u>Step 1</u>: Count all words with three
or more syllables in the text.   Total # of polysyllabic words = 10

<u>Step 2</u>: Count the number of   Total # of sentences = 20
sentences.

<u>Step 3</u>: Find the average number of   Average = <u>Total # of polysyllabic words</u> =
polysyllabic words per sentence.   Total # of sentenses (20)   .5

<u>Step 4</u>: Multiply the <u>average</u> by the   Average (.5) x 10 (# of sentences) = 5
number of sentences short of 30   short of 30
in the handout.

<u>Step 5:</u> Add that figure to the total   5 + 10 (Total # of polysyllabic words) =
number of polysyllabic words.   15

<u>Step 6:</u> Find the square root and add   N 15 = 3.8 + 3 = 6.8 Grade level
a constant of 3.

B.   <u>SENTENCE STRUCTURE</u>

   1. Sentences should vary in
      length with an average 8-12
      words.

                      Ex: <u>Wash</u> your feet daily with mild
   2. Verbs should be active, not   soap and lukewarm water.
      passive.

                      Not: <u>Feet should be washed</u> daily with
   3. Paragraphs should be limited   mild soap and lukewarm water.
      to one idea each.

C.   <u>TERMINOLOGY</u>

   1. Common terms should be used in-
      stead of medical terms whenever
      possible.
                      Ex: The following are signs of
   2. If medical or technical terms   hypoglycemia (low blood sugar).
      are used they should be
      immediately clarified i.e. in   The Coronary (heart) arteries
      parenthesis following the   supply the heart muscle with
      medical term.   oxygen.

   3. Avoid abbreviations.

Figure 15-4, continued

III. APPEARANCE/FORMAT

GUIDELINES   EXAMPLES

A. TYPE

1. Type should be 10 point or 12   1.   This is a sample of the 10 point type.
    point size.
                                               This is a sample of the 12 point type.

2. Use serif typeface. Serif has   2.   This is serif typeface.
    tiny lines built into the characters.

3. Do not use script, italics or
    stylized typefaces.

4. Upper and lower case letters
    are easier to read than all
    capital letters. Low literacy
    patients need the characteristic
    humps and bumps above and below
    the line of lower case letters
    in order to recognize them.

B. COLOR

1. Written pamphlets should use   1.   Black print or white
    sharp contrast of the print   background is best. Shades
    on the background material.   of the same color are
                                               difficult to read, i.e.,
C. LAYOUT   brown or beige; green on
                                               green.
1. The "ragged right" margin (uneven
    right margin) is more informal
    and easy to read.

2. Lines consisting of approximately
    40 characters are best. The
    width of the line is best.
    The short line results in longer
    eye fixations on it, which helps
    comprehension; the longer line
    results in eye difficulty on
    the return sweep to the next
    line.

3. Material should be organized
    chronologically.

4. Use subtitles or headings to
    alert the reader as to what
    is coming and to focus on your
    intended message.

5. Use lots of "white space".
    Many readers will glance and
    skip through tightly packed
    pages.

Figure 15-4, continued

D. ILLUSTRATIONS/VISUALS

Visuals reduce the amount of reading
in the text, emphasize key points
in your instructions, and motivate
patients to use the materials.

1. To show anatomical relationships,
    draw enough of the body to be
    sure that people can recognize
    what is shown; do not cut off
    arms and legs; do not omit significant
    body parts.

2. Do not use figures that are
    irrelevant to the message.

3. Visuals can be used to differentiate
    sizes, shapes and positions.

4. Visuals are helpful to illustrate
    body positions or exercises.

5. Visuals can be used to teach
    a series of steps in a specific
    sequence. Place the visuals
    in sequence along with the text.
    The captions and drawings should
    be placed in a left to right
    order and down the page in a
    normal reading order.

6. Illustrations/photographs should
    maintain a consistent viewing
    angle; show the users point
    of view.

7. Avoid using an unnumbered matrix
    design of illustrations. The
    reader does not know in which
    direction he should read and
    his eyes can travel around the
    page without a sense of order
    or sequence.

8. Visuals are helpful:

    A. If you want to contrast
        normal and abnormal conditions.

    B. If you want to dramatize
        a behavior use a visual
        to reinforce a message.

Figure 15-4, continued

C. To provide motivation.

D. To break a long line of text.

9. Tips to improve visuals.

    A. Include captions and titles to explain illustrations.

    B. Be sure captions are brief - 10 words or less.

    C. Be sure the visuals are consistent in their message.

    D. Always emphasize the correct behavior.

    E. Do not use too many cues; such as underlining, arrows and circles.

    F. Avoid overloaded visuals.

Figure 15-4, continued

Chapter 16

Tomorrow's Nursing Profession: The Entrepreneurial Life

One of the most powerful and important ideas in the belief system of nursing is the idea of attaining professional status. Some view nursing as a semi-profession, a subprofession, or a marginal profession (Etzioni 1969), others use the title of professional because of courtesy and tradition, and still others report claims of its attainment as an accomplished fact (Stuart 1981).

Nursing's interest in professional status is not a new issue. Quite the contrary—concern has been expressed in the literature over a number of years (American Nursing Association 1979). It is, however, an issue of renewed interest. Today's health care system offers nurses opportunities to identify needs in the marketplace and respond with innovative and creative responses.

Professionals occupy important positions in our society. To gain recognition, individuals must engage in activities designed to bring them prestige, status, and respectability. It is a tedious process requiring commitment, competency, opportunity, and time. The nurses featured in this chapter reflect characteristics commonly associated with professional behavior. They also illustrate the best in innovation and entrepreneurship.

Peter Drucker has said, "Entrepreneurs see change as the norm and as healthy. Usually, they do not bring about the change themselves, but (and this defines entrepreneur and entrepreneurship) the entrepreneur always searches for change, responds to it and exploits it as an opportunity" (Drucker 1985). Entrepreneurs are energetic, visionary, confident, intense, imaginative, optimistic, and courageous. They demonstrate a purposeful, single-minded orienta-

485

tion, determination, total involvement, exquisite judgment, and a unique kind of peripheral vision that permits them to identify marketplace opportunities (Silver 1986).

As the experiences of the individuals highlighted in this chapter are described, patterns emerge. Each communicates a level of dissatisfaction with her career path, not her chosen field. As a result of this "irritation" each makes a decision to strike out on her own, in order to make a contribution to nursing and society that will make the health care system a better place for all. This experience is typical of the entrepreneurial life (Silver 1986).

Each individual emphasizes the importance of professional organizations and organizational activity in promoting her cause, the role of nurse and nonnurse mentors in her development, the necessity of keeping current in one's field, the importance of making professional contacts through networking, her commitment to the nursing profession, and her need for autonomy.

"The entrepreneur makes a choice between head and heart and chooses heart. The head can distinguish right from wrong, but the heart will not permit a wrongful act. The head can perceive a wrongful act. The head can perceive incompetencies and inaccuracies . . . but it takes the heart to reject them" (Silver 1986). When the budding entrepreneur goes through her period of dissatisfaction with the world around her she is getting her heart back. Ruth Theken, Nan Goddard, Dee Alford and Janet Moll, Margaret O'Brien, and Sallyan Sohr are registered nurses with a lot of heart.

Search Consultant Entrepreneurism

Ruth Tucker Theken
President, Theken Associates
Nashua, New Hampshire

The Beginning

Serendipity was at least partially responsible for Ruth Theken's initial interest in the executive search field. "Following graduate school, I worked as a clinical coordinator in a major Boston teaching hospital. Just about the time I became disillusioned with hospital nursing, an executive search firm contacted me about an international ambulatory nurse consultant position with a for-profit hospital corporation. It was an outstanding professional opportunity — I decided to pursue the position."

Ruth found every aspect of working with the search consultant a stimulating experience. "I was impressed with the detailed screening process, how the consultant helped me understand the position's responsibilities, how thoroughly my questions were answered, and how I was coached to sharpen my interviewing skills." When the process concluded, she felt prepared for a smooth transition into her new role.

Although the position was based in New Orleans, almost all of Ruth's time was spent abroad. As expected, 2 years of rigorous international travel was about all she could physically tolerate. The experience, however, proved enormously beneficial. "Besides affirming my ability to function as an independent thinker and team player, the position provided me an opportunity to demonstrate skill in using a consultant model to set up programs and make systems work. I discovered how much I enjoyed the flexibility, diversity, and creative thinking associated with the consultant role."

Following her resignation, Ruth remained in New Orleans for about a year as a consultant to a professional standards review organization. When she made the decision to leave New Orleans and return to her home in New England, she contacted the search firm and expressed an interest in obtaining another position. "I learned, to my surprise, that my placement had been a fluke, as the company did little placement work in health care." Ruth's contact with the firm's manager, however, sparked an idea. Ruth was asked to join the business and develop a health care practice.

"My primary goal in accepting the search firm's offer was to learn the field. I was interested in starting my own executive search company. A prior friendship with an entrepreneur and role model enabled me to see myself as a risk taker with a variety of marketable skills. With a belief in myself and a strong need to control my destiny, I moved forward. As the months went by, my success in the nursing marketplace grew, but the firm evidenced little commitment to nursing. I felt like an appendage, rather than an integrated business product line."

Several of Ruth's clients encouraged her to set out on her own. They felt, and Ruth agreed, that she would be able to offer clients a more personalized service without big company constraints. "By this time, I had learned that there was no existing search firm that focused exclusively on nursing executives. Thus, in January 1980,

7 months after entering the search consulting field, with two guaranteed clients and $7,000 in personal savings, I opened Theken Associates."

"From the beginning," Ruth asserts, "I committed to provide a consulting service that reflected my values about the dignity and worth of each individual. I was confident my philosophy would be visible through my actions and interactions and would attract clients with similar values, attitudes, and beliefs. Meanwhile, the need to cover living expenses, including a mortgage, necessitated my working out of my home and the aggressive pursuit of business. I had no formal marketing plan, but intuitively knew my first priority was to identify target markets and develop realistic marketing strategies."

A Well-Defined Market

Ruth decided to limit her practice to the placement of top and mid-level nursing executives. The need existed, and the markets were large enough to accommodate a full-time effort. In time, several benefits resulted from this decision. "By concentrating on top and mid-level nurse executives, I was able to identify for myself, and then for others, the qualities that set Theken Associates apart from the competition: expertise in nursing issues and the highly personal service that only a small firm can offer."

"I identified my competitors and educated myself about their work. I also identified and contacted noncompetitive firms with whom I could develop referral relationships. A commitment to nurse executive searches also helped me avoid the time drain associated with developing multiple markets simultaneously."

Strategies to Generate Referrals

Ruth argues that if you ask any search firm consultant how business is most frequently generated, the response will be, "through personal referral." Companies and executives recognize that consultants impact organizations; thus, it is not surprising that they want to ensure that the consultant has an exemplary track record.

"When I formed Theken Associates, I understood the importance of referrals and being recognized as a professional, ethical, discreet, and diplomatic expert in my field. All my marketing efforts are directed at building ongoing sources of referral. For that reason, I have not diverted time, energy, and money into brochure development, advertising, and direct mail campaigns. I did, however, design classically simple business cards and stationery to reinforce the professional image I wanted to establish." Word of mouth is a powerful force in the business world. Ruth's strategy was to differentiate her firm in the marketplace, so that it generated referrals on the personal recommendation of one executive to another.

Building a Base of Support

"The most important step I took in developing a referral base was to form an advisory board. I wanted access to a small group of well-known and respected nursing executives, hospital administrators, and executive search professionals." These individuals, Ruth felt, provided two vital ingredients in her formula for success. First, they offered expert guidance in developing a business plan and marketing strategies, as well as assistance in more concrete areas, such as developing letters of agreement. Second, through working closely with her, the group would be well acquainted with her ability and therefore could testify for her in the marketplace.

"I had worked with Anne Black, Vice-President for Nursing at Boston Children's Hospital, and Sonya Healy, Director of Nursing at St. Joseph's Hospital in Nashua. Because they found my approach to search work efficient, effective, and economic, they supported establishment of my business and were willing to serve on the advisory board. Carl Wathne, my graduate school preceptor; Walter Allen, a community hospital administrator; Ken Bloem, Associate Dean, Boston University College of Health Sciences; Tom Battles, a well-known physician recruiter; and Richard Lee, a teaching hospital administrator, rounded out the group."

Each Board member gave Ruth vital assistance, without compensation! "I think their interest in helping me stemmed from seeing the need for a business like mine and because they each knew how very much I respected their knowledge and skill. I made a point of not taking undue advantage of their time. The quarterly meetings were well planned and we stuck to business. To show my appreciation, I provided a special meal after the meeting concluded." Ruth discontinued the advisory board after 2 years, in order to avoid possible conflicts of interest, and because her client load had grown.

Collegial Relationships

"When I went out on my own," Ruth says, "I joined organizations that increased my contacts and furthered my education." For example, Ruth regularly attends meetings of the American Organization of Nurse Executives. This keeps her in touch with nursing issues, and participation as an exhibitor provides an opportunity to communicate the fact that the firm is composed of human resource professionals and nursing peers.

The American Association of Healthcare Consultants (AAHC) is also a valuable resource for Ruth. Through it she gains further insight into mechanisms that increase referrals, improve consultation skills, and analyze issues in other areas of the health care marketplace. "For example," reports Ruth, "I often refer individuals to search consultants I respect in other specialty fields, and they do the same for me. Through contacts I make as a part of my organizational activities, I am able to arrange speaking engagements on topics from contemporary career issues to resume development. These activities not only meet marketplace demand but create an impression, particularly about our approach to the executive search process."

Each meeting Ruth attends is preceded by a planning period. "I think about who will be there and who I want to meet. Ideally, I ask a contact to introduce me. If this approach is not workable, I ask to join groups where the individual is having lunch, dinner, or cocktails." Ruth also sponsors events that increase her professional and personal exposure. "For important meetings, such as the American Organization of Nurse Executives and the American College of Healthcare Executives, I sponsor hospitality suites. In the early years, when funds were limited, I restricted the number of attendees by sending formal invitations. As a further cost-cutting measure, I shared hospitality expenses with other search professionals, such as Tom Battles. This not only reduced cost but increased the number of personal contacts I was able to make."

Over the years, Ruth has found that others are just as interested in meeting her as she them. "I am able to provide a national perspective on salaries, benefits, and career issues that are of interest to individuals in leadership positions. I have a policy to contact each colleague at least once a year. My network is very valuable to me — maintenance mandates that you stay in touch."

Making Every Contact Work for You

Building a reputation for excellence requires a lot of hard work. "Every contact," asserts Ruth, "must work for you. The catch-22 of consulting is that in order to generate referrals you must demonstrate consulting skill. For that reason, I seek to capitalize on every opportunity to prove my effectiveness in working with individuals and organizations. Initially, this meant I spent time on referrals that had no immediate payoff other than personal satisfaction."

In the beginning, nurse executives and hospital administrators requested that Ruth work with friends, employees, and colleagues who were experiencing career problems. For example, Ruth worked with a nurse executive who had been terminated. Particular attention was directed at helping her deal with the anger she felt and retrospectively evaluate the experience to see how a similar situation could be avoided in the future. Ultimately, Ruth placed this individual in a position of equal status. She has been a source of several referrals over the years.

Existing clients are another referral source. Theken Associates enters into a collaborative arrangement with each client to learn about its mission, corporate structure, current issues, and future plans. At the conclusion of this assessment, process search guidelines are established. The firm conducts exhaustive research, multiple interviews, and reference audits, and participates in compensation negotiations. "In other words, we do everything possible to structure a smooth transaction for the organization and the nurse executive alike. Our letter of agreement establishes mutual expectations—there are no surprises. Clarity is essential in fostering ongoing relationships." The entrepreneur strives, at all costs, to avoid dissatisfied clients.

Taking Action

Proactive response is essential to building a successful business. When Ruth first established her firm, she recognized that clients would not beat a path to her door. "Through contacts, I learned of organizations with executive-level nursing vacancies. I contacted the administrator conducting the search and described Theken Associates' personalized service, giving specifics on what I could do for the organization. I asked to make a presentation to the search committee and furnished references that might be particularly meaningful to the administrator. To some extent, I still operate that way, after 8 years in the business."

Taking action also means that each representative of Theken Associates is important to the firm's overall marketing effort. "Each of us is concerned with how, for example, telephone manners and correspondence affect professional image. As our skills improve, potential clients are more receptive to our marketing efforts. In effect, by taking direct action, we generate many of our own referrals. While this form of marketing is difficult at first, it is a very effective method, one I would recommend to others."

Screening Potential Clients

"Experience has taught me that not all potential clients make good clients," states Ruth, "regardless of how much I would like their business. In some situations we are not the right firm to handle their needs, and in other situations they are not the right kind of client for Theken Associates." Before accepting a client, Ruth conducts a marketing assessment of key individuals in the organization. Five criteria are used to structure the review.

First, do prevailing attitudes of the medical staff, nursing staff, and hospital administration support a positive integration of a candidate Theken Associates might place? Second, is an honest appraisal of organizational problems communicated? Third, does the organization have realistic expectations regarding solutions and turnaround time frames? Does the organization plan an appropriate compensation and benefit package for the skill and experience required? Finally, is the organization open to candid dialogue between the candidate and all relevant organizational constituents? If these conditions are not present, I am not reluctant to decline the offer. In the long run, this protects Theken Associates' most important asset — our reputation and credibility with health care organizations and potential clients."

Reflection

Ruth was asked to look back over her entrepreneurial experience and reflect on what she might have done differently. "Generally, I am pleased with the way my original marketing plan worked out. I sought the advice of good people and thought each step through before taking action. If I were starting out all over again, however, there are a few areas I would handle differently.

"In an effort to provide a full range of related services, I asked by husband, a well-known human resources and labor relations executive, to join the firm as a part-time associate. This strategy did not work for a variety of reasons. First, we had different opinions about the nurse executive marketplace, and we encountered control issues. Neither of us anticipated how a husband-and-wife team might be perceived. Thinking we would be augmenting one another's practice, we actually turned off several potential clients who saw us as a 'mom-and-pop' operation. Once we recognized that these attitudes interfered with our personal relationship, as well as the progress of the firm, we agreed that he should leave the business. Based on this experience, I would caution others to give careful consideration before involving a spouse.

"In the beginning, I also charged less for the firm's services than the competition. Although my fee structure reflected the same percentage as other firms, I based it on the midpoint of the proposed salary range, rather than on a higher figure. In actual experience, the nurse executives we placed commanded higher level salaries than the midpoint.

"Lastly, I realize that early on I should have placed more emphasis on promoting myself and the business directly to chief executive officers, since they are key in selecting search consultants. I started with nursing administrators, probably because I felt more comfortable with them. This activity paid off in recognition for the firm and its principles, but did not get our message to the decision-makers. We are focusing on this area in our current marketing plan. Even though Theken Associates is firmly established, we've learned the importance of periodically updating our marketing plan and strategies."

Ruth Theken's entrepreneurial experience in establishing a search firm and her use of marketing philosophy and science have served her well. In 1980, she began her business with two customers. In 1987 she served 34.

Nurse Educator as Entrepreneur

Nannette L. Goddard, R.N., M.S.
President, Goddard Management Resources
Houston, Texas

After graduating from Adelphi University School of Nursing, Nan Goddard accepted a staff nurse position at the Loeb Center for Nursing and Rehabilitation at Montefiore Medical Center, New York City. A promotion to senior staff nurse (head nurse) 1 year later encouraged her to pursue a graduate degree. At Russell Sage College in upstate New York, Nan worked as a clinical instructor while earning her master's degree in nursing.

Following completion of her course work in 1978, she moved to Miami, Florida, where she worked with Baptist Hospital and Mount Sinai Medical Center as a consultant on the implementation of a primary nursing delivery system. She was offered a permanent position at Sinai, and over the next 2 years she advanced from Assistant Director to Associate Director and finally to Director of Nursing, Administrative Services. This position involved responsibility for 1,000 full-time equivalent employees and a $35 million budget. During her tenure at Mount Sinai it was chosen as one of the nation's 30 magnet hospitals by the National Commission on Nursing.

Answering both an entrepreneurial call and a proposal of marriage, Nan relocated to Houston, Texas, in 1983 and formed her own company. In her capacity as Senior Partner, Goddard Management Resources, she is called upon by hospitals and long-term care facilities to deliver a wide range of services from revision of staffing and budgetary systems to total departmental analysis and redirection. She is frequently asked to provide lectures and workshops on a variety of topics including financial planning and budgeting, organizational development, leadership education, negotiating skills, staffing and scheduling, productivity and management information reporting, patient classification, primary nursing, computer applications, and intra/entrepreneurship. Nan has published several articles on financial management and holds adjunct faculty appointments at the Medical University of South Carolina and the University of Texas/Galveston.

The preceding paragraphs present the facts, but Nan credits the people she met along the way as substantially responsible for shaping her entrepreneurial career path. "Faculty at Adelphi and Russell Sage gave me a sense of professional belonging and a drive to fully achieve my potential. I have also been fortunate to work with progressive nursing departments, who, of course, had progressive nursing leaders."My experience with primary nursing at Loeb placed me in a position of advantage when I competed for the consulting position at Baptist. My performance there helped me expand my primary nurse consulting activities to Mount Sinai, where I became part of their progressive nursing department, one vitally interested in the development of sophisticated nursing management systems.

"I soon recognized that interdisciplinary collaboration was necessary in order to establish the modern applications Sinai wanted. The management engineering department and the finance department at Sinai worked with nursing to develop staffing and fiscal systems that were ahead of their time. After we were selected as a magnet hospital, I received many inquiries about consulting. It was difficult to 'mind the store' and respond to the number of opportunities available, so I arranged for many of those interested in our management systems to visit at Mount Sinai.

"Just about this time, I made a decision to marry. It meant a move to Houston, Texas. The prospect of moving and starting all over again caused me to sit down and take stock of where I was and where I wanted to go. During my 10 years in nursing, I had developed a lot of contacts. I felt that it was time to make a major move in my career. I love consulting, teaching, and working with nursing administrators. My husband encouraged me to explore the idea of starting a consulting firm of my own.

"Needless to say, I liked the idea and felt that the time was right. I didn't have the professional contacts in Houston that I had in other parts of the country. I knew it would take time to establish myself in the nursing community. I was convinced that I could invest the energy required to develop a business if I didn't have the demands of a new position. It was a good breakpoint for me.

"This is where my experience in recruitment, public relations, strategic planning, and marketing at Mount Sinai really paid off. At Sinai, I interviewed a number of nursing students in graduate programs who were interested in positions with us. Based on interviews and subsequent experience with some individuals we hired, I knew there was a big void—they didn't, for example, know how to plan staffing over 7 days, and many had never touched a nursing budget. I was concerned about the lack of integration between concept and operation.

"Experiences such as these made it clear to me that there was a need out there — I wanted to fill it! In order to verify my judgment, I interviewed graduate students, chief operating officers, chief executive officers, and nursing administrators across the nation. Now that I look back, I know there are more scientific methods for market research, but at the time I relied on interviews and networking. Fortunately, the risk I took worked out.

"I focused on the development of three products. First, a broad range of consulting services for nursing departments, centering on organizational development, management systems, and financial planning. Second, continuing education in financial management. And third, the development of academic preparation in finance."

Educational Entrepreneurship

Today, Nan Goddard works out of her home in Houston. She continues to develop and promote the three original products she identified in 1983. Her educational product lines are unique. This example of educational entrepreneurship focuses on two aspects of her business: continuing education and graduate education. It describes the assessment, planning, and promotional activities she conducted to build her business.

Continuing Education

Opportunity and Product Development. The need for information and education in financial management is spurred by revisions in health care pricing and reimbursement enacted during the Reagan administration. Traditionally, nurse executives have been excluded from discussions and decision-making centering on finance. One of the principal reasons is that health care executives tend to view nursing administrators as clinical managers, not as financial managers.

The need for nursing managers to understand and speak the language of accounting and financial planning is a top priority in today's health care system. Graduate programs for preparation in nursing service administration frequently do not include financial course requirements. In addition, many nursing managers do not meet the academic requirements for graduate school admission or cannot commit the time and resources necessary to further their formal education.

The development of appropriate learning opportunities for nursing personnel who require financial management education is a wide-open field. The continuing education services of Goddard Management Resources are designed to promote development in financial management. A 2-day seminar entitled "Financial Planning, Staffing, and Budgeting for Nursing" targets nurse managers, leaders, educators, and administrators. The program objectives and course content are based on interviews Nan conducted with 200 hospital administrators, nursing executives and managers, and graduate school faculty and students across the country. Teaching strategies and program design are developed around the 1984 American Nurses' Association Standards for Continuing Education in Nursing.

Product Promotion and Pricing. The seminar's first presentation was in Houston on January 16 and 17, 1985. During development, Goddard Management Resources retained the services of graphic artists, computer experts, photographers, and media specialists to assist with slides, teaching tools, and handouts for students. Meeting facilities and catering resources were arranged at a highly visible and well-known convention hotel. Supplementary clerical support assisted with details, served as a liaison with the hotel, and summarized seminar evaluation forms. A brochure detailing the program was completed with the assistance of commercial and graphic artists, printers, and continuing education experts.

Nan obtained from the Greater Houston Hospital Council a mailing list of all the hospitals in a 15-country area surrounding Houston. Two brochures were mailed to each of the 100 institutions — one to the Director of Nursing and the other to the Continuing Education Coordinator. One hundred additional brochures were sent to nursing leaders across Texas who had recently attended a national meeting of the American Organization of Nurse Executives, and to local nursing colleagues known to Nan. Personal selling was also used as a promotional technique. Individual appointments with community-based nursing administrators and educators offered an opportunity to further Nan's professional contacts in the community and distribute the brochure.

Pricing decisions were based on a careful review of fee structures for other national, state, and local workshops addressing management topics. Nan found that nationally based professional organization fees ranged from $75 to $150 per day. Local organizations were able to charge somewhat less — $50 to $85 — by obtaining the support of hospitals and hospital supply companies. With these points in mind, the 2-day Goddard financial seminar was priced at $225. A group rate of $200 per person for institutions sending three or more individuals was offered. The tuition covered all materials, daily continental breakfast, lunch, and refreshment breaks.

The expenses related to developing the workshop were not fully recovered from the first offering. Nan made contacts for further distribution in Florida, Georgia, and South Carolina. She found that distribution channels varied in each state, and she adjusted her promotional efforts accordingly. In Florida, the statewide nursing administration association is the key. Contact with its officers was instrumental in arranging seminar sites and generating mailing lists. In South Carolina, the continuing education function in nursing is organized around seven regions, each led by a full-time coordinator, who serves all the health care institutions in the region by organizing and sponsoring pertinent events. In Georgia, the State Hospital Association sponsors educational services for all hospitals in its jurisdiction. These channels are critical to sales. By the conclusion of the second seminar, the firm was in the black.

"The principal responsibility of the business," states Nan, "is to make contact with nursing and health care colleagues in each state, determine the extent of their continuing education needs, develop quality responses in the firm's area of expertise, identify key distribution channels, and effectively promote the product. This process involves many networking contacts."

Nursing conventions and conferences also play a vital role in meeting business objectives. They enhance personal selling opportunities, expand networks, and generate ideas, but most of all they provide a "keep-current" opportunity, so that the firm can stay on top of developments in the field.

Since January 1985, Nan Goddard has conducted 25 seminars in 10 states. That's educational marketing success!

Graduate Education

Opportunity and Product Development. As mentioned earlier, Nan's prior contact with graduate students led her to identify a need for curriculum development in financial management. Shortly after arriving in Houston, she contacted nursing educators at Texas Woman's University in Houston. She learned that the school was developing a graduate program in nursing service administration. Nan met with members of the faculty and shared her experiences, views, and evolving course outline. In the spring of 1984, Nan was selected to teach financial management at Texas Woman's University.

"I also wanted to talk with other nursing educators, in order to learn more about educational program development in administration. Through colleagues, I identified an organization that seemed to meet my need—the Council for Graduate Education for Administration in Nursing (CGEAN). I did not meet membership requirements at the time, but by contacting selected members, I secured permission to attend the organization's upcoming meeting in June 1984.

"Some CGEAN members responded to my ideas and proposals negatively. On the other hand, there were several who were most encouraging. Grace Peterson, who taught nursing administration at DePaul University in Chicago for 27 years, really made a big difference in my life at the CGEAN meeting. Grace took me to lunch and expressed her belief that there was a major need for the curriculum I advocated. Another educator told me to copyright my course outline. On the basis of my experience, I decided to move ahead."

As Nan developed the course outline, she thought of herself as a visiting professor. "At the CGEAN meeting, I met Linda Hodges of the Medical University of South Carolina. She was developing a program in nursing service administration and needed someone who could teach financial content. Together we managed to work things out." In the spring of 1985, Nan Goddard began teaching financial management in the nursing service administration program at Medical University of South Carolina. The course is offered over a 3-week period during a summer session. Since its initiation, student evaluations have been outstanding.

Product Promotion and Pricing. Nan has promoted the graduate course in financial management by word of mouth, personal selling, and organizational contacts. Since 1985, she has developed teaching relationships with the University of Texas at Galveston, the University of Texas at Arlington, the University of Texas at Houston, George Mason University in Fairfax, Virginia, and most recently

Azusa Pacific University in Azusa, California, in addition to others mentioned earlier.

Teaching schedules and course content are shaped to meet the needs of the environment. For example, Nan sometimes includes course content in using business software such as Lotus 1-2-3. Other nursing programs prefer to leave computer skill development for a later date. What Nan's service fee will be is addressed as the instructional contract is developed.

"This particular product will, in all probability, grow in relation to curriculum development," states Nan. "In education, this process is *slow*. 'Have Course — Will Travel,' I believe, has great promise. Entrepreneurial product lines are traditionally a waiting game."

The Future

Nan Goddard plans to continue developing her educational product lines and management consulting activities. She finds her endeavors rewarding and reports that she is heartened by comments from workshop participants and students alike. "I frequently receive letters and cards from participants recounting how they have put theory to use in the real world. I need to know that I make a difference in patient care delivery systems."

Nan is committed to her profession and her firm. One means of keeping in touch and responding to her clients is through her telephone answering machine, which she can access from anywhere in the country. Her message is unique. The reader might want to give her a call, just to hear how she actually greets colleagues and potential customers:

Thank you for calling Goddard Management Resources. Our professional staff members are unavailable to receive your call at this moment. However, it is being monitored and recorded so that we may respond to your message as soon as it is feasible. The voice-activated recorder will give you as much time as you would like to explain the reason for your call. Because the date and time of your call are logged automatically, you may begin your message upon hearing the tone. Thanks so much.

That's marketing!

Entrepreneurship in Clinical Practice

Dolores M. Alford, M.S.N..
R.N., F.A.A.N.
Nursing Associates
Dallas, Texas

Janet A. Moll, M.S., R.N.
G.N.P.
Nursing Associates
Dallas, Texas

Nursing Associates was established in 1974 by Dolores Alford and Janet Moll. Together they designed and implemented a unique model of primary nursing care that has come to be recognized and respected nationally and internationally.

A Partnership Is Formed

When Dee Alford and Janet Moll made their decision to establish an independent nursing practice, many health care professionals, including nurses, expressed severe reservations. "Our major barrier was that imposed by nurses. They didn't appreciate or support the idea of nurses in private practice, nor were many able to identify with the independent health care services nurses can provide." Dee and Janet established their partnership for two primary reasons. First, Dee was teaching geriatric nurse practitioner students at Texas Woman's University. She felt a model practice would facilitate achievement of the program's objectives. Janet, a graduate of Dee's first class, wanted to offer primary health care to older adults. A shared philosophy, entrepreneurial zeal, and clinical commitment brought them together.

"We believe nurses can deliver primary health care. Nurses must fully utilize the practice scope authorized in Nurse Practice Acts, and nurses are capable of managing their own business. Nurses have specialized knowledge and skills, and the services that flow from these can be directly marketed to the consumer. In 1974, we were confident we could live our values, attitudes, and beliefs through private nursing practice. In 1988 we know we have succeeded."

Planning — The First Step

After Dee and Janet made their decision, they spent almost 9 months developing their business plan. "We have never regretted the time we took to plan. Initial decisions revolved around target markets, the services we would offer, charges, and promotional techniques. Our health assessment, health teaching, and counseling skills were marketable to all adults, though our primary target group was the older client.

"Since our practice was such a new idea, we developed a brochure describing our services. It helped people understand who and what Nursing Associates represented and how they could use our expertise. We also established a fee structure. In 1974, we charged $20 an hour. Today we receive $50 an hour."

Product Lines

Nursing Associates' business plan provides for five client services.

Health Promotion Service. The goal of this service is to promote the client's physical, mental, and spiritual well-being. The nursing activities that support achievement of that goal are a comprehensive health history, physical examination, and laboratory studies; development of a client-centered plan to promote wellness via lifestyle changes; health counseling and education for children, adolescents, adults, and seniors; development of stress management skills; and assistance in identifying and utilizing community and health care resources.

Nursing Clinics. Nursing Associates provides health promotion services in the office and at satellite locations such as senior centers, retirement centers, business offices, schools, and apartment complexes. Currently, Nursing Associates clinics are located in Richardson, Irving, Dallas, and Plano, Texas.

Family Consultation. This service assists families in developing family living skills, maintaining independent living for aged parents or older family members, selecting alternative living arrangements for older adults, and promoting functional family status.

Educational Services. Programs are provided for health care professionals and members of the community at large on a variety of topics related to Nursing Associates services, including:

Primary ambulatory care

Physical assessment

Gerontic nursing

Drug use by the older adult

Wellness concepts

Holistic health

Legal aspects of nursing.

Professional Consultation. Nursing Associates offers a team of nurse experts in research, administration, maternal and child health, holistic health, health promotion, and educational media.

Promotional Efforts

Dee and Janet use a variety of marketing techniques. The following sections describe their primary promotional activities.

Identity. "We selected an ancient symbol of longevity as our logo [Figure 16-1]. This never-beginning-or-ending group of squares configured in a diamond shape appears on our letterhead, brochures, cards, and labels. We sometimes wear a handcrafted silver pendant of the symbol, and our office reception area features a wall hanging of the symbol, made by one of our clients."

Brochure Promotion. "Our first brochure was an in-house production. We designed it, used logo artwork donated by a relative, wrote the content, typed it, and had 500 offset copies run off. The brochures were not slick, but they were neat, readable, and adequately described our services.

"The brochure has changed as our practice has changed. Today it reflects the diversity of our practice — direct care, consultations, and educational programs. It is consistent in type style and design with our letterhead and business cards." When it is revised, updated photos of Dee and Janet are included.

"Our brochure is an effective communication mechanism. We always take a number with us on speaking engagements or when meeting a potential client. It has been our experience that people will take the brochure home, put it away, and a year or so later call for an appointment. It is often surprising how the brochure shapes the referral process. We try not to miss an opportunity to enhance visibility. Older clients like to show family and friends our pictures.

**NURSING
ASSOCIATES**

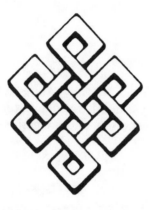

Figure 16-1 The Nursing Associates — company logo.

'That's *my* nurse,' they will say." Brochures offer the elderly something tangible to share in recounting their daily experiences: "I saw my nurse today . . . ."

"A second brochure is designed for and available at each of our clinic sites. It includes information on location, hours of operation, available services, and a brief biographical sketch describing the clinic nurse, Nursing Associates, and the clinic sponsor. At public housing clinics, brochures are given to each resident, and apartment managers are encouraged to give them to new tenants. Landlords find that the brochure is often the clincher in persuading prospective elderly tenants to rent one housing unit rather than another."

Business Cards. "We carry business cards with us wherever we go; they are an ideal promotional tool. We even take them to the restroom. While waiting in line, one can make great contacts. We offer business cards to receptionists when arriving for an appointment, and we enclose business cards in inquiry letters. and other correspondence. We also place cards and brochures in our reception area for clients to take for friends and relatives."

Newsletters. Housing complexes, churches, and senior centers publish calendars and newsletters reminding tenants and participants of available health services. This medium is used as a means of reminding clients when health care screening services are offered.

Newspaper Promotion. "When we began our practice, a dear friend, working on the women's page of a local newspaper, wrote a feature story on Nursing Associates. It focused on women as emerging entrepreneurs. We also wrote our own press release announcing our opening and sent it to all papers within a 100-mile radius of the office. We were pleased to see it printed in several papers. Suburban newspapers, which serve clinic communities, periodically feature a clinic and its services. They also include the clinic's hours and location in the community calendar.

"Our most satisfying newspaper study appeared just as we were preparing a press release recognizing the tenth anniversary of our practice. Dee had just received the American Nurses' Association Honorary Nursing Practice Award. Naturally, ANA sent a press release to the local papers, and a reporter called about the award. We advised her we were developing an announcement, highlighting our 10 years of practice. She extended the interview beyond the award and included a photographer. The result was an extensive article about our practice, featuring a color picture of Dee working in a clinic setting. We received several clients as a result."

Radio Promotion. "We periodically participate on talk shows that encourage listeners to call in with questions. We are also called on intermittently to 'come quickly,' when a scheduled guest is unable to participate. Initially, we developed a topic on the way to the radio station. Now, having learned from our experience, we have ready-to-go subject matter and proactively communicate our willingness to help out. These programs always bring us one or two clients. One gentleman, who lived 500 miles away, called in while we were still on the air and requested appointments for his entire family."

Television Promotion. "Television offers exposure as talk show participants, panel members, and as news reactors. Our friends in television call, asking our opinion on current events — a report or story published in the morning paper. We are frequently asked to comment on the statements of others. Once, a reporter and camera crew called from the lobby of our office building and appeared moments later in the office. Media exposure of any kind means you must remain up to date on current events. For example, reading the morning paper is crucial. Image is affected by how knowledgeable you seem on professional issues, clinical advancements, and the local scene. Expectation and opportunity go hand in hand."

Marketing Wellness Centers

"When our practice opened, we identified a significant barrier to our business objectives. Medicare did not reimburse for our services, and many elderly clients could not afford the out-of-pocket expense." Rather than approach the problem from a "can't do" perspective, Dee and Janet demonstrated the "can do" entrepreneurial spirit. They examined alternative funding arrangements and developed a center sponsor strategy.

"Our first sponsors were three Presbyterian churches in Richardson, a suburb of Dallas. One of the churches had a senior group meeting twice a week. The church identified a need for enhanced health care and spearheaded offering our services as a part of their outreach mission. Our first contract was signed in 1978. The fee was $100 for 6 hours of service.

"Word of our unique form of geriatric care spread. A neighboring suburb contacted us to speak at a church cluster meeting. In less than a year, another contract was signed. Our standard agreement requires sponsors to provide a clinic site and all capital equipment — exam table, chairs, scales, desks, etc. Nursing Associates provides staff and all expendable clinic and office supplies. Except for fee structure, the original contracts we formulated remain substantially unchanged today."

Each clinic is the result of networking activities among professionals and laypersons. "We currently operate four clinic sites in addition to our main office. One clinic is in a public housing complex owned by the Unitarian Church. Nursing Associates reports directly to the Trust Board, which oversees the housing units. A Nursing Associates' representative works with the management company and its employees to ensure an efficient and effective operation. Our second center is located on the vast campus of the Dallas Home for the Jewish Aged. All residents, in public and private housing, are able to take advantage of the clinic. The nurse manager reports to the home's director of nursing. She also has strong interactive lines with the various building managers. Nursing Associates and its representatives recognize and respond to each building manager's unique situation. This approach serves as a means of facilitating referrals and wellness center support. Our fourth senior center is located in Plano, a suburb of Dallas. It is staffed by a geriatric nurse practitioner, who sees elderly clients twice a week by appointment.

"Our sponsors are pleased with the contractual arrangements. They recognize our expertise in managing the clinics and in providing primary health care services to seniors. Clinic nurses secure all clinical and office supplies through our main office, monitor current literature, develop handouts, and order educational material for the clinics. Secretarial services are handled through Nursing Associates. Wellness center sponsors incur little overhead, yet receive recognition for the health care provided. We are proud of the sponsors who have helped us pioneer wellness centers for older adults."

Service Fees

Professional fees are established through cost accounting procedures and by cost-benefit analysis. Dee and Janet focus on indirect expense reductions, to allow for maximum return on investment. Increases in supplies, rent, and purchased services are recovered by fee adjustment.

"We have experienced some difficulty with individuals who do not expect to pay for services rendered. One of the most perplexing problems is inappropriate telephone consultation. We discourage this. Care by telephone is risky at best. We also find individuals who want to observe our practice and are surprised when a consultation fee is mentioned. Fee-for-service arrangements in nursing are new. As nursing grows and develops, acceptance will increase."

Networking

Nurse Networking. "In the beginning, nurses were our major practice barrier. We are pleased to report that this is no longer true. As we grew, so did they. Nurses come to us for care and refer others to us. Frequently, we find ourselves doing health assessments or health maintenance updates during holiday and vacation times, when older family members come to Dallas. Nurses also refer the media to us for information.

"One colleague in particular has been influential in securing two clinic contracts. This dedicated nurse is our advocate in many ways—promoting the nurse practitioner role and educational programs we offer. Other nurse supporters acknowledge our work at meetings and conferences during their own presentations. They also give out cards and brochures."

Physician Networking. "As we expected, some physicians were threatened by our practice. On the other hand, many welcomed us and we formed a collegial relationship. When we identify client health care problems requiring medical attention, we refer them back to their own physician, or help them find a physician who is competent and sensitive to the needs of the elderly.

"We use a variety of communication tools to help physicians understand who we are and what we are. For example, each client receives a health diary. It includes information that assists clients in managing various aspects of the health care system. For example, a hypertension flow sheet and a drug list are important diary components. We include information in the health diary that the client should report or obtain from the physician, and the nurse associate questions the physician through diary entries. Physicians also communicate through the diary and often photocopy diary information for their records."

Dee and Janet report that clients cherish their diaries. "One new client came to a clinic because she felt left out of her social group's diary-sharing activities. " 'My nurse wants me to . . . ,' we hear clients tell one another, as they review goals, instructions, and recommendations documented in their diaries.

"We also teach our clients how to talk to physicians, so that the physician-patient relationship is strengthened. We network with physicians and discuss various approaches to client care and follow-up. These interprofessional interactions demonstrate how well physicians and nurses use their unique expertise to enhance client care. Referrals, in both directions, occur as a result. Physicians, dentists, and podiatrists also donate their time to clinic screening activities and work with us to promote health and health maintenance services."

Referral Patterns. Traditional and nontraditional referral activities also provide Dee and Janet with clients. "One never knows how referral patterns will operate. The telephone company has patched seniors needing assistance into our phone system, and individuals in other states, who see us on TV, contact the office for care. The

Chamber of Commerce, the Public Library, Aging Information Services, university gerontology programs, churches with aging services, public relations personnel, and, of course, various health professionals all refer to us.

"Businesses such as hearing aid companies, real estate firms, printers, and office supply vendors have also referred clients as they learn about our services. We have professional relationships with many vendors, who know they can stop in our office to visit, make a telephone call, or get a cup of coffee. These people pass the word. Personal selling is a vital marketing technique."

Image

Office Location, Decor, and Operation. Nursing Associates is located in a professional building in a large shopping and office complex. "Our location offers many advantages. The building has valet parking, and while clients are seen, family members or drivers can shop. Clients can visit other health care providers in the complex, eat in one of the fine restaurants, or shop in one of the more than 80 stores. The office is also near a bus line and the tollway.

"Decor is a critical marketing tool. Our office is comfortable and attractive, with lots of bright colors for aging eyes. We make certain that magazines and health teaching materials are current. We pride ourselves on having a reception area, not a waiting room. Clients are seen on time, and those individuals who accompany are always offered coffee or tea. On occasion, clients just drop in for a hug, a cup of tea, or for rest while shopping. These services also help promote referrals."

Dress. "No matter how clients dress, they expect us to meet their idea of professional attire. In response, we dress in career-style clothes — dresses, skirts, and blouses or suits. Jewelry which interferes with work is avoided. Shoes are low- or midheeled, look smart, and offer stability. We wear blue or green lab coats, mainly because we need pockets and a place for our name tags."

Diversification — A Key to Success

"The wellness centers represent a major part of our practice, but we also see private clients, of all ages, in our main office for primary health care services. We counsel adult children of aging parents and

nurses who need assistance with their career goals and objectives."
Dee and Janet consult with nurses interested in private practice and
with nursing schools planning nurse-managed centers.

Educational programs and workshops represent one Nursing
Associates product line. "Most of our educational programs are
provided through the Institute of Gerontic Nursing, Inc., a not-for-
profit corporate subsidiary of Nursing Associates dedicated to research, education, and consultation in gerontic nursing. These
programs allow us to pursue contemporary developments in the
health care market."

Future Directions

Untapped markets offer Nursing Associates a bright future. As
the elderly population expands, the demand for services will increase. "We are fortunate—we don't lack for opportunities. There
are not enough hours in the day. The services we currently offer
take priority. They are complex and enormously rewarding. There is
no greater feeling than having a client who conveys a message of
service satisfaction. That is the absolute best marketing we have."

A Home Health Care Entrepreneur

Margaret Y. O'Brien, R.N., M.S.
President, Margaret Y. O'Brien, Inc.
Woodbine, Maryland

In 1981, Margaret Y. O'Brien was the frustrated employee of a
large health maintenance organization in Washington, D.C. "I had a
need for autonomy and control. In my job, I felt I was beating my
head against a brick wall." Margaret was responsible for the
management and coordination of a 24-hour HMO patient care unit
servicing a base of 130,000 clients. "The unit provided emergency
care and included a six-bed holding area. The purpose of the unit
was to avoid, whenever possible, the high cost of emergency rooms
and inpatient hospitalization."

Margaret recognized that she was headed for professional burnout. "I felt I had a lot to contribute to nursing and the health care
system, but I knew I had to make a change. A combination of factors
led me to establish my own consulting business. First, I was living in
the Washington, D.C., area. Consulting is a D.C. way of life. The at-

mosphere was there. Second, I had encouragement from professional colleagues and some limited experience with the consulting process. Most of all, I had a supportive husband who encouraged me to give it a try.

"Without any advance planning—a business plan in particular—I notified my employer that I was leaving. At the same time, however, knowing that it would take several months to replace me, I offered my consulting services to focus on the strategic planning and marketing projects I never could get to as an employee. To my surprise, they agreed. Thus, in the spring of 1981, with one firm engagement, I began a new phase in my professional career. My field had always been ambulatory health care, and it was where I felt the health care system was going. When I look back, after 7 years of experience, I took quite a risk. I must have been a little crazy!"

Building the Business

"As the end of my first engagement approached, I faced reality. I didn't have another client. It was a sobering time. I spent the next 2 years establishing myself. It required a lot of hard work, with little return on investment, in the way of revenue—1982 and 1983 were lean."

During this period, Margaret concentrated on developmental and promotional opportunities. She established linkages with community-based health care agencies, actively participated in professional organizations, and listened closely to what potential clients expressed as needs. "Promotion is promotion of self. You must be visible. You never know when a contact will pay off.

"It is absolutely critical that anyone trying to build a business remain current in their field, be on top of client need, satisfy client expectations, and develop the business skills to support your expertise." Margaret spent time in the library mastering the knowledge base required to develop business plans, product lines, proposals, feasibility studies, contracts, professional portfolio design, and reading the literature.

"I worked out of my home, using such basic communication tools as business cards and a telephone answering machine. I set a goal to publish one article a year, not only to enhance my visibility, but to meet the higher order professional requirement of contributing to the knowledge base. This goal also helped me keep current. Though these 2 years were difficult and at times discouraging, I grew as an individual and successfully competed for two clients. Toward the end of 1983, my big opportunity hit. All the preparation, study, and sacrifice paid off."

In response to the changing health care environment, Maryland passed legislation offering hospitals the opportunity to develop home health care services without going through the certificate-of-need process. The incentive, established by the need to reduce length of stay, was there, and the enabling legislation opened the door. Margaret was positioned in the marketplace to take full advantage of the opportunity. Hospitals wanted to develop home care services, and Margaret was ready, willing, and able to provide the expertise required to assist them in achieving their business goals. Her original belief, that the wave of the future was in community-based care, and her own entrepreneurial spirit had paid off.

"I worked harder in 1984 than I ever believed I could or would. It was overwhelming. I was still a solo consultant, but I set aside time for professional activities and continuing education. Closing yourself off, by just working on engagements, defeats business development objectives in the long run. It was so nice to be needed!"

In 1985, the business continued to grow. During this time, Margaret took on a full-time associate, secured what she describes as a major contract, developed a business brochure, hired a secretary/receptionist, and accepted speaking engagements from state and national associations for home care. "I found that my commitment to satisfied customers paid off. My best sources of referral are former clients."

"As time went by and my client base grew, I gave serious consideration to media promotion. In 1986, I decided to give it a try. My husband, who is in broadcasting, helped me find a small, two-woman advertising agency. I was reluctant to work with the big firms. I felt more secure with the personal service they offered." Margaret placed six ads, one every other month, in a major community health care journal. The total bill was several thousand dollars. Although she did not receive any specific referrals from the ads, she feels strongly that the campaign served image building goals and sent a signal to others regarding the firm's growth and development. Margaret is currently planning her 1988 ad campaign.

In 1981, Margaret O'Brien had one client. Today, her client lists exceeds 100 agencies for whom she has completed one or more engagements. Three rooms in her home are now devoted to the business, and she has seven nurse consultants with whom she works various engagements. "Our incentive plan offers each O'Brien consultant a percentage of any contract they secure. On other jobs, the firm operates on a fee-for-service basis. I have continued to limit permanent employees because of the continuing financial commitment they require."

The entrepreneurial zeal and professional commitment that Margaret O'Brien demonstrated in 1981 have provided a substantial return on investment. When asked what pointers she would give to other nurses who might consider such a move, Margaret offered the following:

"You are always on center stage. The impressions you leave with people, visual or otherwise, play a major role in business development. The reputation you *earn* is critical. Reputation is built on factors other than the quality of your work. Attention to detail cannot be overemphasized. Executives make judgments about your capabilities based on how you and your employees answer the phone, the grammar and punctuation used in correspondence, how you dress, and whether you're on time for appointments. Image development is a constant and ongoing phenomenon. Pay attention!

"People often say to me that because I am in business for myself I can work as little or as much as I want. That may be true, but in the beginning and as the company develops, it is difficult to pass up business. When you know you can do the job, particularly after you have a few tough years, it is hard to turn your back on opportunity. I'm still hungry. The desire to compete, grow, and move forward is always there.

"When you are fortunate enough to have clients, there are deadlines, expectations, and unexpected demands. These expectations are even more pressing than those I experienced as an employee. When I make a business decision, the future of the company is affected. I guess I'm trying to say that while it appears your time is your own, you really don't have the flexibility, in relation to choice, as those looking in from the outside may think.

"One of the most important lessons an entrepreneur learns," asserts Margaret, "is how to deal with rejection. Unaccepted proposals or the loss of a former client is part of doing business. It's one thing to verbalize the facts of business life. The emotion of it is another matter entirely. When a venture is not successful, try and find out why the proposal was passed over. Executives are usually willing to share information about their decision-making process, particularly when they know you are just getting started. Above all else, remember that a business rejection is not a repudiation of self.

"Finally, to coin an old saying, I would say that it is better to have tried and failed than never to have tried at all. I encourage entrepreneurial activity by nurses. The rewards far outweigh the costs. I feel good about my company, its products and services, and about myself. I make a difference in the delivery of quality health care, and I am contributing to the development of my profession. It is a very satisfying feeling."

Entrepreneurship and Multiple Product Lines

Sallyan Sohr, R.N., M.B.A.
President, Sallyan Sohr Health
    Associates, Inc.
Galesville, Maryland

Sallyan Sohr Health Associates, Inc. (SASHA) provides educational, management, consultative, and automated management information services to the health care industry. Primary target markets are clinical nurses and departments of nursing in the acute care setting. Designed to meet the unique and changing needs of the health care system, SASHA was established as a holistic health care service firm, offering a wide range of integrated educational, consultation, and information services.

The company was founded in July 1980 by Sallyan Sohr. While working in the health care industry, Sallyan recognized the need for advanced education, management, and organizational and fiscal services in health care. Over the last 8 years SASHA has served hundreds of institutions, agencies, associations, and thousands of individuals. The firm's success is primarily related to the commitment, hard work, and skill of its leader. Her career path played a major role in her decision to form the company.

Following completion of a baccalaureate degree in nursing at the University of Maryland in 1967, Sallyan held a variety of positions including labor and delivery head nurse, nurse training specialist, and head nurse at a shock trauma unit, emergency department nurse chairman, and nurse coordinator for the State of Maryland. She founded her company in 1980, 5 years after she accepted the nurse coordinator position. Her work in that position played a major role in shaping her career path.

Sallyan Sohr was the first nurse coordinator in the State of Maryland. When she left the position in 1980 there were seven. Her primary responsibility was the upgrading of nursing practice throughout the state by facilitating the development of standards of care and through coordination of activities across the state in acute care facilities.

She helped develop and implement emergency medicine standards for levels of care; designed and coordinated modular health care training programs in multiple trauma, spinal cord injury, burn management, sudden infant death syndrome, sexual assault, crisis intervention, management training, and stress management; and completed a 6-month research project on human asset accounting — a method of reducing cost and increasing productivity in the workforce by job redesign and humanistic training. This project was tremendously successful, documenting hundreds of thousands of dollars in direct cost reductions.

As a result of her work with the state, Sallyan received requests to consult outside Maryland. As she traveled from hospital to hospital, she saw a major need to actualize nursing potential. After 3 years with the state, she began studying at the University of Baltimore for a Master's in Business Administration. Upon completing her degree, she established SASHA.

"I opened my business for three reasons. First, a personal need for growth. Second, I felt it would serve as a means of going beyond the barriers commonly experienced by nurses and nursing in actualizing the potential contribution of our discipline. I have a boundless love for nursing and respect for what it can contribute to health care, particularly if some of the system blockages are removed. Finally, my experience as a state coordinator convinced me there was opportunity, and I had the educational preparation I needed to get the job done. It was a natural progression — as I look back, I can't see my career developing in any other way.

"My decision was not supported by the majority of my nursing colleagues. In fact, some of them felt it was irresponsible, primarily because I was a single parent. I had been with the State of Maryland for a number of years, and my salary and benefits were very good. I did, however, receive support from the faculty at the University of Baltimore. They encouraged me to be anything that I wanted to be."

As graduation approached, Sallyan completed a readiness assessment. She had been able to put together some venture capital and had several clients requesting her services. "You must have tremendous faith in yourself to start your own corporation. Of course, the prospect of no paycheck every 2 weeks also generates a great deal of incentive!"

Educational Division

Sallyan Sohr's original business plan identified three corporate product lines. The first product line that she concentrated on developing was the educational division. "As a state coordinator, I saw a significant need for continuing education, and no reason why that need should ever decrease. Hospitals did not seem to have the interest or capacity to respond." Because of current changes taking place in the health care system, Sallyan feels that this need is even greater than when she started the corporation. SASHA's educational department meets the unique and changing needs of the health care system for training and development. To meet this challenge SASHA offers both "set" and customized programs.

In the customized programs, the customer identifies desired outcomes and SASHA develops a presentation that provides the information and exercises that support the desired behaviors. The set programs consist of 24 educational workshops offered by SASHA in seven program areas. The prospective client is provided with the workshop's behavioral objectives, a content summary, and information about the instructor. Workshops vary in length according to need, the target audience, and agency resources. Participants receive a workbook, a posttest instrument that can be self-administered, and continuing education credit. A description of SASHA's seven program areas follows.

Fiscal Management. This program is designed for individuals who have responsibility for budgeting, staffing system design, and decision-making, such as nursing managers and personnel directors, among others. The participants are provided with an overall understanding of how new cost-containment regulations might affect the viability of their institutions and the quality of patient care. The attendees are provided with concrete approaches for meeting the cost-containment challenge while maintaining quality of care. This program area gives nurse managers the tools to develop the fiscal skills and knowledge demanded in their roles.

Crisis Intervention. This 3-day program meets the needs of those working with patients and/or families who present with any of the following crisis situations: sudden death, sexual assault, family violence, violent patient behavior, suicide, or drug and alcohol crisis.

Stress Management and Burnout Prevention. This workshop is addressed to individuals working in acute and chronic health care settings. Methods for identifying and differentiating stressful and distressful situations are extensively explored. Signs and symptoms of organizational and individual maladaptation are reviewed with a focus on recognition, management, and prevention. Self-assessment and stress reduction techniques are demonstrated.

Assertiveness Training. This 6-hour workshop is offered to nurses who want to increase their effectiveness in communication with physicians, peers, supervisors, and patients. Participants learn assertive communication methods as opposed to aggressive, passive, or passive-aggressive communication techniques. The main focus is on honest and effective communication, without loss of esteem.

Time Management. Participants in this workshop learn to analyze their time utilization patterns, identify time-saving methods for effective crisis intervention, and learn basic principles for maximizing time management.

Management Series. This program is for the middle manager. At its conclusion, the nurse manager should be comfortable with contingency management theories and practices. The participant learns to identify leadership styles and their relative merits; learns about management roles, goals, and functions; and gains a practical awareness of selected management skills.

Advanced Management. This program's target audience is the experienced top-level manager. It enhances development in the utilization of human resources, the growth of middle managers, stress management, utilization of fiscal resources, and the art of influence and manipulation.

SASHA's programs are presented across the nation. To date, participants number in the thousands. Three hundred directors and assistant directors of nursing have participated in the advanced management programs.

Consultation Division

SASHA's consultation services range from those requiring a high level of specific technological knowledge to those of a more general operational nature. This division was built on the 60 successful engagements Sallyan had as a state employee.

Among the consultations SASHA has completed are job-description and criteria-based evaluation development; creative staffing and scheduling designs; patient and nurse classification systems; productivity and workload analysis; quality assurance program development and implementation; recruitment and retention strategies; fiscal system development; and the creation of automated managerial information systems.

On one occasion, SASHA accepted a project that established a pediatric respiratory intensive care unit. It required coordination and supervision of architectural renovation, equipment selection, purchase agreements, advertising, interviewing and hiring staff, policy and procedure development, and a grand opening cocktail party.

Management Services Division

SASHA's management division establishes agreements with health care organizations for the day-to-day operation of units and/or agencies. This arm of the business has experienced the slowest growth rate. "I believe it is a viable service, but of course, it requires strong administrative support in order to achieve successful implementation. It may be" asserts Sallyan Sohr, "an even more attractive arrangement for organizations seeking effective responses to the nursing shortage."

The educational division has been the corporation's most profitable product line. "I started with what I knew best and what was needed in the marketplace. Certification preparation programs for emergency room and critical care nurses opened communication in the clinical areas I knew best."

The consulting division also provides a good return on investment. "We are bottom line oriented. We don't engage in activities which cannot pay for themselves outright, or as part of another project. For example, we make the smallest profit on the SASHA Patient Classification System. However, its installation sometimes results in an ongoing relationship between SASHA and the agency. This helps justify the minimal margins."

Information Systems

In 1984, Sallyan Sohr began to study the feasibility of adding a fourth product line to her business. "Everything pointed to the development of computerized hospital informational systems. In my own immediate office environment, I investigated and subsequently invested in computers. I was mailing out a half-million pieces of promotional literature a year. The mailing list was quite large and required hours to manage, and the accounting and financial functions of the business were demanding increased resources.

"When I set out to explore the field, my own lack of knowledge was a handicap. It took me almost a year to make an office computer system decision. The questions and need for information were endless. How do you develop computer systems? What is the capacity of computers? How could I acquire the programming skills necessary to produce products? It took 3 years to develop the first SASHA computer application. I spent tens of thousands of dollars and learned many valuable lessons along the way."

Sallyan's new product line was developed in a joint venture with systems engineers. SASHA's automated information systems now include a nursing care plan operating system; acuity-based patient classification; calculation of nursing care charges per patient based on patient acuity; productivity reporting that compares budgeted, actual, and required staffing on a daily, monthly, and yearly basis; and staff scheduling systems, which include an employee information data base containing biographical data and data on employee experience, expertise, area, and shift preference, as well as on nursing care hours and skill mix required. The system also screens staff and identifies nurses who meet variable staffing pool needs. "We are continually adding on new modules to our computer system. In fall 1988, our bedside computer units will be installed. The future looks bright. I expect this arm of the corporation to return the greatest profit, and although our major focus is increasingly with information systems, the education and consulting divisions will continue."

Pricing the Product

As Sallyan was developing her 1980 business plan, questions regarding product pricing arose. Her approach was basic and pragmatic. "In order to establish consulting division rates, I estimated what take-home pay I needed to put food on the table and make mortgage payments. Next, I conservatively estimated the number of days per month I thought I might consult and divided one number into the other. I charged $500 a day when I opened the business. To my knowledge, I lost only one job because of the rate. Over the years I have developed a more complex pricing structure that ranges from $700 to $1,000 a day. Customers who have been with me since the beginning are billed at their initial rate. They stood by me — I will stand by them."

Seminar pricing has also changed during the years Sallyan has been in business. "I began by offering a no-frills seminar at $40 a day, but quickly found that due to the benefits of our programs registration remained the same at twice the rate. The driving force is need. We require 12 to 13 participants for a typical staff nurse-level seminar to break even. I try and structure presentations for upper-level management so that attendance is limited. Registration fees of $125 to $150 provide a financial breakeven at six attendees." SASHA also offers fee reductions to agencies who send more than one participant.

"Information system pricing is largely driven by the competition. Promotional cost is, of course, significant, as are those associated with the educational effort necessary to successfully install a system. My basic goal is to offer high-quality services at a profit — one that meets my needs, those of our employees, and the ongoing research and development costs associated with maintaining established products and funding new ventures."

Promoting the Product

Since SASHA's incorporation, Sallyan Sohr has used a variety of methods to promote company products. In the beginning she used her name as a marketing tool. "During my 5 years as a nursing coordinator, I traveled across the state and consulted in various parts of the country. My name was my primary asset — it promoted the business to past contacts." Today, Sallyan believes that the name SASHA may hinder the information system product line because they seemingly bear little relationship to each other. It's a problem, however, she is willing to live with.

"The single most important promotion factor, I believe, is achieved by living your business philosophy. When we price a job, we do so to make a profit, but we don't leave a job until the customer is completely satisfied with the service SASHA provides, even if that means a loss. I advertise, on a fairly regular basis, in *Nursing Management* and the *Journal of Nursing Administration*. The ads always pay for themselves through engagements returned. The reader response services of these journals are outstanding.

"SASHA employees are also marketing agents, from the manner in which they answer the phone to the individual expertise of each consulting team member." Sallyan has four permanent employees and more than 20 nurse experts she uses from time to time on projects. "I like to use people who are actively practicing in the field. It provides a special focus and lends credibility to our recommendations." During the past 2 years, SASHA has taken on several full-time programmers in order to provide for product line growth.

A Backward Glance

In the first year Sallyan was in business she grossed $82,000. She expects to gross $1.3 million this year and $20 million by 1992. "The kind of money we gross sounds terrific, but until you've lived through the experience of establishing a business, you can't appreciate the investment required to get there. First, any individual who is thinking about going into business should be prepared to *work*. I was always a hard worker, but my personal experience during graduate school prepared me for the real world. I was working for the state full-time and going to school full-time. I got up every morning at 5 a.m. and studied until 7. I learned to use every single minute. I made lists of things to do on a daily basis and didn't go to bed until everything was done.

"Effectively organizing workload is a skill that is learned by doing. Entrepreneurship requires it! Self-discipline is a key attribute. The only money I take out of the company is that required to meet basic needs. The remainder is plowed back into the company so that we can remain competitive. When developing a business you must constantly prepare for the future. If I hadn't managed in this manner, the information systems product development would still be a dream. The ability to tolerate delayed gratification is important. Success does not come easily.

"Entrepreneurship requires that you read everything in sight, develop extensive professional networks, participate in professional organizations, and listen, listen, and listen. Whatever you do in business, it must meet a need. Entrepreneurs should see the need before the people who are talking are able to articulate them."

SASHA's future is promising. Sallyan is approached from time to time with offers to buy her corporation. "A number of the offers have been very attractive, but I'm not ready to let go. My business plan calls for expansion in the West over the next 5 years. Currently, 90% of our consulting is in the East. In the beginning, we limited ourselves to the East in order to reduce expenses. Inquiries, however, outside our traditional marketplace continue to grow. We are planning to move into those areas and take advantage of the opportunity they offer." If past success is any indicator—watch out, California, here comes SASHA!

References

American Nurses' Association. 1979. *A case for baccalaureate preparation in nursing.* Kansas City: American Nurses' Association.

Drucker, P.F. 1985. *Innovation and entrepreneurship: practice and principles.* pp. 27, 28. New York: Harper & Row.

Etzioni, A. 1969. *The semi-professions and their organization.* New York: The Free Press.

Silver, D.A. 1986. *The entrepreneurial life: how to go for it and get it.* pp. 26-30, 227, 230, 244. New York: John Wiley.

Stuart, G.W. 1981. How professional is nursing? *Image* 13:18-23.

Review Questions

1. After briefly reviewing Chapters 7 through 9, select any two of the nurse entrepreneurs in this chapter and discuss how they avoided the pitfalls that make many new services fail.

2. Review the decision-making process of each nurse entrepreneur to venture out on her own. What common characteristics are there and how do they compare with

attributes commonly associated with an entrepreneurial experience?

3. What promotional mechanisms did the nurse entrepreneurs utilize. Which were the most successful and why?

4. After reviewing the first part of Chapter 3, select any one of the nurse entrepreneurs in this chapter and identify their "customers," "consumers," "influentials," and so forth who play a role in deciding to utilize her services.

Glossary of Common Marketing Terms

Acceptance surveys: Customer surveys to assess their likely acceptance of a new service in circumstances where actual market testing seems impractical.

Affordable approach: An approach to estimating the marketing budget for existing or new services, that assesses what the provider can afford while still leaving an acceptable surplus revenue. As this approach takes no account of the level of marketing that may actually be needed for effectiveness, it is less desirable than other approaches.

Advertising: Any form of paid, nonpersonal marketing communication by a provider.

Agent: A person who works on behalf of a provider, identifying, advising, persuading, and introducing new customers. Also known as a representative or salesperson.

AIDA: A four-step approach to personal selling: creating *awareness*, establishing *interest, demonstrating* the service, and securing *action* by the prospect.

Backward integration: An action by a provider to become more directly involved in the source of supply of materials used (e.g., home care agencies setting up durable medical equipment businesses). See also *forward integration.*

Benefit: An advantage that a consumer gains by using a service (e.g., staying alive or being better informed).

Benefit bundles: A combination of benefits that a customer seeks in a service (e.g., relief from pain plus information plus a short visit). See also *extended service.*

Brand loyalty: The determination of users of a service to select it again if the same need arises. See also *satisfaction*.

Breakeven: The point at which revenue from a service covers the cost of providing it.

Buyers' market: A situation in which more of a service is available than customers want, allowing customers to be selective among providers.

Cell: In market research, a subset of the sample (e.g., oncology patients within a survey of all patients).

Cold canvassing: Sales approaches to potential customers whose level of interest in the service has not been previously established. See also *hot lead*.

Competitive approach: An approach to estimating marketing budgets for existing or new services by matching or surpassing what competitors appear to be spending to market equivalent services.

Concurrence process: A formal procedure in an organization to have each key function agree that a new service concept is worth pursuing.

Conversion rates: The percentage of people seen by a salesperson who become customers, or of people following up on a marketing communication who become service users.

Cognitive dissonance: A state of mental discomfort or confusion that arises when a service encounter fails to meet expectations, and the mental image built beforehand clashes with that acquired on experiencing the service.

Communications effects: One of the two most measurable areas of the results of marketing communications, which explores how well recipients have received the message. See also *sales effects*.

Confidence interval: A term used in statistics to describe the range of possible error around a value (e.g., 45% plus or minus 5%). See also *level of confidence*.

Consumer: The person who uses a service and benefits from it. See also *customer*.

Customer: The person who initiates use of a service, decides which provider to use, arranges for usage, and pays for it. The customer may not be the consumer. Also, several people may share in these customer activities.

Decline phase: The fourth stage of a service life-cycle, usually characterized by falling volume as new replacement services take over the market.

Demand generation: Marketing activities intended to influence people to recognize that they have certain needs.

Demographics: Information about customers or potential customers relating to such factors as sex, or education. See also *psychographics*.

Differentiation: The translation of a service's positioning strategy into different marketing messages to appeal to different target segments. (Some authors use *positioning* to describe both positioning and differentiation, but they are really two separate tasks.)

Discounts: A reduction in normal prices (e.g., volume discounts for large buyers).

Distribution channel: The means by which a service connects with its customers (e.g., via referring physicians or employers).

Distribution channel compatibility: The degree to which a proposed service would rely on channels that the provider already uses for existing services.

Diversification: The addition of new services designed for markets the provider does not currently serve.

Entitlement: The legal and/or social doctrine that consumers have a right to certain services.

Extended service: The deliberate design of a service to offer extra benefits to consumers (e.g., "help with medical emergencies *plus short waits*").

Forward integration: An action by a provider to become more directly involved with the final consumer of the service. This concept sometimes causes confusion when applied to health care, since both a hospital that buys physician practices and one that buys a nursing home are undertaking forward integration. See also *backward integration*.

Frequency: The number of times that a customer will be exposed to a particular marketing communication.

Gatekeeper: A person who limits the choices available to a customer but does not make the final choice for him or her.

Generic service: The main benefit that a provider offers customers (e.g., "a longer life"). See also *tangible service* and *extended service*.

Gravity model: A concept used to predict consumer flow to a service center on the basis of the size and distance of nearby communities.

Growth phase: The second stage of a service life-cycle, usually characterized by rapid growth and the entry of competitive providers.

Hierarchy of effects: The four steps through which a marketing communication must move the audience to produce a customer: capturing attention, creating awareness, creating preference, and motivating action.

Hierarchy of needs: A concept, developed by Abraham Maslow, that people first satisfy basic human needs, then safety needs, then social needs, then esteem needs, and then self-actualization needs. Different health services focus on satisfying different needs.

Hot lead: A potential customer whose interest in a service has been established. See also *cold canvassing*.

Image conflict: A situation in which a receiver of a marketing communication regards it as incongruent with his or her image of its source (e.g., as in "I am calling from the Internal Revenue Service and I want to help you!")

Incomplete message: A style of marketing communication that deliberately leaves the recipient to fill in part of the message, on the theory that this task is more involving.

Industrial concentration: The extent to which provision of a particular service is in the hands of a few very large providers or scattered among many small providers.

Influencer: A person who shapes the preferences of a customer or consumer but plays no role in either the purchase or the service encounter (e.g., a friend).

Information search: The second step in a customer's service selection process.

Internal competition: A situation in which one provider offers two services that are substitutes for each other.

Introductory phase: The first stage in the life-cycle of a service, usually characterized by slow growth as the service gains recognition among customers.

Inventory paradox: The likelihood that, as competition increases, a provider may have to increase availability (e.g., office hours) to remain competitive, contrary to the initial thought that he or she should reduce availability to cut costs.

"I'm-the-expert" orientation: A belief on the part of service providers that they know what is best for customers, rather than investigating what preferences customers have.

Level of confidence: In statistics, the degree of certainty (e.g., 95%) that a value lies within a certain range (or confidence interval). Also referred to as a *coefficient of confidence*.

Life-cycle: The tendency of all services to start with an introductory phase, followed by a growth phase, followed by a mature phase, followed by a phase of decline.

Maintenance marketing: Marketing to protect existing services. See also *missionary marketing*.

Management technology: The know-how and/or equipment needed to manage and market a service. See also *service technology* and *process technology*.

Market dependence: The percentage of a provider's customers who come from a certain geographical area. See also *market share*.

Market development: Taking existing services to new markets.

Market guidance: Marketing activities intended to steer customers toward a provider and away from competitors.

Marketing myopia: The danger that providers will define their area of competence too narrowly and fail to anticipate, or accommodate to, substitute services that remove the need for their service.

Market penetration: Providing more of an existing service to an existing market.

Market penetrator: A provider who has a large market share in a restricted service area. See also *market skimmer*.

Marketing philosophy: A belief that a matching of goals should form the basis of transactions between providers and consumers.

Marketing presbyopia: The danger that providers may interpret their area of competence too broadly and fail to have a sufficient focus to their planning.

Market share: The percentage of consumers with a particular need in a particular geographical area who use a given provider.

Market skimmer: A provider who has a low market share but a wide service area. See also *market penetrator*.

Mature phase: The third stage of a service life-cycle, usually characterized by no growth and the presence of a multiple competitors.

Missionary marketing: Marketing to introduce new services. See also *maintenance marketing*.

Mission statement: A brief statement of a provider's area of interest and goals that gives a focus to planning.

Multimeaning profile: The total image conveyed to recipients of marketing communications by words and/or visuals that they interpret as having various connotations (e.g., a healthy baby in an obstetrical ad may imply both that the service usually delivers healthy babies and that it recognizes that this is the mother's main concern).

Need recognition: The first step in the service selection process.

New entrant: A new provider in an established field of service.

Niche: A small, but possibly attractive, piece of a broader market.

Noise: In marketing communication, all other messages to which the audience is exposed and which compete for its attention with a given message.

Normal distribution: A statistical pattern in which certain natural phenomena, including consumer attitudes, may be expected to fall. Its practical application is that sample information becomes "statistically significant" if it does not accord with this expected pattern.

Objective-and-task approach: An approach to estimating a marketing budget for existing or new services, by developing a specific plan and costing out each line item.

Parameter: An item of data concerning a population. See also *statistic*.

Payback: The point at which accumulated revenue from a service covers all costs incurred to date.

Penetration pricing: Pricing a service low enough to capture a large market share quickly.

Percentage-of-sales approach: An approach to estimating the marketing budget for existing or new services, by looking at the percentage of total revenue that the provider has spent on marketing in the past for equivalent services that were successfully marketed.

Personal selling: Personal and oral marketing communication.

Plowback approach: An approach to estimating marketing budgets for existing or new services, by establishing an initial budget related to a target revenue, but agreeing that this budget will be increased periodically (e.g., each quarter) if revenues exceed target. Also known as the *response-and-decay approach*.

Process technology: The know-how and/or equipment needed to deliver a service efficiently and economically. See also *service technology* and *management technology*.

Point of service: The physical place in which a service is rendered. May also be referred to as point of sales.

Point-of-service promotion: Promotion activities that occur at the place where service is rendered.

Population: In statistics, the entire universe (e.g., U.S. adults) from which a sample is drawn.

Positioning: The process of designing a service to have maximum appeal to selected market segments. See also *differentiation*.

Position statement: A brief summary of the image that a provider wants customers to have of the provider compared with competitors.

Postuse evaluation: The final step in a customer's service selection process, in which he or she assesses the service encounter.

Preneed: A special type of benefit that customers may seek now to protect themselves against some future situation (e.g., buying insurance).

Prestige pricing: Establishing a high price for a service in the belief that some customers regard higher price as evidence of higher quality.

Price skimming: Starting a service with a high price and lowering it in stages as the market segment willing to pay each price appears to have been exhausted.

Privatization: Official agencies contracting with private providers to provide services that they previously provided themselves, or the sale of government-owned enterprises to the public.

Production orientation: A focus by providers on services that they want to offer, without consideration of whether enough customers want them to make them viable.

Psychographics: Information about what customers think, prefer, want, and how they behave in certain situations. (See also *demographics*.

Publicity: Efforts to obtain favorable media coverage of a service.

Reach: The number of customers likely to see or hear a particular marketing communication or campaign.

Recall: The degree to which recipients of marketing communications can remember their content.

Respondent bias: The possibility that respondents to a survey do not accurately represent the views of nonrespondents.

Response-and-decay approach: See *plowback approach*.

Response rate: The percentage of people surveyed in a market research study who actually reply.

Sales effects: One of the two measurable areas of results from marketing communications, focusing on actual service usage by message recipients. See also *communications effects*.

Sales orientation: A focus by a service provider on selling existing services, rather than investigating how they might have to be modified to maximize their appeal.

Sales promotion: All forms of marketing communication that are not advertising, publicity, or personal selling.

Sales territories: Subdivisions of a service area.

Sample: A subset of a population.

Satisfaction: A consumer's state of mind when a service encounter meets or surpasses the consumer's expectations of it. See also *brand loyalty*.

Segment: A subset of customers defined by either demographics or psychographics.

Sellers' market: A situation in which customers want more of a service than is available, resulting typically in waits for service and relatively undemanding customers.

Service area: The geographical area from which a provider draws most of its customers.

Service compatibility: The extent to which the market for a proposed service coincides with that for existing services.

Service development: Offering new services to existing markets.

Service innovation process: The six-step process through which service innovation occurs: concept generation, concept screening, feasibility assessment, service development, service testing, and service launch. If pursued rigorously, some concepts will be abandoned at each step as nonviable.

Service mix: The range of distinct services that a provider offers.

Service selection process: The five steps that customers go through in using a service: need recognition, information search, usage decision, use, postusage evaluation.

Service technology: The equipment and/or know-how needed to make a service work technically. See also *management technology* and *process technology*.

Seven-step model: An approach to writing direct mail letters.

Spill-out: The reach of a marketing communication beyond its intended audience.

Statistic: An item of data concerning a sample. In common usage, *statistic* is often incorrectly used instead of *parameter* to describe an item of data about the population as a whole.

Substitute service: A service that provides consumers with the same benefits as another service but by a different method.

Surrogate: A person whom a customer allows to select a service for him. See also *gatekeeper*.

Symbolism: The tendency for words and images to have associations for their audience beyond their simple literal meaning (e.g., for black to be associated with death).

Tangible service: The process that a provider uses to deliver benefits to customers (e.g., radiation therapy). See also *generic service* and *extended service*.

Target audience: The desired recipients of a marketing communication.

Technological advantage: A competitive lead that a provider has in hardware (equipment), know-how, or both.

Technology diffusion: The process through which an innovation spreads beyond its initial inventor into the hands of other providers.

Transformation: The conversion of existing customers into loyal future customers.

Unique selling proposition (USP): A theme that distinguishes a service from its competitors, and that is both desirable to consumers and believable by them.

Values and lifestyles (VALS): A method of segmenting markets into groups of people with similar "mindsets."

Venturesomeness: The degree to which customers are likely to try new services or providers.

Index